MW00352679

"A breathtakingly comprehensive work of depth and substance. As a yoga educator I recommend this book become a staple of yoga therapy training reading lists."

—Leslie Kaminoff, co-author of Yoga Anatomy,
Founder of The Breathing Project

"Evan Soroka has done a great service to the community of people diagnosed with diabetes, as well as the therapists whose job it is to support them in finding ways that they can better manage their own condition. This book is a welcome contribution to the growing body of literature that makes these ancient healing modalities accessible."

—Gary Kraftsow, Founder/Director of American Viniyoga Institute, LLC, author of Yoga for Wellness

"I am very impressed by the book that Evan has written. The intersections of yoga, stress management, and diabetes control are illuminated through this wonderful text that spans from scientific theory to practice."

—Michael C. Riddell, Ph.D, Professor School of Kinesiology and Health Science, Muscle Health Research Center, York University, Toronto, Canada

"Diabetes impacts every aspect of life. One needs to balance diet and exercise, and appropriately use medications to control glucose—which one must monitor and adjust life to achieve desired results. The person with diabetes needs to be aware of everything they do, eat, feel, and think to enable management of the diabetes. Evan Soroka has used yoga to do that for herself and has developed yoga practices to help others do that for themselves.

She focuses on using yoga therapy to help with diabetes. However, in doing so, she shows that yoga can be used to help with all aspects of life. And her insights into diabetes are profound."

—Jay S. Skyler, MD, MACP, Professor of Medicine, Paediatrics and Psychology, Deputy Director, Diabetes Research Institute, University of Miami Miller School of Medicine

of related interest

Yoga Therapy for Insomnia and Sleep Recovery
An Integrated Approach to Supporting Healthy Sleep and Sustaining Energy All Day
Lisa Sanfilippo
ISBN 978 1 84819 391 8
eISBN 978 0 85701 348 4

Yoga Therapy for Stroke
A Handbook for Yoga Therapists and Healthcare Professionals
Arlene A. Schmid and Marieke Van Puymbroeck
Forewords by Matthew J. Taylor and Linda Williams
ISBN 978 1 84819 369 7
eISBN 978 0 85701 327 9

Yoga Therapy for Fear
Treating Anxiety, Depression and Rage with the Vagus Nerve and Other Techniques
Beth Spindler
ISBN 978 1 84819 374 1
eISBN 978 0 85701 331 6

Yoga Therapy for Digestive Health
Charlotte Watts
ISBN 978 1 84819 354 3
eISBN 978 0 85701 312 5

Yoga Therapy as a Creative Response to Pain
Matthew J. Taylor
Foreword by John Kepner
ISBN 978 1 84819 356 7
eISBN 978 0 85701 315 6

Yoga Therapy for Diabetes

EVAN SOROKA

Illustrated by Kirsteen Wright

SINGING DRAGON
LONDON AND PHILADELPHIA

First published in Great Britain in 2021 by Singing Dragon, an imprint of Jessica Kingsley Publishers
An Hachette Company

1

Front cover image source: Lydia Mann.

The information contained in this book is not intended to replace the services of trained medical professionals or to be a substitute for medical advice. The complementary therapy described in this book may not be suitable for everyone to follow. You are advised to consult a doctor before embarking on any complementary therapy programme and on any matters relating to your health, and in particular on any matters that may require diagnosis or medical attention.

Recipe on pp.151–152 reproduced with kind permission of The Ayurvedic Press.

A CIP catalogue record for this title is available from the British Library and the Library of Congress

ISBN 978 1 78775 261 0
eISBN 978 1 78775 262 7

Printed and bound in the United States by Integrated Books International

Jessica Kingsley Publishers' policy is to use papers that are natural, renewable and recyclable products and made from wood grown in sustainable forests. The logging and manufacturing processes are expected to conform to the environmental regulations of the country of origin.

Jessica Kingsley Publishers
Carmelite House
50 Victoria Embankment
London EC4Y 0DZ

www.singingdragon.com

The wound is where the light enters you.

Rumi

Contents

Introduction

We All Have a Story to Tell

This is mine, at least part of it, for now. It is a story that I wrote under the influence of diabetes. Every word is imbued with the lived experience of diabetes in me. I write from that place but also from beyond that place. As it is part of me, but not really me.

My story is not particularly unique or special, but it is mine. I could have been another statistic, a victim of diabetes, but instead, I am here sharing this story with you. I hope that my diabetes journey can show others that you are never alone with diabetes, even when it feels like no one gets it. You are never really alone.

I'm a Colorado girl; being in nature has always been part of my life and upbringing, so it is fitting that this is where I figured out I had diabetes. It was the summer between seventh and eighth grade. I was on the cusp of adolescence, a pivotal time in anyone's life. The months leading up to my diagnosis were foreboded with the typical warning signs of diabetes, and looking back, it was too close to see.

All I remember is the feeling: a violent thirst like a hungry wolf would pull me up out of bed every night. I wet the bed the night before my bat mitzvah; gosh, if the other kids only knew. For the most part, I kept all of the warning signs to myself. I knew something was wrong, but I chose to ignore it with the hope it would go away. That intuitive whisper never got louder; but it never went away, and when things were quiet, I could hear it calling me.

That year was the eighth-grade solo, a trip we excitedly anticipated and secretly dreaded. The apex was an unofficial rite of passage into high school, a 24-hour solo excursion with just a candy bar, a bottle of water, and a tarp. Our camp was at treeline above 11,000 ft, high in the Colorado mountain tundra. A valley of alpine flowers meets jagged ominous peaks. The ground is soft and slightly moist from the snowmelt. I found a sheltered overlook laden with trees, perfect for my new abode. Below was a high alpine stream, the only sound perceivable to my young ears.

Within the first hour, I drank my entire water supply. Too proud to ask for help, I toughed it out for the remaining 23 hours. All I remember was the sound of that stream and the feeling inside like an evil gremlin possessing me.

Silence allows you to listen. In the silence of the mountains, for the first time in my life, completely alone, I could finally hear what my body had been telling me for months. Something was terribly wrong; I could not ignore it any longer. It was more than a feeling; it was a deep calling from my soul to take action.

A few days later, in the hospital, my blood sugar was off the charts. They told me I had something called juvenile diabetes and said that it was an anomaly I was still alive. My parents were shocked and ridden with guilt for not having seen the visible signs of diabetes. But how could they? I hid my suffering so well. I should have been devastated; instead, I was relieved.

You lie there in bed, people come to see you. Family, doctors, nurses, friends, everyone looks at you like you're sick. It's like you've got to handle their pain for them. I'm fine, I've got this. Friends come to visit. They say they are sorry and bring you chocolate. Everyone has something to say, nobody gets it. Learn this, do that. You're expected to absorb it somehow. But nothing can prepare you for a life with diabetes. Nothing except doing it. Not a single thing you learn from a book makes sense until you apply it in your life. Diabetes proficiency is gained by living it.

Any diagnosis is stressful, but as a pre-teen, you are just trying to figure out who you are. All of a sudden, you are required to be highly disciplined and aware of everything that you are doing, as it relates to your health. You are supposed to keep your blood sugars in a tight range of 80–180 mg/dL (4.4–10.0 mmol/L) and inject insulin several times a day.

Suddenly you have to think about food. There is good food, bad food, and everyone has an opinion about what that is. Everything you do now has to be considered through a diabetes lens; it feels suffocating.

The moment I was diagnosed, I fervently rejected any attempts by my parents or others to help me do diabetes. I wanted the responsibility to fall entirely on my shoulders. The first time my parents tried to inject me, their trepidation was palpable. Their hands shook with fear of hurting me. It was the first and only time I let them.

On the one hand, the declaration of independence was a positive attribute, and on the other hand, it produced unnecessary drama in my life. I just wanted everyone to let me be and allow me to take care of diabetes on my own. I did not want extra attention, I just wanted to be normal. Anytime I was to go over to a friend's house, their parents would receive an instruction manual about how to take care of me. I hated the spotlight and was annoyed that special measures had to be made for me when I knew how to take care of myself.

My parents and I fought a lot. I resisted, rebelled, and retaliated every time there was a question about my blood glucose (BG), what I was eating, or what I should do. That is an excellent way of saying I gave them a lot of reason to worry; I was a wreck.

My behavior was more than teenage angst, it was a product of diabetes and stress. I was so insecure about my body, overwhelmed by diabetes management, and frustrated by adults looming over every decision that I made. It was at a boiling point, and I did not have any outlets for the emotional overflow. Hope was not all lost; underneath the guise of rebellion was a person who cared deeply about her health and wellbeing. I am lucky, and I think that the only reason why I do not have any complications is that no matter what I did, I always tested my BG and tried to correct it if it was off.

My weight fluctuated, as food had become an object of desire; I wanted the things I could not have. When my BG was low, I would binge eat and spend the entire next day abstaining from food in punishment. Eating disorders are a common effect of type 1 diabetes (T1D). Controlling what we put in our bodies gives us a false sense of control when everything else in our lives seems so out of control. I was so uncomfortable in my body that the thought of someone touching me was enough to scream. My A1c (BG average) lingered in the high eights. I tried to work out, but only met frustration when the weight would not budge or my BG would fall.

In junior year of high school, I convinced my parents to let me move to Brazil for a year. In all honesty, I do not think I gave them a choice. Brazil was incredible for me. I was free to make my own decisions with no one looming over me. It boosted my confidence and awakened a curiosity within me to experience as much of life as possible.

Returning in one piece helped me prove to my parents that I could do it on my own, but I still lacked appropriate coping tools and strategies to offset the emotional cost of diabetes. I had turned to smoking and drinking like a lot of teens, but I was relying on it to cope. Diabetes was taking a toll on me, and I could not see it.

One day, my best friend at the time went to a yoga class. We met up afterwards, and she was a different person. Glowing and happy, she did not want to participate in the usual debauchery that the others and I were into. Naturally, I was intrigued, and the next week I went to a class on my own to see what it was about.

All I can say is that I was uncomfortable and awkward. Every position made me want to scream and run away, but for some reason, I stayed. I remember lying in a pool of sweat at the end of the first class, feeling euphoric. It was unlike anything I had felt in my entire life. I was alive, at ease, and complete. All of the distractions, discomfort, angst melted away for a moment.

I kept going back to yoga, even when I did not want to. There were times when I hated it. I wanted to leave and run away. But I stayed, and when I did, I was rewarded. We do not realize how much we are suffering until we experience the opposite. Yoga showed me that the way I was living was not sustainable and awakened an interest in self-discovery, health, and wellness.

Those first years of intense physical practice helped purify my body, mind, and senses and prepared me for what was next: transformation. I learned how to love myself more, cherish my body, and practice self-care. I felt more equipped and confident to handle diabetes challenges.

Yoga taught me that I was more than the experience of diabetes, more than my emotions, fears, and discomfort. I learned that if I took time to practice, I always felt better, and when I felt better, I was more myself. That was the beginning of the rest of my life. I thought I was practicing for my physical appearance, but as time went on, yoga began to inform my whole life. It was what I did to feel whole again, to give myself space to just be present. When I practiced, I felt better. All of my relationships improved and, most importantly, so did my relationship with myself. This relationship is fluid, continually growing, and evolving. I became a teacher and started to share my experiences with others.

About five years into practice, I herniated a disc in my back. I had to completely stop the way I was practicing. It was the first time in my life I sustained an injury like that—where I could not walk. Like a diabetes diagnosis, an injury is a wake-up call to change your direction. I wanted to continue the feeling I once achieved in yoga āsana, but my practice motivation had to shift. I began to look deeper into the philosophy and psychology of yoga and went on to complete my studies in yoga therapy with Gary Kraftsow and the American Viniyoga Institute. I learned how to work with the breath and sequence for energetics, specifically the autonomic nervous system.

I noticed that when my energy was low, I could do a practice to build it back up. If my energy was too high, or I was anxious or nervous, I could practice to calm myself down. I noticed that these qualities of energy could be applied to specific diabetes challenges, addressing short-term needs, and reducing long-term complications. If my blood sugar was running high, I could practice increasing circulation and lowering the number. Even if the number did not come down, the practice helped me have more energy for the rest of my day. I could go about my day with more vitality.

I am so grateful to have the opportunity to share with you my life experience of practicing for and with diabetes. I am not here as an expert and do not claim that yoga is the answer to diabetes. Yoga is a self-care strategy which improves diabetes management and builds resilience against diabetes risks.

This book is an amalgamation of my science experiments with yoga therapy for diabetes. All the practices are informed by science and yoga tradition. I am sharing what works for me and for those I work with.

Yoga and diabetes are complementary practices. They both teach you how to be the observer of the experience and watch your thoughts, sensations, emotions, and actions as an observer. Whenever I inject my body, I do not think I am injecting my body. I do it without identification.

When I sit in meditation and witness my mind having a tantrum, I learn how to stay and not get involved. This informs the way I take care of diabetes. If I test my BG and do not like what I see, I have a choice. I can freak out, blame myself, or something else, or I can see the number and respond appropriately. If I still cannot figure it out, I have a practice that always nourishes my system, calms my mind, and purifies my body. I know that no matter what diabetes or life throws at me, I always have what I need.

Diabetes still throws me curveballs from time to time. I do not profess to be perfect at it. I still have highs and lows. I make mistakes sometimes and get frustrated, and that is okay. Yoga has equipped me with the skills to be aware of my needs, identify the imbalances, and choose appropriate practices to reestablish equilibrium. I feel confident in my ability to manage diabetes and equipped with an understanding that although I am in charge, I am not the master of everything I do. I can let go of things that cannot be changed (diabetes) and focus on what I can change (feeling well). This skillset trickles into every avenue of my life and is what I most enjoy sharing with others.

CHAPTER 1

It's Time to Change the Narrative

When you think about the word *diabetes*, what images come to your mind? Very rarely do we hear *diabetes* and have a positive association. Call me crazy, but I see it differently. I believe that diabetes can be synonymous with health.

I feel this way because of what yoga practice has taught me and continues to teach me. It is my primary source of self-care, support, and inspiration. It is what works for me, and I wrote this book to share it with you.

The problem is that diabetes is hard, and although we've been given a lot of tools to help manage this thing, it is always changing; we never know which way it is going to turn. We've got to be shape-shifters, moving like the wind with every ebb and turn diabetes throws at us. But to do that, we have to really understand diabetes and, of course, understand ourselves, because it shows up differently in everyone who has it. The experience of diabetes is a metaphor for all of life, and yoga is the metaphor for practice. Practice shows us how to create a protective buffer to turn risk into a benefit.

Let me take a step back and say: I am by no means perfect at diabetes. I still strive to improve and have days when it gets me down. But I also know that I would not be half the person I am today without it. It has taught me what it means to appreciate life and persevere.

As a young yogi growing up and trying to link yoga with diabetes, I was always disappointed with the information out there, one-dimensional and limited to āsana for type 2 diabetes (T2D). No one was talking about T1D. No one was talking about the energetics and the real culprit in diabetes: the mind; how understanding the mind governs nourishment at every level of the *person*. Yoga and diabetes were presented as being side by side but separate. That's fine, but it is not yoga. I thought that there had to be a better way.

I wrote this book to share with you, with yoga therapists and people with diabetes alike, that yoga is more than a life preserver; it's the wings that help you to rise up and soar above diabetes. Let's remember that this is the aim of yoga for everyone, regardless of diabetes. What makes this book so special is that I've distilled the information down so that it can complement diabetes as a whole.

Fascinated with the science of human behavior since I was a child, I have always been interested in humans to the extent that I majored in anthropology and languages in college. I've always been curious about how and why we do what we do and the science behind it. I did not want to limit this book to yoga because it would not give you ample context for why and how to practice the art and science of yoga therapy for diabetes. I have created an *ethnography* of yoga for diabetes in the spirit of the study of human behavior and the creativity of personal empowerment.

I want to dispel the misinformation about diabetes, and to educate the therapists and even the people living with diabetes about diabetes. You will find comprehensive information merging Western science, Eastern tradition, and evidence-based research with anecdotal experience of diabetes. I hope to provide a context where you can formulate your own ideas and get creative.

It is said that the best offense is a good defense; I've created strategies to address the primary diabetes challenges and their effects. There is a short-term benefit: to reduce immediate suffering and decrease risk by helping someone feel better right away. The long-term benefit of these practices is to create a protective buffer against the duration of diabetes, safeguarding the body's organs and regulatory systems, and truly empower people to feel like they have some say in their lives.

The practices engender self-awareness, adaptability, and confidence. When people feel better, they are inspired to take better care of themselves. With practice, people see what they are doing that is harmful and what is helpful. They choose better. This promotes resilience against inevitable diabetes risks and setbacks. By and large, the basic motivating blocks getting in the way of individuals achieving this realization are experiential, and the experience is only obtained through practice. This is why Patañjali said that yoga needs to be practiced over a long time with no breaks. Meaning: don't take days off. A little bit every day goes a long way.

As diabetes is a self-care disease, with a majority share beholden to individual responsibility, it presents various challenges that make it difficult to manage without support. I will call these challenges "pain-points," which vary from type of diabetes, duration of disease, the unique constitution, and psycho-emotional state.

The pain-points include, but are not limited to:

- the burden of daily management requirements
- BG levels in the short and long term
- physiological imbalances as a result of said BG fluctuations and management requirements
- gastrointestinal problems
- other co-morbidities from long-term diabetes: heart disease and neuropathy
- psycho-emotional challenges from unresolved stress, burnout, distress, anxiety, and depression
- sleep disturbances
- triggers, habits, unhealthy patterns
- an inability to separate one's essential self from the experience of diabetes.

There are three main orientations for practice, and you will find that most of the methods combine all three in some way, shape, or form.

Physical: Reduce suffering from BG and diabetes physical effects, balance the autonomic nervous system, and improve energy levels.

Mental: This is where the nervous and endocrine systems meet behavioral psychology and yoga philosophy. We take a deep dive into neuroanatomy and yoga psychology 101. Learn to witness the triggers behind stress responses and rewire them with awareness and practice.

Beyond diabetes: A connection with a higher self, a place untouched by the effect of diabetes, a place of deep meaning and inherent support.

I must stress that the practices outlined in this book are *descriptive* and not prescriptive. My goal is to show yoga therapists and people with diabetes alike how to provide a direct understanding of "I am whole, I am not diabetes" through the practices of yoga therapy. Yoga is just one way to practice self-care. It is what I do, and I think it is one of the greatest gifts to mankind. I am not here to write a book about a cure or offer holistic platitudes that yoga is the answer. It is just one part, yet a vital part, of the equation.

The goal of *Yoga Therapy for Diabetes* is to help people with every type of diabetes embrace their condition as an opportunity for personal growth and optimal wellbeing. Of course, the practice does not stop at diabetes but uses diabetes as a launchpad for yoga's real aim, self-mastery.

CHAPTER 2

The Diabetes Problem and Solution

Diabetes is one of the fastest-growing health challenges of the 21st century.[1] According to the World Health Organization diabetes is the seventh leading cause of death in the world.[2] The number of people with diabetes worldwide has risen from 108 million in 1980 to 422 million in 2014.[3] In 2016, an estimated 1.6 million deaths were directly caused by diabetes, and another 2.2 million deaths were attributable to high BG in 2012.[4] The numbers for diabetes are expected to grow worldwide, especially in industrialized low-income countries.

A 2018 report by the American Diabetes Association (ADA) stated that over 34.2 million Americans, 10.5% of the population, had diabetes and 88 million had prediabetes.[5] Of this total, about 1.6 million Americans have T1D, including about 187,000 children.[6] T2D constitutes about 90–95% of all diabetes diagnoses.[7]

The exponential growth of diabetes worldwide is attributable to a complex

1 International Diabetes Federation (2019) *IDF Diabetes Atlas*. Ninth edition. Accessed on 30/06/20 at: https://diabetesatlas.org/en/sections/worldwide-toll-of-diabetes.html.

2 World Health Organization (2018) *The Top 10 Causes of Death*. Accessed on 30/06/20 at: www.who.int/news-room/fact-sheets/detail/the-top-10-causes-of-death.

3 World Health Organization (2020) *Diabetes*. Accessed on 26/08/20 at: www.who.int/news-room/fact-sheets/detail/diabetes.

4 World Health Organization (2020) *Diabetes*. Accessed on 26/08/20 at: www.who.int/news-room/fact-sheets/detail/diabetes.

5 American Diabetes Association (n.d.) *Statistics About Diabetes*. Accessed on 26/08/20 at: www.diabetes.org/resources/statistics/statistics-about-diabetes.

6 American Diabetes Association (n.d.) *Statistics About Diabetes*. Accessed on 26/08/20 at: www.diabetes.org/resources/statistics/statistics-about-diabetes.

7 Centers for Disease Control and Prevention (2019) *Type 2 Diabetes*. Accessed on 26/08/20 at: www.cdc.gov/diabetes/basics/type2.html.

web of socioeconomic, demographic, environmental, and genetic factors; each type has its own set of causative risk factors.[8]

T1D is generally diagnosed in childhood, although adults can also develop T1D. It develops in children quite rapidly and people tend to be quite sick upon diagnosis. The first wave of diagnosis occurs between 4 and 7 years old, and the second peak between 10 and 14 years old.[9] Genetics, family history, environmental contaminants, and geography are all T1D risk factors. Interestingly, the further away from the equator, the higher the incidence of T1D. People in Finland and Sardinia have the highest rate of T1D: 400 times the rate of an equatorial country like Venezuela.[10] Other risk factors have also been researched, although none have been proven. Some of these theories suggest the introduction of antibiotics[11] and exposure to viruses like Epstein-Barr,[12] Coxsackie, and the mumps.

T2D is generally developed later in adulthood, although children are now developing T2D at an astounding rate. T2D is caused by a combination of genetic, socioeconomic, and behavioral risk factors. People with T2D are more likely than those with T1D to have a family history or close relative with T2D. Obesity, lack of exercise, and unhealthy eating behaviors are all attributable risks to the development of insulin resistance, prediabetes, and eventually T2D. However, not everyone with T2D fits the stereotype and we cannot attribute the development of T2D solely to behavioral factors.

The causes and risks are distinct but the result of uncontrolled hyperglycemia is similar no matter the type of diabetes. Diabetes significantly increases the risk of developing other diseases, like cardiovascular disease, microvascular complications like peripheral and autonomic retinopathy, kidney disease, Alzheimer's disease, stroke, and various heart conditions.[13] Hyperglycemia

8 International Diabetes Federation (2020) *Worldwide Toll of Diabetes*. Accessed on 26/08/20 at: www.diabetesatlas.org/en/sections/worldwide-toll-of-diabetes.html.

9 Tirumalesh, M. (2008) *Stress, Psychology, Wellbeing and Quality of Life Among Diabetes Mellitus Patients*. Tirupati: Mangalapalli Tirumalesh. p.67.

10 Tirumalesh, M. (2008) *Stress, Psychology, Wellbeing and Quality of Life Among Diabetes Mellitus Patients*. Tirupati: Mangalapalli Tirumalesh. p.67.

11 Zhang, X.-S., Li, J., Krautkramer, K. A., Badri, M., *et al.* (2018) "Antibiotic-induced acceleration of type 1 diabetes alters maturation of innate intestinal immunity." *eLife*, doi: 10.7554/eLife.37816.

12 Schneider, L. K. (2018) "Diabetes risk increases with exposure to Epstein-Barr virus." *Endocrine Web*. Accessed on 30/06/20 at: www.endocrineweb.com/professional/endocrinology/diabetes-risk-increases-exposure-epstein-barr-virus.

13 Innes, K. E. (2016) "Yoga Therapy for Diabetes." In *The Principles and Practice of Yoga in Healthcare*. Pencaitland: Handspring Publishing. p.209.

may be the cause of co-morbidity and organ damage. Most people do not die of high BG, but rather of heart disease, and the risk of heart complications is even higher in T2D than in T1D.[14]

Diabetes imposes a staggering financial burden on society. The cost of diabetes continues to rise, and is one of the most expensive strains on the global healthcare system. In 2018, the ADA estimated that the total cost of diagnosed diabetes rose from $245 billion in 2012 to $327 billion in 2017 in America alone; a 26% increase in just five years.[15] These numbers do not include the cost of diabetes on work productivity, increased absenteeism, and co-morbid disorders attributed to diabetes complications. The expense of the financial and societal burden of diabetes is expected to rise to $490 billion by 2030.[16] By 2050, it is estimated that one in three people in America will be affected by diabetes.[17] A diabetes diagnosis puts the individual at a severe financial disadvantage; the personal cost of diabetes in America alone averaged $16,752 annually; about 2.3 times more than the cost in the absence of diabetes.[18] T2D gets most of the credit for the surge in the cost and growth of diabetes thanks to increased modernization, mass-produced food, and lack of physical movement.

What is Diabetes?

Diabetes mellitus is a metabolic disorder where a person cannot metabolize glucose (sugar) and it remains in the bloodstream (hyperglycemia), damaging blood vessels and organs. Hyperglycemia is caused by insufficient insulin production, or its absence, and insulin resistance, where the cells do not respond to insulin. All types of diabetes are represented by high BG, and although the effect that high BG has on a person's physiology and its long-term complications are similar, the treatment, management requirements, and etiology of each condition are very different.

---

14 WebMD (2019) *Heart Disease and Diabetes.* Accessed on 30/06/20 at: webmd.com/diabetes/heart-blood-disease.

15 American Diabetes Association (n.d.) *Statistics About Diabetes.* Accessed on 26/08/20 at: www.diabetes.org/resources/statistics/statistics-about-diabetes.

16 American Diabetes Association (2018) *The Cost of Diabetes.* Accessed on 30/06/20 at: www.diabetes.org/resources/statistics/cost-diabetes.

17 Centers for Disease Control and Prevention (2019) *Number of Americans with Diabetes Projected to Double or Triple by 2050.* Accessed on 26/08/20 at: www.cdc.gov/media/pressrel/2010/r101022.html.

18 American Diabetes Association (2018) *The Cost of Diabetes.* Accessed on 30/06/20 at: www.diabetes.org/resources/statistics/cost-diabetes.

The symptoms of undiagnosed diabetes may include: excessive thirst, uncontrolled need to urinate, unexplained weight loss, extreme hunger, vision changes, tingling in the fingers or toes, exhaustion, sores that do not heal, and prolonged illness and infection.

To understand diabetes, what it is, and its underlying causes, it is beneficial to look at the role of metabolism, neuroendocrine responses, and how the body uses the energy from the food we eat to support the function of the brain and organs.

The Role of Metabolism and Evolutionary Biology

Humans first evolved as hunter-gatherers. During this time in our evolutionary history, meals were not consistent or abundant. It was either feast or famine. Our ancestors developed processes to store fuel in times of alimentary surplus and efficiently utilize these stored reserves in times of scarcity. The fuel had to be easily accessible and fast acting. Glucose became the main fuel of choice, especially for quick energy spurts while running from danger during an acute stress response.

The mechanisms became rules of metabolic survival. These rules not only ensured the survival of the individual but also, most importantly, the survival of the species. Those rules, first set by Cahill (1971),[19] are as follows.

- Sustain a tight threshold of glucose levels during feast and famine.
- Create and maintain a storehouse of energetic surplus (glycogen), easily accessed during need, like a "fight-or-flight" response.
- Deliberately store fat and protein in times of abundance.
- Successfully maintain protein reserves.

The most critical players in maintaining the rules of metabolic survival are insulin and glucagon. Think of insulin as the power to uptake and glucagon as the ability to output stored fuel. Insulin, made from pancreatic *b cells*, lowers BG levels in a fed state. It takes the excess glucose in the bloodstream, organizes it, and directs it for immediate use or to a storage location in the liver, muscles,

19 Cahill, G. F. (1971) "Physiology of insulin in man: The Banting Memorial Lecture 1971." *Diabetes 20*, 12, 785– 799.

and adipose tissue. Glucagon, secreted by pancreatic *a cells*, raises BG levels during fasting states and exercise by harvesting glucose directly from storage.

Indeed an artful balancing act, the pancreas works simultaneously with a complex network of diverse metabolic pathways to maintain glucose balance.[20] It is quite an extraordinary mechanism. The pancreas secretes the exact amount of hormones necessary to raise or lower BG levels. The pancreas, part of the endocrine system, is made up of glands and hormones. But its function is mediated by the nervous system.

The hypothalamus part of the structure of the central nervous system (CNS), located in the forebrain, is the link between the nervous and endocrine systems via the pituitary gland. The hypothalamus houses nerve centers that direct specific metabolic processes. It works in a close relationship with the pituitary gland, which is like the conductor of the hypothalamus's requests. The two are so closely related that they are known together as the hypothalamic-pituitary-adrenal (HPA) axis, which you should remember for later discussion. The two work together to either stimulate or inhibit hormones.

In a fed state, after eating a meal, the pancreas produces insulin in a dose-specific manner to metabolize glucose, pulling it out of the bloodstream and into the cells for immediate use or storage.

In a fasting state, there is less insulin and more glucagon to maintain tight control of BG levels. The mechanisms at play are intelligent and efficient; they carefully allocate fuel throughout the body. It is important to note that the brain requires more glucose production than any other part of the body.

Throughout the CNS and peripheral nervous system (PNS) are glucose-sensing neurons specialized in indicating when the body needs insulin or glucagon. In the case of hypoglycemia, when glucose-sensing neurons perceive glycemic levels are dropping, they signal the autonomic nervous system and pancreas to counteract this through a series of physiological hormonal responses.[21]

The first **counterregulatory response** (CRR) is the suspension of insulin production, and the second is the release of **glucagon**. As BG levels reach 80–85 mg/dL (4.4–4.7 mmol/L), the pancreas stops the production of insulin.

20 Hoese, J. (n.d.) "What is Hypoglycemia Unawareness?" *Beyond Type 1*. Accessed on 30/06/20 at: https://beyondtype1.org/hypoglycemia-unawareness-unabridged.

21 McCrimmon, R. J. (2014) "Counterregulatory Deficiencies in Diabetes." In B. M. Freier, S. Heller and R. McCrimmon (eds) *Hypoglycemia in Clinical Diabetes*. Third edition. Chichester: John Wiley & Sons Ltd. p.49.

Suspending insulin production is sometimes enough to inhibit the further decline of BG levels. It is also a necessary first step in the CRR. For glucagon to work its magic, insulin first has to be out of the picture. If BG levels continue to drop to around 65–70 mg/dL (3.6–4.0 mmol/L), the pancreas produces glucagon.

Glucagon's aim is one-pointed: to arrive at the **liver** quickly and convert glycogen into glucose. The liver is the repository of stored energy in the form of **glycogen**. Glucagon is the key that opens the vault of energetic reserves. Glycogen, a carbohydrate, is a fast-acting energy source. Remember the rules of metabolic survival: store fast-acting energy for emergency purposes. Insufficient glucose constitutes an emergency.

When glucagon arrives at the liver, it binds to the surface and opens the storage vault, a process called gluconeogenesis—harvesting glycogen and turning it into glucose. In normal physiology, gluconeogenesis doesn't release the glycogen stores all at once but instead does it slowly and incrementally. It only allocates what is necessary and conserves the rest. This is perfect during prolonged fasting periods and when the body needs fuel, fast.

Activation of the sympathetic nervous system (SNS) is responsible for many of the physical warning signs of hypoglycemia. Symptoms like shaking, sweating, and dizziness help to trigger a behavioral response (eating) but also support the production and circulation of counterregulatory hormones.

The SNS communicates with the HPA axis to produce epinephrine (adrenaline), cortisol, and growth hormone to restore BG.

Epinephrine is an activator. Aside from the physical warning signs of hypoglycemia, it potentiates glucagon, speeding up its arrival at the liver. While epinephrine's effect is automatic because it is stored, the adrenals manufacture cortisol and growth hormone. These secondary hormones act in the same way as epinephrine, providing insulin resistance for hours to come.

In normal non-diabetic physiology, true hypoglycemia is a rare occurrence. In ancient times, during times of plenty and lack, our evolutionary biology developed to be resilient to drastic nutritional fluctuations. The pancreas precisely orchestrates the production of BG inhibiting and stimulating hormones, maintaining glycemic homeostasis. In conjunction with the brain and SNS, the pancreas can keep glucose within very narrow limits and access fast-acting fuel in the form of glucose when needed.

But this is not what happens in diabetes. In T1D, an autoimmune disease, the body attacks its own beta cells, destroying its ability to produce adequate insulin. In T2D, a metabolic disorder, the pancreatic beta cells become overworked due to increased demand to metabolize food. Over time the body's cells become resistant to insulin, and more and more insulin is required to cover the need. T2D is a product of both insufficient insulin production and insulin resistance, which is the dulling of insulin's potency to unlock the door into the cell. When BG rises over time, the cells do not receive the energy they need, and the blood vessels are damaged. In both T1D and T2D, the damage of high BG in the blood cells is what destroys the body and causes horrendous effects, co-morbid disorders, and even death.

There are many types of diabetes that can be subcategorized either as an autoimmune condition or predominantly due to insulin resistance. It is common knowledge that there are two main types of diabetes, but I want to take time to go over the subtypes. As diabetes evolves in the modern age, we are seeing diagnoses of T1D in adults and T2D in children. Although not all of these types are addressed explicitly by practices in this book, it is essential to understand the distinctions, causes, and recommended allopathic treatments.

T1D is an autoimmune condition where the immune system destroys pancreatic beta cells, the cells that produce insulin. The cause of T1D is still debatable but can be correlated with genetic and environmental factors. The onset of T1D is rapid; something can trigger an autoimmune reaction and a person will develop T1D within a short period. I recall in my own diagnosis story first noticing symptoms in June and being diagnosed at the end of August.

During the development of T1D, something triggers the immune system to mistake pancreatic beta cells for hazardous invader cells and destroys their production. People with T1D cannot produce sufficient endogenous (self-produced) insulin required for metabolic function and are required to inject exogenous insulin through a variety of methods. Although the pancreas still makes some insulin, its productivity is dramatically reduced. For a long time, T1D was known as juvenile diabetes, typically diagnosed in childhood or early adolescence.

Before the discovery of insulin in 1921, T1D was a death sentence, with a grim life expectancy of one to two months. There are stories about the discoverers of insulin injecting juvenile patients in the hospital ward of the University of Toronto. Almost immediately, these emaciated children on the brink of death woke up from their comas, and color returned to their faces. The discovery of insulin is arguably one of the more important discoveries of the 20th century, and it remains the only form of treatment for T1D to this day.

Theoretically, people with T1D cannot produce endogenous insulin. If detected early on in the development of the disease and treated with exogenous insulin, people with T1D can retain some level of insulin production, although it is still insufficient.[22] Doctors call the first few months after diagnosis the "honeymoon" phase, where BG levels are less drastic due to some remaining endogenous insulin. Maintaining an A1c under 7.0% can help to decelerate the destruction of what remaining insulin production is intact, but eventually most people with T1D lose their ability to produce their own insulin and all must administer insulin. There is no such thing as "curing" or "reversing" T1D, although certain lifestyle practices can improve insulin absorption and requirements. As T1D is an autoimmune condition, it increases the risk of developing other autoimmune conditions like celiac disease and disorders like hypothyroidism.

All people with T1D are required to administer some form of exogenous insulin through subcutaneous injections or infusions. The top means by which people deliver insulin are via manual daily injections (MDIs) or through subcutaneous injection with an insulin pump. MDIs are a combination of fast-acting and long-release insulin. Typically, individuals need to inject long-acting insulin once or twice a day to cover their basic metabolic needs. Fast-acting insulin is used to cover carbohydrates and to correct high BG readings. Insulin pumps similarly use a basal rate, which is a slow drip of fast-acting insulin to cover metabolic requirements, and a bolus, which is a more significant dose to include food and corrections. Boluses can be altered depending upon the type and quantity of food. For instance, 25g of juice would require one bolus all at once. However, 25g of carbohydrates with 50g of fat and protein would probably need a percentage upfront and the remainder over a one- to three-hour period to replicate the body's digestion rate.

There are a few different types of insulin pump technologies:

- tube: Medtronic and Tandem
- tubeless: Omnipod.

Most modern insulin pumps are made to work in conjunction with a continuous glucose monitor (CGM). Some of these systems possess an intelligent closed loop that monitors BG levels in real time and auto adjusts basal rates.

22 Bernstein, R. K. (2011) *Dr. Bernstein's Diabetes Solution: The Complete Guide to Achieving Normal Blood Sugars*. Fourth edition. Boston, MA: Little Brown Publishers. p.39.

This technology has been shown to be particularly helpful for maintaining tighter control and reducing nocturnal hyper and hypoglycemia.

However, new technologies have limitations. They are incredibly expensive, even with health insurance, and not covered by all plans. They do not account for human error, miscalculations, sickness, hormonal changes, and exercise. At this point, T1D is still a disease that must be attended to and managed by the individual 24/7.

T1D is a severe and relentless condition. It requires a lot of daily work on the part of the individual to maintain glucose homeostasis. By taking better care, people with T1D can also improve their insulin sensitivity so that the insulin that they administer subcutaneously works more efficiently and reduces short- and long-term complications.

It is a constant math equation with infinite variables. Individuals must be intensely involved, proactive, and capable of anticipating problems and solving existing problems. T1D is physically and mentally exhausting, so self-care is an essential part of managing it successfully. The methods outlined in this book will help individuals with T1D identify their habits and challenges, manage real-time complications, and potentially prevent future ones.

Type 1.5 diabetes (LADA) is a relatively recent discovery. Latent Autoimmune Diabetes in Adults (LADA) is a subtype of T1D. Like T1D, LADA is an autoimmune condition that destroys insulin-producing beta cells. It is diagnosed in individuals over the age of 30 and has a slow onset, generally over five to ten years.[23] For many, the symptoms of LADA go unnoticed by healthcare providers. They may show slightly elevated numbers, only confounding doctors because they do not fit into the classic T2D model. Exercise can mask the symptoms of LADA for many years. Many are misdiagnosed with T2D, only to struggle with glucose control despite their efforts. They may be initially placed on T2D oral medications only to find that the medication is not working. It is essential to recognize this subset of diabetes, as its rate and incidence in the diabetes population are increasing. By understanding its symptoms in others or ourselves, we can possibly avoid years of living with misdiagnosis and the damage that comes from it. The implications and risks of poorly managed LADA are the same as T1D. It is necessary for people with LADA to try to

---

23 Khambatta, C. and Barbaro, R. (2020) *Mastering Diabetes: The Revolutionary Method to Reverse Insulin Resistance Permanently in Type 1, Type 1.5, Type 2, Prediabetes, and Gestational Diabetes.* New York: Avery Publishing.

maintain what beta-cell function they do possess to reduce common diabetes complications once diagnosed.

Due to its slow onset, the treatment of LADA may seem like a mild version of T1D at first, with adjustments to diet, exercise, and a small amount of insulin needed. If diagnosed early enough, people with LADA can maintain a higher rate of endogenous insulin production, making BG potentially more manageable. Over time, endogenous insulin weakens and must follow similar treatment protocols to T1D.

Prediabetes is a serious but preventable and reversible health condition where people have higher than normal BG levels that are not high enough to be diagnosed as diabetes. Prediabetes is diagnosed when your fasting BG values are between 100 and 125 mg/dL (5.5 and 7.0 mmol/L) or when the A1c value is between 5.7% and 6.4%.[24] It is estimated that of the 88 million American adults who have prediabetes, more than 80% of them do not know they have it.[25]

The cause of prediabetes is ineffective insulin production and inadequate response. The cells in the body do not respond to the effects of insulin in the same way as in a non-prediabetes person. The pancreas needs to make more insulin to cover demand, but it cannot keep up. Unless the multifactorial causes of insulin resistance are reduced or eliminated, in all likelihood the person will develop T2D later on. The application of yoga therapy for diabetes can be applied to individuals with prediabetes, helping them offset diabetes risk by improving self-care practices, managing stress levels, and metabolic control.

T2D is a progressive, slow onset, metabolic condition represented by insulin resistance and inadequate insulin production.[26] It is a member of the cluster of metabolic diseases known as Syndrome X or metabolic syndrome, including heart disease, obesity, high cholesterol, high blood pressure, and stroke. T2D is caused by a combination of genetic, behavioral, socioeconomic, and environmental factors but has a secure link to age and obesity. T2D was

24 Khambatta, C. and Barbaro, R. (2020) *Mastering Diabetes: The Revolutionary Method to Reverse Insulin Resistance Permanently in Type 1, Type 1.5, Type 2, Prediabetes, and Gestational Diabetes.* New York: Avery Publishing.

25 CDC (2020) *Prediabetes: Your Chance to Prevent Type 2 Diabetes.* Accessed on 30/06/20 at: www.cdc.gov/diabetes/basics/prediabetes.html.

26 Bernstein, R. K. (2011) *Dr. Bernstein's Diabetes Solution: The Complete Guide to Achieving Normal Blood Sugars.* Fourth edition. Boston, MA: Little Brown Publishers. p.106.

traditionally called adult-onset diabetes but is presently diagnosed in children at a rapidly growing rate, potentially due to the rise in childhood obesity.[27]

Sometimes people with T2D still produce sufficient insulin and can treat their condition with lifestyle interventions and oral medications alone. Should they follow through on behavioral and lifestyle recommendations, resolve insulin resistance, and lower their A1c, they can reverse T2D altogether. But not everyone can apply such radical lifestyle changes, especially when the behaviors are potentially contributing factors to the onset of the condition in the first place.

Over the long duration of T2D, beta-cell production can be compromised, requiring some to take additional insulin to compensate for what the pancreas cannot produce. These individuals need medications to help achieve target BG levels, in addition to healthy lifestyle choices. Sometimes a single drug is sufficient; in other cases, a mix of medicines works better.[28] As any type 2 diagnosis is represented by an A1c over 6.5%, non-insulin-dependent people with T2D are still at a higher risk for diabetes complications.

The goal of a self-care practice is to empower individuals with T2D to reduce or eliminate their need for medications by addressing the underlying mechanisms behind the causes and physiological problems of their condition.

Gestational diabetes typically affects women in the later stages of pregnancy and generally disappears after birth, although they have an increased likelihood of developing T2D within five to ten years.[29] Like prediabetes and T2D, gestational diabetes can develop when the woman develops insulin resistance. Women with gestational diabetes can treat their condition by watching their diet and staying active.

What is Complete Diabetes Health?

Diabetes is not just a disease; it is part of a person and can adversely affect their wellbeing and quality of life unless they learn how to manage it. Health in

27 Mayo Clinic (2019) *Type 2 Diabetes*. Accessed on 30/06/20 at: www.mayoclinic.org/diseases-conditions/type-2-diabetes/symptoms-causes/syc-20351193.

28 Mayo Clinic (2018) *Diabetes Treatment: Type 2 Diabetes Medications*. Accessed on 30/06/20 at: www.mayoclinic.org/diseases-conditions/type-2-diabetes/in-depth/diabetes-treatment/art-20051004.

29 Tirumalesh, M. (2008) *Stress, Psychology, Wellbeing and Quality of Life Among Diabetes Mellitus Patients*. Tirupati: Mangalapalli Tirumalesh. p.49.

diabetes is not just about a number; it is about being resilient and adaptive to an illness that is always changing.

There is a deep connection between the biological, psychological, and behavioral components of diabetes. Since the 1990s, we've seen a dramatic shift in the design of diabetes health models to represent a need to address the link between the body, mind, and self-management compliance. However, despite the information out there, people are still falling short. Why is that?

The Western view on diabetes healthcare recommends several important, if not essential, pillars for optimal diabetes care but lacks precise methods for one to fully undertake such requirements: *diet, exercise, behavioral adaptiveness, mental and emotional health, relationships support, energy management, rest, and sleep.*

But the Western view does not really say how to do this nor can a method be prescribed, because everyone is different. It is not enough to encourage people to maintain a healthy lifestyle; many actually do. But where most people are falling short is in the self-care, mental, and emotional spectrum of diabetes management. They need to be shown how and why taking time to prioritize this will change their lives.

Many think they are doing everything they can; they are exercising and eating right but are still experiencing anxiety, sleeplessness, depression, and negative attitudes about diabetes. They live in fear of hyperglycemia and hypoglycemia, doctors, and needles. They struggle with the day-to-day management or harbor harmful coping mechanisms to "deal" with the burden of a relentless illness.

For the individual with T1D, generally diagnosed in childhood or adolescence, diabetes self-care requires both discipline and maturity, something that a child may not yet possess. The burden can be passed on to parents who cannot, despite their concerted efforts, fully understand the experience of diabetes. Children and teens notoriously rebuke suggestions imposed by superiors, creating a schism between parent and child, and deflecting the individual's self-responsibility and personal growth. Mistakes are inevitable, as one learns along the way, and such errors can leave deep grooves of fear, beliefs, and attachments to how diabetes should be done. The mistakes appropriated in childhood set the tone for the relationship one has with diabetes in adulthood.

The reason why people are struggling is not that they do not care, it is because diabetes requires you to dive deep into yourself and look at your patterns, habits, and beliefs. People aren't always ready to do that, nor do they even know that it is possible. It implores us to look within, and unless we turn to face ourselves, using diabetes as a medium for self-study, the illness will always take the driver's seat.

As most diabetes control is about self-management, it requires discipline, knowledge, patience, persistence, and practice. These are qualities we learn through life experience, but with or without diabetes, if you are not provided with the tools, encouragement, and support, it is easy to fall short or give up. Education about an illness and its complications only goes so far. People who live with diabetes need to have a vested interest in their self-management to succeed with diabetes.

As T2D is often diagnosed in adulthood, a person can already be formed in their personality, beliefs, and habits when they get their diagnosis. The development of T2D and its treatment are primarily related to how people care for themselves. This requires an enormous lifestyle shift, which can only happen if a person makes a 180-degree pivot. As behavior is wrapped up in biology and psychology, a strategy is needed to, in effect, shake things up, and awaken the individual to their responsibility and potential.

Starting one mindful behavior sets the motions for subsequent positive behavioral changes. Yoga is a kind of gateway for people. They start with one type of practice, which can ignite a curiosity in other wellness practices, and they inquire more about who they are and what makes them happy.

Yoga can be a starting point for that.

What helps me more than anything, and what I hope to provide to others like me, is space. Self-care practice gives me room to take care of diabetes by treating myself. Strategies like yoga, meditation, and relaxation help people improve their BG levels, metabolic outcomes, and quality of life.

Self-care is what I do to unwind, nourish my body, and release the chaos. It is more than sleeping or taking a lavender bath; it is an intimate connection with myself. It empowers me to feel like I am in control, or at least more in control, and relaxed when diabetes is in the driver's seat. Through the practices of self-care, I also learn how to respond and adapt better. When you get quiet, the chaos surrounding you slows down, and you can perceive more clearly. Taking time out of your regular routine to practice self-care requires effort, patience, dedication, and faith, but when the pain point is so great, as with diabetes, there are no other options.[30]

---

30 Rubin, R. R. (2009) "Psychotherapy and Counselling in Diabetes Mellitus." In F. J. Snoek and C. T. J. Skinner (eds) *Psychology in Diabetes Care*. Chichester: Wiley & Sons Ltd. p.237.

The information presented in this book is nothing new. I am simply supporting what yoga and Āyurveda have said for thousands of years about health as longevity, and what behavioral psychologists and scientists now support.

Much of this book is about how to use yoga therapy as a reliable and ever-evolving form of diabetes self-care and personal empowerment. But what it requires is *action*.

Yoga shows us how to take action for the health of our whole person, body, mind, and spirit, and by considering the whole person we can improve our relationship with diabetes as it also impacts the whole person.

A person may not initially know what that is, but if they follow a practice such as the ones outlined in ancient yoga and Āyurveda texts, the world is their oyster.

There is no end to growth. Yoga and Āyurveda provide self-care practices that complement the recommendations set by healthcare providers for optimal diabetes wellbeing. Suddenly, individuals with diabetes have a precise method to adapt to their ever-changing needs and, in turn, feel more empowered and efficacious in their management of diabetes. The motivation does not come from a doctor, parent, or spouse but from within. This is the only place it can come from.

Summary

Diabetes is a global epidemic crisis with two major types: type 1 is an autoimmune condition with an absolute need for insulin; type 2 is a progressive metabolic condition caused by various factors and includes 90–95% of the population with diabetes.[31] T2D can be treated with diet, exercise, and oral medication. Sometimes, people with T2D need to take insulin as well, although, unlike those with T1D, this not always for the rest of their lives. The causes are different; the treatment is similar but also different. What unites all kinds of diabetes is high BG and a need for effective self-care strategies.

Although the metabolic and physiological conditions of T1D and T2D are similar to the causes, preventative practices and treatments vary. Understanding

31 Centers for Disease Control and Prevention (2019) *Type 2 Diabetes*. Accessed on 26/08/20 at: www.cdc.gov/diabetes/basics/type2.html.

these distinctions will help inform your own application of yoga therapy for diabetes, whether in yourself or in a professional yoga therapy setting.

Part of the global diabetes crisis problem is that diabetes needs to be managed by the individual. When a person leaves the doctor's office, it is up to them to fulfill their self-management requirements. Compliance is challenging as the very causes of diabetes, aggravating factors responsible for complications and personal behaviors, are intertwined. People need effective strategies to overcome their habits, and feel empowered and inspired to take care of diabetes from a place of love of life instead of obligation.

Doctors recommend mindful, stress-reduction strategies as part of an effective diabetes management protocol, yet the methods are not clearly outlined. People say, "Manage your energy, take care of your mind, sleep better, relax, meditate, and such," but no one is saying exactly how to do these things and how to consider them as they relate to the lived experience of diabetes. Complete diabetes care goes much deeper than a number. Diabetes affects the whole person, and unless we look at its treatment through the entire person, those who have diabetes will not be able to rise above it.

This book aims to address the how and the why. Yoga provides a cost-effective, multidimensional intervention strategy for people with all types of diabetes to address and balance the physiological, psychological, and behavioral components to diabetes self-management through reliable and applicable self-care strategies.

CHAPTER 3

Stress and Diabetes

Diabetes is a self-management disease, meaning that a large majority of success with diabetes has to do with how a person is taking care of themselves and the choices that they make in every moment of the day. Decisions are informed by how we think and feel. This presents a challenge for people with diabetes, because BG changes and fluctuations impact the energetic condition, and the energetic condition governs our emotions. If a person does not feel well, it is hard to make the right decisions with regard to diabetes management. It can be stressful to always be thinking about diabetes while living life. When BG levels are swinging high or low, the physiological experience impacts emotion, perception, and how a person feels. The mix of not feeling well, constant bombardment of self-management requirements, and simultaneously living life is a lot for the body and the mind to handle. Without clear and consistent protective practices to down-regulate stress responses, people with diabetes are at an increased risk of co-morbid disorders like heart disease, depression, and reduction of quality of life.

As a type 1 diabetic, I have to think about and consider diabetes in just about every moment of the day. The choices I make, the activities I partake in, and how productive I am are all dependent on how well I am managing diabetes. It is hard to prioritize diabetes as the number one focus in a way that does not make you either feel crazy or like you are not living the life you want to live. The psychological burden of diabetes is invisible and challenging to see when you live it every day.

Diabetes-related stress is a risk to a person's health, longevity, and quality of life, which diminishes self-management and leads to suboptimal control of BG. The perception of diabetes as a constant and debilitating threat diminishes self-care by leading to psychological conditions like diabetes distress, anxiety, burnout, and behavioral problems,[1] reducing quality of life. Stress affects metabolic control directly by its increase of cortisol and other catabolic hormones that interfere with insulin metabolism, and may also affect metabolic control by interfering with an individual's self-care tasks.[2] This is why stress management and modulating the psychophysiological responses to stress are essential steps in cultivating diabetes resilience.

By understanding what stress is and how it manifests both physiologically and psychologically in the lived experience of diabetes, we can potentially modulate negative stress with yoga practices and empower people to take charge of their condition. Yoga is shown to be a reliable and effective intervention strategy to reduce psychological stress through āsana, prāṇāyāma, meditation, and other yogic-based practices. The cumulative effect of yoga is self-awareness, efficacy, and physical and mental fitness, pivotal for enhanced quality of life and perception of self-worth. When a person feels good, they are less likely to react when a stressor occurs. They may have a non-reaction. With a condition like diabetes, especially T1D, that requires such intense self-management requirements, yoga is a way for individuals to process their stress and increase the negative feedback loops that turn off the stress response. Yoga regulates levels of hormones and neurotransmitters that affect physiological functions responsible for the stress response.[3] Breathing practices are especially helpful with this.

It was important to me to take time to explain the science and psychology of stress. Having this context in the background of your understanding as we move into the nitty gritty practices of yoga therapy for diabetes means you will understand what the practices do and why. This will transform your understanding so that you can take the practices and begin to use them with your own creativity and flavor.

Let's Talk About Stress

Defining stress is almost as crazy as explaining consciousness. It was stressful to write this chapter, let me tell you! Stress is one of the most misunderstood

---

1 Hilliard, M. E., Harris, M. A. and Weissberg-Benchell, J. (2012) "Diabetes resilience: a model of risk and protection in type 1 diabetes." *Current Diabetes Reports 12*, 6, 739–748. p.747.

2 Tirumalesh, M. (2008) *Stress, Psychology, Wellbeing and Quality of Life Among Diabetes Mellitus Patients*. Tirupati: Mangalapalli Tirumalesh. p.26.

3 Mahajan, A. S. (2014) "Role of yoga in hormonal homeostasis." *International Journal of Clinical and Experimental Physiology 1*, 3, 173–178. Accessed on 01/07/20 at: www.ijcep.org/index.php/ijcep/article/view/109.

and overused words (not just by me in this chapter). Its meaning is so non-specific and subjective that it defies all reasonable explanations. Stress mostly has a negative connotation—something to be avoided and reduced. Stress is commonly associated with the word diabetes, and it is true that diabetes can be stressful, but that is not necessarily a bad thing. Beautiful things are created out of adversity. While it causes many physical and mental ailments, it is a necessary biological response intended to keep us alive. Maintaining the function of the autonomic stress response is as important to stress management as it is to consciously practicing relaxation exercises. Actually, practicing relaxation will help you respond to stress better by strengthening the stress response.

I want to invite you to take a deep dive into the science and psychology of stress, not only because it is fascinating, but more importantly, because it is the entry point for understanding the cause and cure for most diabetes challenges. Unresolved and mismanaged stress with diabetes can be a recipe for disaster, but understanding why and influencing our response to it is the entry point into transforming the physical, emotional, and behavioral reactions to diabetes.

Stressful Origins

The history and origin of the word stress is one of the reasons why it is largely misunderstood. It originated in the 1600s as a term related to metallurgy—the malleability to shape metal under intense strain.[4] The term "stress" as we know it in a modern context was described as "the non-specific response of the body to any demand for change" by scientist Hans Selye.[5] In the 1930s Selye accidentally "discovered" a link between intense, traumatic, imposed environment strain and the development of ulcers, enlarged adrenal glands, and immune deficiency in animal rat models. As the story goes, Selye was not a laboratory scientist, he had previously been a physician, and was also kind of a klutz when it came to handling rats. He clumsily stuck needles in them, dropped them, chased them around the room with a broom, and exposed them to extreme environmental changes. What he found was that all of his rats, including the control ones injected with saline, developed ulcers,

4 Online Etymology Dictionary (2001–2020) *Stress*. Accessed on 01/07/20 at: www.etymonline.com/word/stress.

5 Tan, S. Y. and Yip, A. (2018) "Hans Selye (1907–1982): founder of the stress theory." *Singapore Medical Journal* 59, 170–171.

entered immune system failure, and eventually died.[6] Selye's accidental finding suggested that external stressors could cause the same diseases, not only in laboratory animals but also in humans.

People were intrigued, and the term stress was latched on to as a novel term for physical or mental strain, trauma, or *anything that happens that you don't want to happen*.[7] No one wanted stress; it was the cause of all suffering to be avoided at all costs. What we did not realize, at least at that point, was that the very act of avoiding stress actually creates the same conditions for stress to occur.

If you look back at Selye's original definition, stress is "the non-specific response of the body to any demand for change," implying *adaptability* in the face of change. There is no mention of negative or positive, it just is. It was not Selye's intention for stress to be demonized as an unfavorable courtesan of doom. To help clarify the distinction, in the 1970s he came up with two new phrases: positive stress (eustress) and negative stress (distress). But it was too late.

The truth is that stress can be an asset or it can be a risk. What largely determines the distinction is our perception of stress as good or bad.

Positive stress is seen as healthy stress. These are positive stressors that encourage adaptability or resilience to challenge in the face of change. Eustress is perceived as being within our coping abilities and as motivating and focusing our attention and performance.

We need stress to develop our immune systems to prevent future illnesses. Stress helps to fuel the fire to accomplish important goals. It promotes courage, mental fortitude, and focus. A reasonable amount of stress helps people grow into well-adapted human beings equipped to respond to life challenges and unforeseen obstacles.

Ingrained in the stress response are vital alarm systems that warn of danger. Adaptively speaking, the stress response helped us survive in times of famine, during temperature changes, and during dehydration. The stress response is an essential part of how our body prevents hypoglycemia, by not only helping BG levels rise but also providing very uncomfortable and momentous symptoms as a signal to respond to the drop in BG with carbohydrates. For people with diabetes, this is a "positive" stress response to retain.

---

6 McGonigal, K. (2015) *The Upside of Stress: Why Stress Is Good for You (and How to Get Good at It)*. New York: Penguin Random House. p.40.

7 McGonigal, K. (2015) *The Upside of Stress: Why Stress Is Good for You (and How to Get Good at It)*. New York: Penguin Random House. p.41.

Another example of good stress is the kind of stress we self-impose. I am not a scary movie fan; watching them is not fun for me. But for some people, sitting for two hours in front of a horror film is fun. Thrill seekers and adrenaline junkies enjoy flinging themselves off cliffs, dropping out of airplanes, going really, really, really fast. These experiences all cause stress, but the differences between this stress and negative stress are: it is temporary, you know it is going to end; you are in charge and you choose it. When we do not choose stress, it is imposed upon us, it can feel like an insurmountable challenge, and we get "stressed out."

Negative stress is distress. You did not choose it, it is imposed on you, and there is seemingly no end in sight. It is like those poor rats in Selye's laboratory subjected to interminable and unpredictable strain. The nervous system has a threshold of how much stress it can take before it exhausts itself and shuts down. Distress can be psychological and can be caused by negative attitudes, overwhelm, sadness, and fear. It can be physical, like chronic pain and illness. It can be behavioral, like repeating the same thing over and over again, expecting a different result (or is that insanity?).

The physiology of eustress and distress are the same, but the result of distress decreases our performance and can lead to mental and physical problems.[8] Loss, death, physical injury, and a life-threatening diagnosis are all examples of distress. The experience of distress can lead to mental health complications like anxiety and depression, increasing risk and decreasing resilience.

Stress and the Stress Response

A stressor is anything in your world that takes your body out of homeostasis, and the *stress response* is the internal processes designed to bring you back into balance. They are part of our natural evolutionary biology. Balance is a relative term; we can have emotional and physical balance, but in this context balance signifies homeostasis: the biological equilibrium as maintained by physiological processes.

A stressor is an "external" event that triggers an internal response; that response is experienced within the body in the form of thoughts, mood, and impulses. External stressors can come from our environment, nature, people,

8 Mills, H., Reiss, N. and Dombeck, M. (1995–2020) "Types of Stressors (Eustress vs. Distress)." *Cascade: A Behavioral Health Agency.* Accessed on 01/07/20 at: www.cascadementalhealth.org/poc/view_doc.php?type=doc&id=15644&cn=117.

or situations. Memories from past experiences or fear about future ones also are stressors. The thoughts we think, emotions we feel, and actions we partake in can all be stressors. Emotions like worry, excitement, or dread activate the same internal physiological mechanisms as an external stressor.

What determines a positive stressor that increases resilience versus a negative stressor that perpetuates risk is the perception of threat and non-threat. A danger in an evolutionary sense is something that jeopardizes our life. Even Patañjali in the Yoga Sūtra-s says that *abhiniveśa*, the fear of death, is the most difficult of obstacles to overcome. Survival is biological imperative número uno. Our interest in yoga therapy is looking at why we perceive certain things to be a threat and why other things do not bother us at all. Every time our mind decides that something is threatening, and consistently so, the adaptive stress response created to turn on and turn off stays on. This is when it becomes a problem.

The process of returning to balance after a stressful event is called *allostasis*. Another way of thinking about allostasis is the power of the body's regulatory processes to adapt amidst change. Our bodies readily adapt, but when under chronic stress, the regulatory systems get worn out. *Allostatic load* is the wear-and-tear of the body's adaptive response mechanisms. The higher the allostatic load, the greater the long-term risk.

Whether or not a stressor is a real threat to life or self-created fear of future events, our physiology does not discriminate. In a modern sense, negative stress is mostly self-created. Most of the time, we are not in immediate danger, but still, we experience stress. Actual and factual stressors create the same internal stress responses. So, it seems rather evident, as I hope you can tell at this point, that the key to transforming stress lies in our perception of it. Not all stress is bad. Our response to it, whether it is positive (adaptive) or negative (harmful), lies in our ability to identify stressors and consciously choose to override them with our mind.

But it is not so simple. Our responses are often so habituated that we are entirely unconscious of them. You would think that the brain could distinguish the difference between an actual stressor and something that's self-created. But it doesn't. Especially when under chronic stress.

Could it be that what and how we think and the attitudes we hold about life's changing circumstances are as detrimental and costly to our vitality as the actual stressor?

The good news is that just as stress is self-created, it can also be evaded by changing our perception. A negative thought is just as powerful in the creation of a stress response as a real event. When the mind no longer perceives something as stressful, there is a non-reaction, and stress is nullified.

Let's look at a simple example of a positive and negative response to a typical diabetes stressor: high BG. Let's say you are going about your business, doing everything you are "supposed" to do to manage diabetes correctly, but upon glancing at your CGM you see that your BG is skyrocketing—triple arrows up. You have a choice in that moment. Option one: Freak out, identify with the number, take *way* too much insulin, stare at the screen every minute until the arrows stop going up, and complain about it in the process. Your BG ends up plummeting later, then you over correct for the low, end up high, and feel both emotionally and physically drained. Option two: You see the number and say to yourself, "My BG is going up quite fast. That is because I just had a shake and maybe the insulin has not had a chance to kick in. I already have adequate insulin on-board. Instead of taking more insulin, I will do five minutes of movement and reduce the spike. I'll remember for next time that I need to take insulin sooner and wait longer before I have the shake."

With both examples there is stress response. The same systems are activated, but there is a distinction between them. In option one, the individual experiences a classic fight-or-flight response: I see a number, I register it as dangerous, and overreact. Option two: I see a number, I register it, there is no emotion, and I respond appropriately. This is a positive stress response—one that encourages correct action, or in this case, in-action.

I know you are getting excited! Me too. Let's enjoy this positive stress response we are experiencing, take that brain fuel, and apply it towards learning! No, really it might sound boring, but unless you've got this science of stress down, the rest of this book will not make any sense.

Like anything involving education, we can begin to attune to these very mechanisms within ourselves and feel when the stress response occurs. Just like we can feel our body move, our spine articulate, and our lungs breathe, we can also attune to the internal experience of stress and the situational factors that contribute to it. With interoceptive (body) and introspective (mind) awareness, we can begin to discern fact from fiction.

The Limbic Brain

Before we dive deeper into stress and diabetes, I want to take a moment to look at the brain's structure and function, as it offers a scientific model for the connection between mind and body.

Stress is a primitive and biological response sparked by an innate desire to survive. Part of mastering diabetes and reducing the impact of allostatic load is rewiring the stress response to perceive threats accurately and control decisions.

How do we do this? Yoga says: practice. Ayurveda says: create an optimal environment so the body can heal. Neuroscience says: look at the limbic system, the center of perception, emotion, and behavior.

The human brain's anatomy has three distinct layers, which all play a part in its evolutionary development and function. The deepest part is the most primitive brain structure, consisting of the brainstem and cerebellum. All animals possess it. The brainstem and cerebellum preside over automatic and involuntary activities, like breathing, sleeping, digestion, the release of hormones and motor functions, and controlled by the autonomic nervous system.[9] This part of the brain does not think; it only does. Its role is to maintain homeostasis and ensure survival. Think of a reptile; it does not snuggle or play. It is always on guard to respond to a potential threat. Given its automatic nature, this part of the brain relies on instinct. In an emergency situation, we do not think. We just respond. Even though we are not running from saber-tooth cats anymore, this ancient part of our neuroanatomy will always be in charge unless we are present.

The brain's outer layer, the cerebrum, is our *thinking* brain. The most recent layer to develop, evolutionarily speaking, the cerebrum, is what makes us human. When Descartes said, "I think; therefore, I am," he referred to the cerebrum. The cerebrum is divided into the right and left hemispheres, and each region comprises four lobes. Responsible for our highest mental processes, like abstract thought, memory, human language development, and consciousness. It helps us assess information from our senses and voluntarily move our body's muscles. The cerebrum is plastic, meaning it is flexible and can learn new and unlearn old things.[10]

---

9 Leopold, C. (2018) "Everything You Need to Know About the Cerebellum." *Medical News Today*. Accessed on 01/07/20 at: www.medicalnewstoday.com/articles/313265#anatomy.

10 The Brain from Top to Bottom (n.d.) *The Evolutionary Layers of the Brain*. Accessed on 01/07/20 at: https://thebrain.mcgill.ca/flash/d/d_05/d_05_cr/d_05_cr_her/d_05_cr_her.html.

Finally, we have the limbic system, the emotional brain, and the star player of our brief discussion on neuroscience. Older than the cerebrum and younger than the brainstem and cerebellum, the limbic brain is the center of emotion, memory, and motivation. Located *structurally* and *functionally* between the brainstem/cerebellum and the cerebrum, it is the only part of the brain that connects automatic responses with higher cognitive reasoning. Structurally it is made up of the amygdala, hippocampus, thalamus, hypothalamus, and basal ganglia.

The *amygdala* and *hippocampus* help us receive information from our senses and relate that information to our memory. The amygdala is responsible for an emotional response from the senses. The hippocampus is like the repository of all memory; it governs learning and information retrieval. It is like the shock absorber of the stress response and a gateway to transforming stress. As humans accumulate memory and life experience, the hippocampus will store that information as threatening and non-threatening. It talks with the amygdala, the emotional center, and validates what it sees and feels.

Interestingly, the size of a person's amygdala reflects how well or poorly they perceive stress. For instance, a larger amygdala is indicative of a more reactive fear response. Studies show that regular meditation and yoga practitioners have a smaller amygdala and better coping mechanisms for stress.[11]

When the amygdala perceives a changing emotional state through the various senses and environment, it signals to another part of the limbic brain, the hypothalamus, to take charge. The hypothalamus is a big player in the nervous and endocrine system and is where the limbic system connects to the automatic processes of the body. The limbic system is basically structured around trying to influence the hypothalamus to do stuff.[12] Think of the hypothalamus like the CEO of the stress response who signals its manager, the pituitary gland—a hormone-secreting gland that sits just below the hypothalamus—to make sure everyone does their work. The pituitary gland signals its minions, the adrenal glands, two triangular-shaped glands located above the kidneys, to produce the first line of stress hormones.

When the limbic brain receives information via the amygdala from the

11 Gotink, R. A., Vernooij, M. W., Ikram, M. A., Niessen, W. J., *et al.* (2018) "Meditation and yoga practice are associated with smaller right amygdala volume: the Rotterdam study." *Brain Imaging and Behavior 12*, 6, 1631–1639.

12 Sapolsky, R. (2010) *Limbic System*. Stanford, CA: Stanford University. Accessed on 27/08/20 at: www.youtube.com/watch?v=CAOnSbDSaOw&t=2822s.

senses, it can "discern" with the hippocampus's help whether or not to sound the alarms. Sometimes, the response bypasses all thought and conscious reasoning[13] and goes directly into a fight-or-flight state.

The limbic system is cross-wired between the parts that govern thought and biological imperatives. Just think about it. If our perception says that something is awry, the nervous and endocrine system responds by secreting hormones to restore homeostasis. When the body is secreting stress hormones, these hormones will impact our physiology (think blood glucose), thoughts, emotions, and subsequent behaviors.

The answer to fixing the stress response and transforming negative stress lies within the limbic system's structure. In a fight-or-flight response, all rational thought goes into hibernation. The reptilian brain makes the majority of the decisions, and we follow along. Our brain signals the nervous system to release a cascade of stress hormones that alter perception and metabolism, impacting blood glucose, and behavior. With discernment developed through self-awareness strategies that down-regulate stress responses, we can modulate the stress response, rewire automatic function, and decrease allostatic load.

Under chronic stress, people can get stuck in a pattern of reaction instead of pausing, assessing, and responding appropriately. The saying "count to ten" holds up today, training higher cognitive discernment to override automatic impulses.

In the pause, we ask ourselves, "*Is this really what I am feeling? Do I need to respond this way? Or can I instead take a deep breath and choose a different way of operating?*" These are all critical questions to ask in the height of the moment. We are usually so identified and wrapped up in the experience of sympathetic overdrive that our impulses far outweigh free will.

The impulsive reaction is terrible for anyone, but especially for people living with diabetes. Since diabetes is about management, meaning a person has to make thousands of in-the-moment decisions regarding their health all day long, there is a need for higher discernment and analytical decision-making skills. Unless individuals can train their brains to pause and strategize, they can get caught up in the vicious cycle of stress, damaging neuroendocrine responses, and making diabetes way harder to manage.

Luckily, there is an answer, and yoga practice is part of the equation.

13 Kraftsow, G. (1999) *Yoga for Wellness*. New York: Penguin Compass. p.304.

Physiology: Stress Response

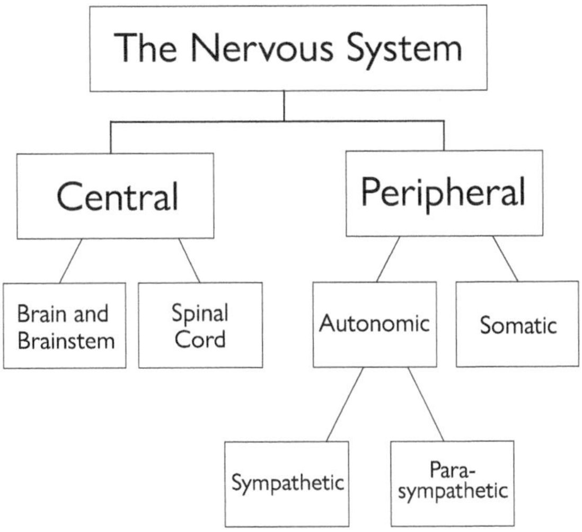

FIGURE 3.1

Stress is a physiological phenomenon that impacts the neuroendocrine responses to restore homeostasis. Whether that has to do with the internal processes involved in maintaining glucose homeostasis or the mental processes that demand action in diabetes management, the physiology is similar. It is an ingrained biological process that ensures our survival.

When we are talking about stress and the stress response, we are talking about the nervous system. The nervous system is a highly complex network coordinating the actions with sensory information. It accomplishes this by transmitting signals (neurotransmitters) from the body to the brain and the brain to parts of the body. The nervous system is one big sensor, which detects environmental changes that impact the body and coordinates simultaneously with the endocrine system.[14] All of these networks work together to promote balance, or internal homeostasis—the equivalent of health and wellbeing on a physical and mental level.

The nervous system is made up of two main systems: the central nervous system (CNS) and peripheral nervous system (PNS). The CNS consists of the brain and spinal cord. The PNS consists of cranial and spinal nerves, connecting the CNS with the rest of the body.[15] Our main focus for adapting

14 Wikipedia (2020) *Nervous System*. Accessed on 01/07/20 at: https://en.wikipedia.org/wiki/Nervous_system.

15 Wikipedia (2020) *Nervous System*. Accessed on 01/07/20 at: https://en.wikipedia.org/wiki/Nervous_system.

the stress response lies within the PNS and its afferent (sensory) and efferent (motor) divisions.

Afferent nerves transport information from somatic and visceral nerves back into the CNS, and efferent nerves transport information from the CNS into our motor fibers, muscles, and glands to cause an effect or action.[16] The PNS is further divided into the somatic (voluntary movement), autonomic (involuntary), and enteric (motility and secretion) systems. Of the three, all you really need to know is the *autonomic nervous system* (ANS) and its two branches: *sympathetic* and *parasympathetic*.

Diabetes affects both the CNS and PNS. Every facet of the nervous system and its supporting structures, from the parts of the brain to all organs involved in neuroendocrine responses, are impacted by complications of diabetes. Diabetes damages the blood vessels, influencing virtually every organ in the body. These involvements are caused by BG changes from hyperglycemia and hypoglycemia and the attempt to regulate them, hyperglycemia-induced metabolic derangements, brain chemistry, and cardiovascular health.[17]

The sympathetic and parasympathetic branches of the ANS are responsible for the activation or pacification of our stress responses and the ANS's connection with the endocrine system. That being said, the inherent connection of our nervous system with our endocrine system governs our metabolism and BG homeostasis. When we are in a fasting state, the sympathetic branch produces glucagon to stave off hypoglycemia. In the fed state, the parasympathetic branch helps us digest our food and produce insulin.

This is why sympathetic activation has been dubbed the "fight-or-flight" response, which is really the get-it-done response, and parasympathetic activation as our "rest-and-digest" response. We need the sympathetic response to allocate energy to take charge throughout our day, and the parasympathetic response to help us recover and build-back our resources. The parasympathetic response acts as the brakes to the sympathetic branch's gas pedal.

The body abides by a rhythm of activation and rest, which is inherent to our ability to derive energy when needed and relax when it is time to rest. Each branch supports the other, and a healthy nervous system is one that can weave seamlessly between the two extremes, both serving an essential purpose. It is like an internal checks-and-balances system. There are times when you need

16 National Cancer Institute (n.d.) *Organization of the Nervous System, SEER Training*. Accessed on 26/08/20 at: https://training.seer.cancer.gov/anatomy/nervous/organization.

17 Harati, Y. (1996) "Diabetes and the nervous system." *Endocrinology and Metabolism Clinics 25*, 2, 325–359.

extra help mobilizing your defenses and other times when it is better to invest in long-term building projects.

When something "stressful" happens to us, the response is mediated by the sympathetic branch. There are two main systems or pathways involved with a stress response: the HPA axis and the sympathoadrenal medullary (SAM) system. They work both together and separately to help us cover the energetic demands of stress. Remember, there are many different kinds of stress to consider: physical exercise, sleep deprivation, hypoglycemia, environmental stresses, trauma, and infection, to name a few.[18] Sometimes we need our responses to be quick and immediate; other times we need energy to help us make it for longer distances. Each pathway produces various hormones to support immediate and long-duration demands.

The SAM system is synonymous with the sympathetic activation. After the amygdala perceives a threat via the senses, it signals to the hypothalamus to activate the sympathetic branch of the ANS through its nerves to the adrenal glands, where it provides the body with fast-acting catecholamines (norepinephrine and epinephrine). Also known as adrenaline, these hormones increase heart rate, blood pressure, and the perception of anxiety. This response prepares us for the short-term, immediate action by turning off the parasympathetic nervous system, responsible for rest, regeneration, and digestion. In a heightened state of arousal, we need all of our energy to go towards survival, not rest. During a fight-or-flight stress response, other physiological functions are turned off because the body needs all of its power to cope with a stressor. Essential anabolic functions like digesting food and building cells will be placed on pause because in an emergency state, or any physiological stress activation, survival is more important.

The HPA axis is another branch in the stress system and is best known for its role in the long-term response to stress. It is the kind of stress response we need to make the long haul. Evolutionarily speaking, we needed this stress response in times of fasting or traveling long distances. Implied by its name, the HPA axis comprises the hypothalamus, pituitary gland, and adrenal glands, and its primary function is to secrete glucocorticoids. The most important of these for you to know about is the steroid hormone *cortisol*.

---

18 Horton, E. S. and Beisel, W. R. (1994) "The Metabolic Responses to Stress and Physical Activity." In B. M. Marriott (ed.) *Food Components to Enhance Performance: An Evaluation of Potential Performance-Enhancing Food Components for Operational Rations.* Washington DC: National Academies Press. Accessed on 01/07/20 at: www.ncbi.nlm.nih.gov/books/NBK209038.

Cortisol is a good thing—in moderation. It buffers out the jittery effects of the SAM system (adrenaline or epinephrine), increasing heart rate, circulation, and adaptive response to immediate stress. Cortisol is a hormone responsible for our energy throughout the day. Ideally, we wake up with abundant cortisol and it tapers off over the day. By evening we have our lowest cortisol levels and are ready to go to bed, where our bodies can regenerate. Changes in cortisol levels can be indicative of mental health disorders like depression and insulin resistance.

The HPA axis provides the body with necessary long-term fuel to cover longer durations of stress. A healthy stress response can turn on and off when it is no longer needed. This is called a negative feedback loop, which is actually a good thing. When cortisol levels reach their peak, this is sensed by the hypothalamus and the hippocampus, and the production of cortisol is turned off.

When the body is always under stress (real or perceived—it doesn't matter), the HPA axis does not recognize when there is too much cortisol, and the negative feedback loop is not efficient. Cortisol reserves are depleted, and the SAM system's release of epinephrine is unfiltered. People feel jittery and anxious, distorting the perception of stress and damaging positive coping. The chronic activation of the HPA axis and cortisol causes fatty acids[19] and glucose to flow into the bloodstream, increasing BG levels and diabetes risk.

Although the activation of the HPA axis and SAM system is part of a normal and healthy stress response, too much of it damages the function of the stress response to adapt to life's changes.

Every stressor and stress response has a cumulative cost, which influences all future responses. If a person is taking good care of themselves, and managing their emotions and energy, every time they incur stress they are able to offset that stress by applying a protective measure, either from the food they eat or the health-providing activities they partake in.

Immunity, Inflammation, and the Stress Response

The immune system is part of our body's defense team. Its role is to distinguish between self and non-self. Very yogic. In this case, "self" is not consciousness,

19 Ross, A. and Michalsen, A. (2016) "Yoga for Prevention and Wellness." In S. B. S. Khalsa, L. Cohen, T. McCall and S. Telles (eds) *The Principles and Practice of Yoga in Healthcare*. Pencaitland: Handspring Publishing. p.472.

but rather the body's native cells. Non-self is "foreign" cells that have entered the body in one way or another. It is the immune system's job to detect foreign cells and destroy them. Sometimes it does a good job and a person is able to fight off a virus or attack a tumor. But the immune system is not perfect and it needs checks and balances to stop it from overworking. Without such a mechanism, the immune system lacks correct discernment. It will mistake the self for non-self, destroying the body's own cells and tissues.[20] This is what happens in T1D. The immune system destroys pancreatic beta cells. Any autoimmune condition is the fundamental misunderstanding by the immune system that the self is the non-self. There is yoga philosophy even in our physiology.

For unknown reasons, in the first hour of an immune response, glucocorticoids actually potentiate immunity, increasing the immune system's activation. But after about an hour, these hormones start to lower the levels of white blood cells, bringing them back to normal. Glucocorticoids supply the body with glucose during a prolonged stressor. They are also a buffer to the immune system's response to "foreign invaders." White blood cells, or lymphocytes, are what the immune system uses to rid the body of a virus, bacteria, and anything that is essentially a threat to internal balance. When the immune system kicks in, just like anything that is regulated by the body, there is a curve of productivity. Initially that curve goes up. White blood cells increase—a greater army to destroy potential invaders. However, as the curve rises, there is also a CRR for keeping the immune system in check, bringing it back to baseline. That is the stress response, the sympathetic branch, and glucocorticoids. Glucocorticoids are released by the adrenals, which help to distribute white blood cells properly and even kill off weak ones. Glucocorticoids are the CRR to the immune system's attack phase. Without this check and balance, immunity will continue to skyrocket and increase the risk of autoimmune diseases, i.e. T1D.

Although there is not yet a clear cause for T1D, what we do know is that something triggers the immune system to mistake pancreatic beta cells for foreign invaders. We also know that the nervous system has an important role in regulating immunity. Without an internal mechanism for checks and balances, the immune system will go on killing cells and tissues indiscriminately. The nervous system helps the immune system return to baseline. When it comes

20 U.S. Department of Health and Human Services, National Institutes of Health (2003) *Understanding the Immune System. How It Works.* Accessed on 01/07/20 at: www.imgt.org/IMGTeducation/Tutorials/ImmuneSystem/UK/the_immune_system.pdf.

to autoimmunity, the stress response is not a bad thing. Cortisol suppresses the inflammatory response, which is the immune system's way of attacking foreign non-self cells. More on this later, as it has a direct effect on BG, insulin sensitivity, and the cause of T1D.

You could say that a weakened release of glucocorticoids could cause an autoimmune condition. It is not uncommon to hear of people experiencing bouts of chronic stress several years before a diagnosis of T1D (although there is still no evidence to corroborate this scientifically). When it functions properly, the stress response is an important check and balance to immunity. Glucocorticoids act as a negative feedback loop (stop) to the immune system. We need glucocorticoids (a healthy stress hormone in this case) to regulate the immune system's attack against foreign invader cells. Without this negative feedback loop, the immune system will continue to attack and is the cause of T1D. Our physiology is not black and white. It is about optimizing its balance.

We have demonized glucocorticoids as the cause of so many health issues when in fact glucocorticoids are not at fault; it is the overproduction of glucocorticoids (during chronic stress) that weakens the production of glucocorticoids. So, overproducing it ends up underproducing it. We need a balanced production of glucocorticoids to help the immune system return to baseline after the threat of infection has subsided, but with too much glucocorticoid the immune system is suppressed. While in the first hour of acute stress the immune system is heightened, if the stress is chronic, the wear and tear of allostatic load also impact the function of the immune system. Chronic stress can both heighten the release of glucocorticoids and weaken their potency.

If autoimmune diseases are a product of insufficient glucocorticoids and an overactive immune system,[21] insulin resistance and T2D are the products of excessive glucocorticoids and an underactive immune system. To best understand the effect of excessive cortisol on insulin resistance, let's look at what happens to a normal non-diabetic person's physiology when they take a cortisone or prednisone shot. These are synthetic versions of cortisol intended to reduce inflammation, but an effect of them is insulin resistance. People tend to gain weight after a shot as a result of insulin resistance. The painful inflammation goes away, but their BG levels will increase. Even though

21 Silverman, M. N. and Sternberg, E. M. (2012) "Glucocorticoid regulation of inflammation and its functional correlates: from HPA axis to glucocorticoid receptor dysfunction." *Annals of the New York Academy of Sciences 1261*, 55–63.

glucocorticoids reduce inflammation, the effect is insulin resistance. Sometimes people will find out that they are type 2 or pre-type 2 after a bout of steroids. It is not advisable for anyone with T1D or T2D to take synthetic steroids because it will make BG even harder to control. I once had a shot after hurting my back and was in so much pain that I decided to have higher blood sugars than be in that pain. I could not bring my numbers below 250 mg/dL (13.9 mmol/L) for several weeks.

The example of synthetic steroids is exemplary of what occurs in a non-diabetic person's physiology when they are under chronic stress. During chronic stress, the HPA axis releases more cortisol to support longer-duration stressors. More stress equals more cortisol. The effect of this is additional glucose in the bloodstream and an increased production of insulin. Over time the body becomes resistant to the effects of insulin, requiring more and more of it to maintain glucose homeostasis. The effect of insulin resistance is weight gain; not the other way around.

People with diabetes are more susceptible to developing infections because high BG levels weaken immune defenses.[22] Excessive glucocorticoids suppress immune function and increase insulin resistance. Many of the effects of unmanaged BG levels are bacterial infections affecting the skin and urinary tract. Other effects like diabetic neuropathy, a damaging of the nerves in the feet in particular, contribute to foot infections as a person may not be able to perceive the infection if they have lost the feeling in their feet. A suppressed immune system makes it more difficult for people with diabetes to fight off infection. But it is important to note that diabetics are only more susceptible when their blood sugars are higher. Being sick also presents a challenge for diabetics. The nature of fighting off a viral or bacterial infection increases glucocorticoids, which raises BG levels. It is not uncommon for diabetics to need additional insulin during times of sickness.

The immune system and nervous system work together to promote immunity. Glucocorticoids are regulated by the HPA axis and act as the buffer to an overactive immune system. Insufficient glucocorticoid release by an impaired HPA axis can be a contributing factor in autoimmune disease. Excessive glucocorticoids, either as a result of unmanaged chronic stress or synthetically applied due to a physical inflammatory stress response, suppress

22 Ross, H. M. (2019) "What infections are you at risk for with diabetes?" *Verywell Health*. Accessed on 01/07/20 at: www.verywellhealth.com/what-are-the-common-infections-with-diabetes-1087622.

immunity and can cause insulin resistance. This can be a cause of prediabetes and also a major management deterrent for BG homeostasis. Stress-induced hyperglycemia causes insulin resistance for both T1D and T2D, also increasing vulnerability by inhibiting immunity.

The Vicious Cycle of Stress

The problem with stress occurs when we cannot shut it off. Professor Robert Sapolsky of Stanford University coined a useful analogy to the insidious cycle of stress and how it impacts an organism's health.

Consider the body and its physiological processes as a country. To be a balanced, functioning society with a good status globally, a country needs to have strong defenses and a robust internal structure built on the inhabitants' health, education, and wellbeing.

When our bodies are under chronic stress, our internal defenses are always on the front line, on guard, and ready for the attack. The body puts all energy into its offenses, not towards its defenses. All of its long-term building projects are placed on hold. Forget about education and healthcare. There is no budget. Stress hormones like epinephrine and norepinephrine (adrenaline) accelerate heart rate and blood pressure, putting the defensive "soldiers" on edge. With jittery hormones pumping through the veins, one false move, and it is easy to misfire, either shooting yourself in the foot or firing on a member of your team. This is what it is like to be in the body of a person whose stress responses are chronically activated. The offenses remain vigilant, unable to turn off their attack mechanisms, leaving little, if any, national investment in the essential building projects that sustain a society's growth and wellbeing.

Diabetes presents its own set of stressors that compound stress. Some of them are temporal, like hyperglycemia or hypoglycemia. You correct them and the stressors go away. But diabetes itself does not go away. The persistent burden of highs and lows, the challenges of self-management, and all that goes into taking care of diabetes, not to mention the effects associated with the long duration of the disease, create a context for the defenses to always be up and on guard. Chronic stress is fueled by the limbic system and the SAM-HPA axis. When something stressful occurs, your body becomes activated. The physical symptoms of sweaty palms and an increased heart rate are interpreted by the limbic system as a threat, triggering more stress-fueled reactions, swelling stress hormones.[23]

Heightened stress hormones increase reactivity to perceived stress and require more effort to return to balance after a stress response. Our stress response systems negotiate the process of *allostasis*. Remember, the stress responses try to restore balance; allostasis is how efficiently we achieve that balance. In the short term, allostasis works well when resolving acute stress. The stressor stops, and we can return to balance.

But everything has a threshold of just how much damage it can put up with, just like Selye's rats. While the physiological mechanisms behind the stress response are adaptive in the short term, every time we bring ourselves back into balance, there is a cost. The process of allostasis impacts our body and organs. Under chronic stress, there is an increased production of long-term stress hormones, particularly cortisol from the HPA axis, resulting in wear and tear on our nervous system, not to mention increasing insulin resistance. Many scientists believe that our nervous system was not designed to withstand constant activation.

Because of this, there is a cumulative cost of repeated neuroendocrine responses resulting from stress. In what would otherwise be a positive response, repeated and prolonged activation of stress responses can lead to dysregulation of multiple physiological systems and deterioration of health.[24, 25] Chronic stress has been linked to heart disease, high blood pressure, high cholesterol, T2D, and depression.[26] Reduced health outcomes increase future sensitivity to stressors. In effect, people get stuck in a loop of stress, reaction, decreased willpower, adverse health outcomes, and increased sensitivity.

You've heard the phrase "Burning the candle at both ends," right? Unless we are applying strategies to offset the cost of stress by training the nervous system, there is a threshold of how much our system can take before it burns out. An example of this is adrenal fatigue, where the adrenal glands are maxed

---

23 Hanson, R. (2009) *Buddha's Brain: The Practical Neuroscience of Happiness, Love and Wisdom.* Oakland, CA: New Harbinger Publications. p.113.

24 Ross, A. and Michalsen, A. (2016) "Yoga for Prevention and Wellness." In S. B. S. Khalsa, L. Cohen, T. McCall and S. Telles (eds) *The Principles and Practice of Yoga in Healthcare.* Pencaitland: Handspring Publishing. p.473.

25 Hilliard, M. E., Yi-Frazier, J. P., Hessler, D., Butler, A. M., Anderson, B. J. and Jaser, S. (2016) "Stress and A1c among people with diabetes across the lifespan." *Current Diabetes Reports 16*, 8, 67.

26 Centre for Studies on Human Stress (CSHS) (2019) *Acute vs. Chronic Stress.* Accessed on 01/07/20 at: https://humanstress.ca/stress/understand-your-stress/acute-vs-chronic-stress.

out by overactivation, and individuals have no buffer to handle any type of stressor. Diabetes is another—the constant wear and tear of physiological and psychological risks of stress chip away resilience.

Just think about it. If we put all of our money into our offenses, there is nothing to put into long-term growth and restoration. There is a limit to how much we can do this before a real imbalance occurs. This in no way means that people are responsible for creating T2D or an autoimmune response that attacks the production of beta cells as it does in T1D. It merely implies that specific actions can buffer and reduce the risk of incurring long-term damage from chronic stress. Individuals who participate in healthy activities and behaviors are protected from chronic stress and susceptibility to genetic and environmental predispositions.

Without protective measures like downregulation of the ANS and increased sympathetic tone, the eventual wear and tear on the internal processes that restore balance loses it bounce-back rate. People become more sensitive to stress, and the cycle of stress perpetuates.

Acute Versus Chronic Stress

Let's take a moment to review the different types of temporal stress related to stress response and diabetes.

Acute Stress

Acute stress is a short-term, sympathoadrenal response produced by the SAM pathway. We typically associate it with a fight-or-flight response. During an acute stress response, the hormones epinephrine and norepinephrine are released, elevating heart rate and blood pressure to respond to an immediate emergency.

This fast-acting response helps us attend to in-the-moment, recent-past, or near-future stressors. It is temporal, meaning it comes on quickly and should evaporate within a few minutes to hours once the stressor has subsided. Some real-life examples are being in a car crash, experiencing airplane turbulence, and starting a race.

Acute Diabetes Stress

The physiological pathos of diabetes contributes to acute stress. That's a fancy way of saying that blood sugar fluctuations cause acute stress. An example of an acute diabetes stressor would be hypoglycemia. The very hormones released by the neuroendocrine systems to respond and counteract hypoglycemia (epinephrine and norepinephrine) are the same hormones released during an acute stress response mediated by the SAM system. Other causes of acute diabetes-related stress are related to management challenges and behavior. From insulin changes to new management devices, any shift in the usual routine can be stressful. New technologies can be an extra cause when they are introduced, with their constant information and alarm systems.

Acute stress impacts glycemic control. Ask anyone who lives with diabetes, and they will tell you BG levels run higher when the body is under acute stress. Both general and diabetes-related acute stress can impact glycemic control. Whenever I present publicly, my BG will spike. Also, after a severe low BG episode, my BG levels sometimes run higher. Both are due to the additional counterregulatory hormones in my system. Whether acute stress has a direct impact on A1c levels is still up for debate. Acute stress temporarily raises glycemic levels, but the increase is not substantial or prolonged enough to impact the A1c. This is perhaps because the glycemic impact is short lived and not sufficient to influence A1c.

Chronic Stress

Chronic stress is a repeated and persistent strain that does not subside. It's the emotional state of feeling like there is no way out and emotional resignation. In a modern sense, chronic stress is a product of the times we live in, the cumulative wear and tear of perceived stressful stimuli. We are not running from lions and tigers anymore; we are running from ourselves. Chronic anxiety, procrastination, fears, and aversions are all faces of chronic stress. The neuroendocrine mechanisms behind chronic stress are the HPA axis, and its most famous hormone, cortisol, is interconnected with chronic stress.

While the physiological mechanisms behind the stress response are adaptive in the short term, there are implications of repeated wear and tear on the body's regulatory systems. Many scientists believe that our nervous system was not designed to withstand constant activation. Because of this, there is a cumulative cost of repeated neuroendocrine responses resulting from chronic stress.

In what would otherwise be a positive response, repeated and prolonged activation of stress responses can lead to dysregulation of multiple physiological systems and deterioration of health.[27] Chronic stress has been linked to heart disease, high blood pressure, high cholesterol, T2D, and depression.[28]

Chronic Diabetes-Related Stress

Chronic diabetes-related stress or "distress" is the emotional stress associated with ongoing worries, burdens, and concerns related to diabetes management. It is an attitude of being always frustrated, overwhelmed, and discouraged by diabetes requirements. For individuals with T1D, stress is most associated with feelings of powerlessness, hypo fears, self-management, and eating. Those with T2D report treatment regimen and the emotional burden as the primary triggers.[29]

Chronic Stress and Glycemic Control

Chronic diabetes stress is associated with significantly higher A1c in T2D, and increases in diabetes-related stress have been associated with decreases in A1c.[30] Research has shown that there is a strong correlation between chronic stress and glycemic outcomes.[31] Chronic stress increases susceptibility to other diabetes-related challenges like diabetes distress, burnout, anxiety, and depression, all of which have a negative effect on cognitions, self-management, and quality of life.

The Antidote

Yoga practices can help attenuate the impact of allostatic load, facilitating adaptive stress responses amid a stressor, and even reverse it by turning off the HPA axis-SAM system's response to stress and decreasing levels of cortisol, epinephrine, norepinephrine, and inflammatory cytokines.[32] It does this by regulating the ANS through parasympathetic activation.

---

27 Ross, A. and Michalsen, A. (2016) "Yoga for Prevention and Wellness." In S. B. S. Khalsa, L. Cohen, T. McCall and S. Telles (eds) *The Principles and Practice of Yoga in Healthcare.* Pencaitland: Handspring Publishing. p.473.

28 Centre for Studies on Human Stress (CSHS) (2019) *Acute vs. Chronic Stress.* Accessed on 01/07/20 at: https://humanstress.ca/stress/understand-your-stress/acute-vs-chronic-stress.

29 Hilliard, M. E., Yi-Frazier, J. P., Hessler, D., Butler, A. M., Anderson, B. J. and Jaser, S. (2016) "Stress and A1c among people with diabetes across the lifespan." *Current Diabetes Reports 16*, 8, 67.

30 Hilliard, M. E., Yi-Frazier, J. P., Hessler, D., Butler, A. M., Anderson, B. J. and Jaser, S. (2016) "Stress and A1c among people with diabetes across the lifespan." *Current Diabetes Reports 16*, 8, 67.

31 Hilliard, M. E., Yi-Frazier, J. P., Hessler, D., Butler, A. M., Anderson, B. J. and Jaser, S. (2016) "Stress and A1c among people with diabetes across the lifespan." *Current Diabetes Reports 16*, 8, 67.

32 Schmalzl, L., Streeter, C. C. and Khalsa, S. B. S. (2016) "Research on the Psychophysiology of Yoga." In S. B. S. Khalsa, L. Cohen, T. McCall and S. Telles (eds) *The Principles and Practice of Yoga in Healthcare.* Pencaitland: Handspring Publishing. p.60.

The stress response is not a bad thing—we need sympathetic activation to function—it just becomes detrimental when we go beyond our ability to cope and return to baseline.[33] Chronic sympathetic overdrive damages the potency of sympathetic responses and increases the wear and tear on the body's protective processes of regeneration. The result is an overactive stress response, increased perception of stress, and decreased self-care behaviors. Yoga-based practices help to restore autonomic function, and prevent metabolic deterioration and inflammation that wreak havoc on diabetes management by modulating between sympathetic and parasympathetic activation.[34]

A potential pathway for shifting the mind's perception of stress is through the vagus nerve. Parasympathetic activation is modulated by the vagus nerve, the tenth cranial nerve, also known as the "great wandering protector"[35] because it regulates autonomic function and extends from the brain to multiple regions of the body, innervating the heart, lungs, and stomach. Parasympathetic activation and the function of the vagus nerve are the primary defense mechanism to counteract the damage of unabated chronic stress and the impact of such stress on every organ system and, in turn, the quality of a person's life.

The vagus nerve is a "mixed" nerve, possessing both afferent (sensory) and efferent (motor) fibers. This means that the vagus nerve carries information from the CNS to the organs it innervates and from these organs back into the CNS.[36] The amygdala (fear detector) and the cerebrum (prefrontal cortex as center of thought and self-regulatory behaviors)[37] are linked via the vagus nerve to the regulation of neuroendocrine responses. Regularly activating the parasympathetic branch tonifies the vagus nerve and acts as a potential modulator for transforming the perception of stress from the senses into the body and vice versa. It provides a moment of "pause" where the higher, discerning mind can assess and decide how to respond, rather than react from impulse.

Just the other day, I was getting ready for a mountain bike ride with my husband and noticed I was feeling anxious. There is a disquieting sensation to

33 Stephens, I. (2017) "Medical yoga therapy." *Children 4*, 2, 12.

34 Stephens, I. (2017) "Medical yoga therapy." *Children 4*, 2, 12.

35 Gerritsen, R. J. S. and Band, G. P. H. (2018) "Breath of life: the respiratory vagal stimulation model of contemplative activity." *Frontiers in Human Neuroscience 12*, 397.

36 Byrne, M. (2020) "Vagus nerve." *Ken Hub.* Accessed on 01/07/20 at: www.kenhub.com/en/library/anatomy/the-vagus-nerve.

37 Schmalzl, L., Streeter, C. C. and Khalsa, S. B. S. (2016) "Research on the Psychophysiology of Yoga." In S. B. S. Khalsa, L. Cohen, T. McCall and S. Telles (eds) *The Principles and Practice of Yoga in Healthcare.* Pencaitland: Handspring Publishing. p.61.

it, a hurry and immediacy of "I've got to get this ride started." I had nothing to be anxious about, we were going on a relatively easy and familiar ride, but when I reflected on it for a moment I realized that the anxiety I was feeling was about exercise and my BG going high or low. It was a completely subconscious psychological stress response; I had not even thought about it. The impulse to worry about my BG was there because it is always a risk. Instead of festering in that feeling, I recognized that I was feeling it, and then I listed everything that was working. My BG levels were in good order. I did not have too much insulin in my system (something that would cause a low). I was okay. The anxiety was completely unfounded. The first step was the recognition of anxiety, the second step was the moment of pause and reflection on the validity of it, the third was the choice. But this has not always been the case. I've been stuck on mountain tops in white-outs, with fogged goggles, low blood sugars, and panic attacks, while hiking. Even in the midst of those, cultivating the pause helps you get through emergency situations.

The effectiveness or strength of a person's vagus nerve to modulate information coming in from the senses to the brain, and the brain back into the body, is called vagal tone. High vagal tone is associated with more adaptive top-town and bottom-up processes such as: attention regulation, affective processing, and flexibility of the nervous system to adapt and respond to the environment.[38] Studies show that vagal control increases self-awareness, self-control, and self-regulation in response to challenges.[39]

We can measure vagal tone by looking at heart rate variability—the more variable our heart rate, the more adaptive our stress response. This means that our heart rate can activate and go up just as easily as it can come down. It does so on every beat and breath.

Conversely, low vagal tone is associated with many conditions that are risk factors for diabetes like anxiety, depression, and other adverse health outcomes.[40] This variability is used as an indicator for physical conditioning,

---

38 Sullivan, M. B., Erb, M., Schmalzl, L., Moonaz, S., Noggle Taylor, J. and Porges, S. W. (2018) "Yoga therapy and polyvagal theory: the convergence of traditional wisdom and contemporary neuroscience for self-regulation and resilience." *Frontiers in Human Neuroscience 12*, 67.

39 Sullivan, M. B., Erb, M., Schmalzl, L., Moonaz, S., Noggle Taylor, J. and Porges, S. W. (2018) "Yoga therapy and polyvagal theory: the convergence of traditional wisdom and contemporary neuroscience for self-regulation and resilience." *Frontiers in Human Neuroscience 12*, 67.

40 Sullivan, M. B., Erb, M., Schmalzl, L., Moonaz, S., Noggle Taylor, J. and Porges, S. W. (2018) "Yoga therapy and polyvagal theory: the convergence of traditional wisdom and contemporary neuroscience for self-regulation and resilience." *Frontiers in Human Neuroscience 12*, 67.

general health, and reactivity to and from high stress levels. The greater the peaks and valleys, the better the variability associated with lower perceived stress levels and better health and disease outcomes.[41] Assessing heart rate variability is an effective way to measure the potential of invisible autonomic complications of diabetes.

We can train the vagus nerve with conscious breathing practices. The vagus nerve is suppressed during inhalation and activated during exhalation and smooth respiratory cycles.[42]

Prāṇāyāma as a breath adaptation in āsana and seated prāṇāyāma practices are important training tools for restoring autonomic function and reducing perceived stress.

By modulating the stress response via vagal stimulation from conscious breathing exercises, people can bolster their resilience to all forms of negative stressors; diabetes is no exception.

A study on respiratory effect on vagal stimulation found that there are two ways that breathing can stimulate the vagus nerve: directly and indirectly. The direct path is focused on lengthening exhalation and abdominal (diaphragm) versus thoracic (chest) breathing. The indirect path is through body awareness and relaxation practices like the preparatory practices for yoga nidrā. This is when the breath is completely involuntary and is a focal point for the mind to rest upon. By just being aware of the breath, and not "doing" the breath, the practitioner enters slower and deeper respiration cycles.[43]

These practices improve heart rate variability, lower the heart rate and blood pressure, inhibit the SNS, and down-regulate the HPA axis, potentially activating an anti-inflammatory pathway and resulting in a decrease of acute stress levels.[44] We can posit that this network of self-regulating properties is the key to unlocking the physiological and psychological challenges associated with diabetes-related stress, if not all stress, in the short and long term.

There is a direct impact on the parasympathetic nervous system during and after practice and a shift in autonomic function over time. As the faculties of

41 Gerritsen, R. J. S. and Band, G. P. H. (2018) "Breath of life: the respiratory vagal stimulation model of contemplative activity." *Frontiers in Human Neuroscience 12*, 397.

42 Gerritsen, R. J. S. and Band, G. P. H. (2018) "Breath of life: the respiratory vagal stimulation model of contemplative activity." *Frontiers in Human Neuroscience 12*, 397.

43 Gerritsen, R. J. S. and Band, G. P. H. (2018) "Breath of life: the respiratory vagal stimulation model of contemplative activity." *Frontiers in Human Neuroscience 12*, 397.

44 Gerritsen, R. J. S. and Band, G. P. H. (2018) "Breath of life: the respiratory vagal stimulation model of contemplative activity." *Frontiers in Human Neuroscience 12*, 397.

the parasympathetic nervous system increase, sympathetic predominance is reduced, attenuating the long-term impact of chronic stress.[45] Remember that sympathetic activation is not harmful; it plays an essential role in how we relate and respond to the world. The problem occurs when the stress responses do not turn off, increasing allostatic load, and heightening the risk of developing stress-related complications.

Individuals with diabetes are at a higher risk of problems stemming from impaired vagal function. High BG levels damage the nerves in the body, and the vagus nerve is no different.

Peripheral neuropathy impairs the nerves in the feet and hands, but autonomic neuropathy harms the ANS and the balance of sympathetic and parasympathetic activation. The ANS governs the nerves responsible for everyday bodily processes like heart rate and digestion. Low vagal tone can debilitate many organ systems, causing more damage than any other nerve.

Issues that involve autonomic neuropathy can include rapid heart rate, sexual dysfunction, and gastroparesis, a delayed stomach emptying. Gastroparesis makes insulin-to-food timing especially challenging for people with diabetes.

By learning to regulate the vagus nerve through yoga-based practices, individuals with diabetes can potentially preserve what pancreatic faculties remain and improve the function that what was once damaged.[46]

A Practice for Vagal Tone

Let's take a moment to pay attention to our breath. Lengthening the exhale activates the parasympathetic branch, decreases the heart rate and blood pressure, and increases heart rate variability. The greater the heart rate variability, the better a person can adapt to stress in a positive way by choosing their response to it or negating it all together.

Go ahead and close your eyes. Spend a moment just noticing your body breathing.

Then begin to progressively deepen your inhale and exhale, making sure to smooth out any tension in your breathing.

---

45 Gerritsen, R. J. S. and Band, G. P. H. (2018) "Breath of life: the respiratory vagal stimulation model of contemplative activity." *Frontiers in Human Neuroscience 12*, 397.

46 Bernstein, R. K. (2011) *Dr. Bernstein's Diabetes Solution: The Complete Guide to Achieving Normal Blood Sugars*. Fourth edition. Boston, MA: Little Brown Publishers. p.65.

Pay attention to the exhalation. Feel its origin deep in the belly as you contract the abdominal muscles, the diaphragm lifts, and the lungs empty.

Slow down the exhale. I like to imagine I am slowly letting the exhale out of my body like I am releasing air from a balloon. It might not sound like you are breathing, but you feel a very slow release of the exhale.

Then, when it feels comfortable, add a slight pause at the end of the exhale. The exhale doesn't have to be "completely" vacating your lungs; this is impossible and will create anxiety. Just give it a brief pause for two seconds, three seconds, and so on until it feels like your breath is mostly pause and could go on forever. The inhale and exhale may be barely there.

When you feel the pause, relax your mind completely. Just let it stop and melt into the inner peace.

Keep it up for about five minutes and notice the space in the mind. It creates a pause, or an inner mental stillness. This is the still point, deep in the mid-brain in the limbic structure. You can visualize it, just imagine it. The amygdala and hippocampus relaxed, and attuned to higher cognitive faculties. Perceiving the senses accurately and clearly. The hypothalamus and all automatic function are in balance. Relax your awareness and return slowly.

Attitude is everything when it comes to diabetes. Yes, all that goes into it is tiring and relentless, but the attitude of it all being terrible stems from the habit of belief. Through yoga-based interventions we can actively strengthen heart rate variability and find clarity even in the midst of a stress response. This is beneficial for all beings, but especially so for those with diabetes.

Developing the pause where the thinking brain can discern a threat from a non-threat allows people to feel the stress but not buy into the reaction that this whole thing is so terrible and awful. That takes time and practice. Now let's look at the potential contributors to diabetes stress in an effort to identify and eventually eradicate the causes of suffering and suboptimal diabetes care.

Identifying Diabetes Stress and Risk

Stress has an enormous impact on diabetes management and care, and the outcomes of diabetes-based interventions are dependent on how well an individual responds to negative stress. Stressors are believed to impact diabetes, affecting the quality of self-management and its outcomes.[47] The ADA highlights the role of stress in fulfilling glycemic objectives for health and longevity.[48]

It is estimated that 20–40% of people with T1D and T2D experience diabetes-related stress,[49] although I would argue that it is more because so many people have suboptimal care. While stress can impact BG levels, stress mostly affects the way an individual takes care of themselves and their perceptions of how effective they are as a metric for self-worth. Stress is an important factor in the cases in which BG cannot be regulated despite medical treatment,[50] so addressing stress through the physical and psychological benefit of yoga is potentially a highly effective medium to identify stress triggers and actually do something about them.

Negative associations with general stress and diabetes-related distress can perpetuate feelings of powerlessness and emotional burden. On the flip side, individuals who are more resilient to stress (less perceived stress) are associated with better glycemic control.[51] Positive associations with diabetes challenges instill feelings of empowerment and self-efficacy in the face of stress, transforming the risk of stress into a personal strength and adaptability.

Identifying the source of negative stress will help to guide personal practice and intervention strategies. I have attempted to outline the varying types of stress, the origins, and the causes of individuals living with diabetes to encourage identification so that improvements can be made.

Three main classifications determine diabetes stress.

The first relates to the physical experience of diabetes itself within the human body. Hyperglycemia, hypoglycemia, and co-morbid disorders are a physical result of diabetes. The tension, body aches, and physical effects of diabetes, like a stomach ache or headache, are all potential contributors to physical stress. How a person feels physically is indicative of their energetic

---

47 Butkiewicz, E., Carbone, A., Green, S., Miano, A. and Wegner, E. (2016) "Diabetes Management." In M. A. Burg and O. Oyama (eds) *Behavioral Health Specialist.* New York: Springer Publishing Company. p.91.

48 Hilliard, M. E., Yi-Frazier, J. P., Hessler, D., Butler, A. M., Anderson, B. J. and Jaser, S. (2016) "Stress and A1c among people with diabetes across the lifespan." *Current Diabetes Reports 16*, 8, 67.

49 Hilliard, M. E., Yi-Frazier, J. P., Hessler, D., Butler, A. M., Anderson, B. J. and Jaser, S. (2016) "Stress and A1c among people with diabetes across the lifespan." *Current Diabetes Reports 16*, 8, 67.

50 Tirumalesh, M. (2008) *Stress, Psychology, Wellbeing and Quality of Life Among Diabetes Mellitus Patients.* Tirupati: Mangalapalli Tirumalesh. p.65.

51 Hilliard, M. E., Yi-Frazier, J. P., Hessler, D., Butler, A. M., Anderson, B. J. and Jaser, S. (2016) "Stress and A1c among people with diabetes across the lifespan." *Current Diabetes Reports 16*, 8, 67.

state, a state that also impacts emotions, thoughts, and subsequent actions as they relate to diabetes management.

The second is stress from diabetes management: the effort required to take care of diabetes, including problem-solving skills and implementation of action-based strategies.

The last, and probably not final, as I am sure someone reading this can come up with more, is the stress of co-managing diabetes with regular life and managing life with diabetes. It would be one thing to do all that has to go into self-management with a single focus, but most people are doing multiple things at the same time. It takes presence and precision to take care of low BG in the midst of pulling two kids to hockey. Or to teach a yoga class while checking your BG and treatment. How about the emotional side of it—having to communicate, "Sorry I've got to deal with this first, you come second"? That is hard for a lot of people. Their priorities get mixed up and diabetes can come later on in the list of importance. But it is just like they say: You have got to put your own mask on before you put one on another. On another side of the coin, stressful life events can make diabetes stressful, or diabetes can make life stressors worse.

Diabetes Stressors

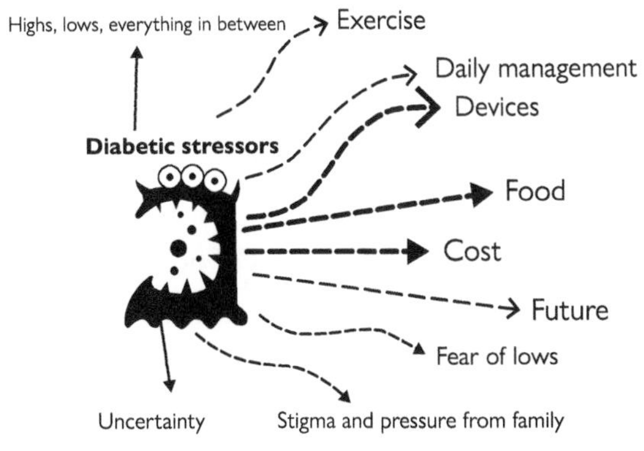

FIGURE 3.2

I think the reason why diabetes can be so stressful is its *unpredictability*. Sometimes it is like it has a mind of its own. With all types of diabetes, the intention is to achieve and maintain optimal BG levels to reduce the risk of diabetes-related complications. But despite our aim and effort, it is not always enough. Diabetes is like a constantly moving target, making it nearly impossible to hit the bullseye all of the time. And yet, people with diabetes put so much pressure on themselves to be on target 24/7 that they can lose sight of the big picture. It is not just about the numbers, it is also about how well you are living with diabetes. Unmanaged, unresolved acute and chronic stress overwhelm and tax a person's resilience when they "miss the mark." Unmanaged stress turns into more insidious conditions, like diabetes distress, burnout, anxiety, and depression; something we will talk about at greater length later in this book (Chapter 11). These conditions make diabetes management really hard to follow through on and compromise the quality of a person's life and wellbeing.

For me, yoga therapy is about showing others that diabetes is a relationship, just as someone would have a relationship with a partner, friend, or even themselves. A relationship is fluid. There is compromise, give and take. But unlike some relationships, diabetes is the kind that you cannot get rid of. It is closer than a family member; it is a part of a person and yet completely separate from them. To make an intentional cognitive separation of subject and object, for example "I am not diabetes," is difficult because it is such a deeply ingrained part of a person's self-identity. They live with it every day and feel its changes. The daily work and effort required to manage diabetes is unpredictable in its predictability. It is like a job where no one pays you or thanks you for your work. That is a hard cross to bear, especially without helpful tools to remind you that you are whole, no matter what diabetes or diabetes-related stressors are telling you.

The nature of diabetes aggravates stress because it influences and permeates every level of a person's sense of self, coloring our moods, emotions, thoughts, and actions. It can seem like infinite variables of potential problems in both the long and short term: immediate worries about the moment and longer-term worries about the future. Effort met with disappointing results can create a stressful hypervigilance (anxiety) or a reluctant fatalism (depression) unless a person can transform their identification to and with diabetes stressors. Unmanaged daily stress and subsequent reactivity to diabetes stressors also add fuel to the stress fire because they increase vulnerability and allostatic load. Daily stress depletes physical and mental resilience, so when benign stressors occur, a person is more susceptible to overreaction and therefore can perpetuate the cycle of stressor, stress hormones, insulin resistance, and wear and tear. Although T1D and T2D are completely separate conditions, and their requirements vary depending upon the severity of the disease, both demand prioritized stress-reduction strategies.

Diabetes is like living with an antenna inside and outside your body. It is exhausting to have to be *that* aware of every little thing occurring inside and outside. I think it is why many of the diabetics that I work with are already much more in tune with their bodies than non-diabetic clients. If people without diabetes could understand how much brainpower is being put into making daily diabetes decisions, they would be more compassionate about our moods. Stress is caused by every aspect of a decision, the possible outcomes of such a decision, and the variable potential problems that could come from the decision. If a person is already under the influence of uncontrolled BG levels, such decisions compound the stress and overwhelm.

I came up with a list of the top diabetes stressors. Let me remind you that this is from my experience of living with T1D, so there may be a bias.

BG: The physiological and neuroendocrine responses to highs and lows are biological imperatives to ensure survival; however, they are uncomfortable and can really deplete a person's energy and cognitive function. Emotions go on high alert and people may experience hypersensitivity when their BG levels are awry. After diagnosis I was very emotional and cried a lot. It could have been a product of being a teenager, being a Pisces with cancer rising, or the fact that blood sugar swings make you really emotional. BG levels impact how a person feels and behaves, and unless they acquire tools to recognize that what they are feeling may be a product of BG changes, or the general burden of diabetes, they will react from emotion rather than discernment. At times, I still have to ask myself, "Am I really feeling this way or is it my BG?" Recognizing the subtle residue of emotionalism caused by BG changes helps a person to gain control over diabetes stress and subsequent behavioral responses.

BG causes another type of stress, one that is created psychologically. The harder a person pushes and forces unrealistic parameters of diabetes perfection, the more stressed out they are about diabetes. The pressure to maintain BG levels of 80–180 mg/dL (4.4–10.0 mmol/L) causes hypervigilance in some people and aversion in others. People can personalize a number as a grade and subsequently create a litany of negative emotions, including frustration, blame, guilt, and anger, further deepening the groove of negative diabetes associations and poor self-care.

Food: When we are told that we cannot have something, we want it more.

If a guru says to you, "Meditate on anything, but a pink elephant," what is the first thing that you think of? A pink elephant. When people are diagnosed with diabetes, they go through a transitional phase where their relationship with food has to change. You no longer see a banana, you see a number: 27g of carbs. Certain beloved foods become "bad" or "off limits" and that creates inner turmoil and obsession. During my first years of diagnosis, my willpower was so low that I asked my parents to lock up my brother's treats in a toolbox. All I could think about when I came home from school was that toolbox. I found a way to slip my hand in between the cracks and grab a cookie. It is not healthy to make things off limits; this creates obsession and binge eating. A common problem for many people is night eating. They go all day doing the right thing, only to make it home and graze for hours into the night.

Food and diabetes requires willpower, strategic planning, and a lot of crunching of numbers. Understanding how food impacts BG and how to eat with diabetes takes years and years of trial and error. The biggest impetus to abstain from food that will challenge diabetes metabolic control and encourage foods that make metabolic control easier is the understanding of how a food will make you feel afterwards. Cultivating a healthy relationship with food happens with stress management. When a person feels better, they are encouraged to eat better. They are not eating to fill an anxious void, or because of some obsession with something that they can't have. They are eating for nourishment. Still, for people who have to take insulin to cover for the food they eat, food remains a source of distress, even with healthy food associations.

Insulin: As a type 1 diabetic with little to no insulin production I must time my meals appropriately with insulin and activity. Time of day, nutrient contents of food, current BG, prevision of subsequent activity, and even my hormonal cycles all go into my thought process when I am administering insulin for food. Insulin is administered to correct hyperglycemia, eat a meal, and maintain glucose levels throughout the day and night. I must make adjustments to my insulin if I am eating a high fat meal, going to exercise, or running high or low. Dosing the correct amount of insulin is highly intuitive and not an exact science. There is a lot of room for error which can be a trigger for anxiety.

Fear of lows: We will dive into hypoglycemia or "lows" in greater detail later on in this book (Chapter 9). Just know that hypoglycemia creates two responses: one is a sympathetic fight-or-flight response, releasing catecholamine hormones from the adrenal glands and creating a litany of uncomfortable sensations in the body. The other is absence of glucose to the brain, making a person loopy and confused. Untreated, it can be fatal. Hypos can come on really fast and sometimes several times a day. There is often an underlying fear of hypoglycemia for people who take insulin and are active.

Relationships: Diabetes is isolating and lonely at times. It can feel like no one understands you. Your friends and family care and say they get it but they don't. How can they? They are not living with it. It is part of our responsibility as people who live with diabetes to educate our friends and loved ones about diabetes and to communicate our needs. There are friends who get it. They always ask how your BG is. Others couldn't care less. I have friends for specific things. There are the ones I know and trust that I can adventure with them. These are the ones who wait for you when you are low. Those are the real friends. I have broken up with a friend (not just for this reason) because he did not make me feel safe when my BG was low or I was having an off day. The nice thing is that sometimes diabetes weeds out the bad apples for you. But sometimes we do not have a choice. From family to friends, co-workers, and even doctors. It can feel like you are being judged, unheard, and misunderstood.

Financial burden: The cost of diabetes is astronomical, at least in America. Yes, it can be done at a lower cost, but cutting corners when it comes to diabetes care never pays off. This is not a reality for many of the world's diabetics who do not have access to devices or cannot afford the exorbitant cost of insulin (which is really the issue in America). Most of the diabetics around the world do not have access to the same quality of diabetes technology that we have in the Western world, so I hope that I am not coming off in a negative way. I do appreciate what I have, but I pay for it. Health insurance in America is not yet a national right. As a yoga teacher who works for herself, with a husband who works for himself as a private contractor, our premiums and deductibles are extremely high. But I will not do without good coverage. I will just work harder for it, but that is not the reality for many Americans who work just as hard as me and still cannot cover the bill of health insurance. Rationing or minimizing the use of insulin to just stay alive, because a person cannot foot the bill, is the reality for many people. Just as I am writing this, the United States Supreme Court has approved a bill attempting to repeal the required coverage by health insurance companies of pre-existing conditions like diabetes. We live in turbulent times. Remember how psychologically induced stress is caused by perceived threat? Healthcare and the cost of insulin and supplies is one of the deepest-seated fears.

Security and stability for immediate survival. For me, the cost and coverage of diabetes is one of the most stress-triggering circumstances. I spent years at a job that I wanted to leave for fear of risking it on my own and not being able to pay the bills.

Devices: These are stressful variables. From malfunctions to wearability and self-consciousness around the symbol of disease (it is like wearing a billboard for diabetes on your body), the very devices people use to reduce diabetes stress are a cause for stress. I did not used to be like this as a teenager, but as an adult I am over prepared. When I travel, I have Plan A, Plan B, and even Plan C. Being organized and prepared for potential technological difficulties at all times provides a reassurance and stability that people need. It takes time for people to truly absorb this. Perhaps it requires people to have experienced circumstances in which their pump fails or their insulin gets damaged by temperature extremes.

Recently I wrote an article in *Yoga Journal* about diabetes technology as a source of stress. I wish we had a metric for people pre and post CGM to see if people felt less stressed after starting using one. I am torn. While I admit that a CGM is a very useful tool and I would never consider living without one as it helps me keep my numbers in range, I question how much is too much information. Being constantly plugged in can aggravate a hypervigilant type A (not me?!) personality to constantly be involved with every fluctuation and arrow. It ceases to be feedback and becomes a competitive game for perfect numbers fueled by fear. Whether that fear comes from an inherent need to have the best numbers possible, fear of hypos or hypers, or future fear from complications, these factors all create stress. There is a fine line between responding and "rage" bolusing. The constant connection with a number, and the fact that many people's CGMs are actually linked to a cell phone, encourages a level of dependency, attenuating individual perception and sensitivity to diabetes.

There was once a time when a diabetes diagnosis meant that you would not live a long and healthy life, even after the discovery of therapeutic insulin. Everyone with diabetes has some level of fear about what will happen further down the road in the background of their mind. Who knows what all those years of unregulated numbers will do? Kidney failure, retinopathy, nerve damage, and heart disease are all but some of the effects of a lifetime of diabetes. Even if a person has been able to achieve an A1c under 7.0% for the majority of the duration of their diabetes, there is still an unforeseen cost. No one is able to predict their future with or without diabetes, but it does not make it any less stressful when a person's blood sugars will not come down from 300 because of any of the other factors mentioned previously. It is an existential crisis of uncertainty. Caring about future health is essential; worrying does not change the fact of diagnosis.

Sleep: Rather, sleepless. Just last night my BG was hovering at 80 mg/dL (4.4 mmol/L). I did not want to treat it with any glucose because I knew that it would skyrocket. But because of this, my CGM kept buzzing all night long to remind me that I was going low. This feeds into the device difficulties, but the result was a sleepless night. Sleeplessness is common with people with diabetes because they are wound up or cannot get comfortable. There is a looming fear of falling asleep and not waking up. I think many of us sleep lightly just in case we have to wake up for a BG emergency. For those of us who have CGMs, knowing there is an alarm can help us sleep a little better, unless that alarm is a false alarm that you cannot turn off because of the programming. Lack of sleep increases stress by de-regulating our circadian rhythm, producing cortisol, and never allowing the body and mind adequate time to restore and rebuild.

Exercise: Exercise is a physical and mental stressor. Even though exercise strengthens our muscles and trains our heart, it is a physiological stress response. To keep BG levels up, the body uses the SNS to employ immediate energy. Just as exercise is beneficial, exercise without adequate rest and compensatory practices will also deplete vitality, increasing allostatic load.

Psychologically, exercise can be a stressor because it can affect BG levels quite rapidly.

Aerobic activity can potentiate exogenous (injected) insulin and increases the risk of exercise-induced hypoglycemia. Anaerobic exercise can raise BG levels, but not for everyone. And mix this with timing. For instance, let's say I go on a two-hour mountain-bike ride. As I live in the Rocky Mountains, this usually means I am going straight up a mountain and then straight down. In the first hour of climbing, I need very little insulin and must fuel with some carbs to keep my BG from getting low. But as soon as I get to the top, with adrenaline and cortisol pumping, my BG levels are likely to increase because of the lack of insulin on-board and stress hormones potentiating an increase in CRR.

It is possible that the fear of lows on the uphill exertion portion is more stressful, but if BG spikes high on the way down, it defeats the purpose of the exercise.

I find that many type 1 diabetics need more recovery time after intense activity, especially if the exercise made the numbers jumble. Some people with diabetes may avoid doing fun things like longer duration exercise because of the fear of going low, going high, or the extra tax on their neuroendocrine responses. Exercise is essential for both types of diabetes; it improves insulin absorption, heart health, and mental health. It can, however, be an extra variable and cause for stress if people do not understand how to manage their BG levels during, before, and after exercise. Preparation for the event, organization of emergency supplies, and conscious snacking all work together to ensure that exercise is a positive experience for diabetics.

How to Change the Stress Response

Everything we feel, think, and do is intimately connected with our perception of who we are. This is called the *self-concept* and comprises our thoughts, emotions, physical sensations, and impulses. All of these guys work together to formulate our opinion of ourselves. Emotions impact thought, thoughts sway our behaviors. There is not really a starting point: one will always impact the other, and over the duration of a life this creates a persona of likes, dislikes, beliefs, triggers, and actions. In the structure of the brain, this is like a dance that goes on in the limbic system between the amygdala, hippocampus, and hypothalamus.

The interesting, or maybe hilarious, thing is that all of the chaos is created by external stressors. These are things, circumstances, people, and conditions that trigger a stress response. According to this model, anything outside of the self-concept (thought, emotion, behavior) from our physiology, anatomy, relationships, and environment can be a source of stress.

We've established at this point that stress is created by our perception of it. If all we see in diabetes is stress, that is how we will respond to it. But if we can shift the perception, we can change our response. So now you have identified a stressor, but it continues to stress you out. How does one defuse the charge? To rewire the stress response, we first need to establish an awareness of what we are thinking, feeling, and doing.

Everything that goes on with diabetes impacts our thoughts, emotions, and subsequent actions, right? The closer that stressor is to my self-concept, the more intrinsic the response. For instance, a physiological neuroendocrine response is pretty close to my self-concept because it is part of the body. I feel my body heat up and my heart rate increase, how can I *not* identify with what I feel in my body as part of who I am?

If my BG is moving in a direction that I did not anticipate, there are physical sensations, thoughts, emotions, and a response.

Take another stressor, a device for example. You test your BG or glance at a CGM and see that the number is not what you want it to be. Even though the device is outside of you, you see the number and it is felt in the self-concept. Thoughts, for example "That is good or that is bad," emotions or sensations, for example a "rapid heartbeat," and action take waaayyy too much insulin.

The next layer could be a person in your life, let's say your spouse. They are always telling you how to do diabetes, or they lack compassion for your circumstances. They say or do things that impact your thoughts and emotions and influence your behaviors. You may react outwardly or internalize inwardly. Unless we have a way to offload, process, and assimilate the stress, it turns into future stress.

The answer in transforming a negative stressor into a positive one lies within the recognition of these associations. When we can perceive a source of stress, we can begin to look at it objectively. This is what yoga is all about.

As we will see in the next chapter, all negative emotions are based in a misunderstanding. The misunderstanding is that *we are* the *stress*, *we are* the *changes* of *diabetes*. We know that we are not the highs and lows, but when we feel the emotions, it is hard not to identify and react.

Stress is a form of pain that we can liberate ourselves from by recognizing it, addressing it, and applying protective processes that buffer the negative impact of repeated exposure to stressful situations. There are physiological stressors from the lived experience of diabetes in the body, psychological stressors from emotions, triggers, and impulses in response to diabetes, and behavioral stressors from improper coping, strategizing, and lack of willpower.

Diabetes stress isolates, aggravates, and perpetuates negative self-management behaviors, dampening the quality of a person's life and increasing the likelihood for mental health problems, as we will address later on in this book (Chapter 11).

Stress management contributes to the overall success of diabetes defined not only by an A1c number but also by the quality of a person's life—how well they can manage diabetes and also live in the way that they want to, *with* diabetes, not *despite* it. It is in our interest as yogis, therapists, and people who live with diabetes to educate ourselves about what stress is and how it manifests with diabetes if we are going to help others, if not ourselves, to live freely.

There is a need for effective therapies to assist people in dealing with the daily demands of diabetes. I hope that through the practices and psychology of yoga therapy we can help people identify stressors, reduce the stress response, and radically improve self-care by transforming the perception of daily diabetes management from a burden to an act of self-empowerment. As we move into the next chapter, we will dive into the practice and philosophy of yoga as it informs our foundation for all yoga therapy for diabetes practices.

CHAPTER 4

The Inner Practices of Yoga for Diabetes

The Windshield of the Mind

Picture yourself on a road-trip through a vast and spectacular desert landscape. Red rocks, giant spires, and the epic, open, blue desert sky highlight your pristine view.

Like on all trips, grime splatters on your windshield and you cannot see the view as well as you once could. Despite your efforts to spray washer fluid, the windshield remains streaky, clouded by a residue of dirt and grime. Along the journey, you adapt to perceiving the world through a dirty windshield, never fully experiencing the view, sun, and sky in their true splendor. From your perspective, the scenery outside becomes more and more obstructed, and eventually you forget what a clear view even was.

This is what happens to us over our lives. The hazards of the journey smudge up our view and we go through the motions, never fully seeing what is really there.

Unless you take the time to stop and clean your windshield regularly, you'll never see the world from a clear perspective.

Living with diabetes is a lot like driving on the same road but through a blizzard. There are no breaks, and even when it stops snowing, there's still mud on the ground to splash over your windshield. It may seem silly to spend the time and money washing your car when it is just going to get dirty again. But with so much accumulation, it is even more important to do the work to prevent long-term corrosion and deterioration.

Yoga practice clears the windshield of the mind so you can see from a different vantage point. Without it, we see everything through a sullied filter. Shadows are tigers, rope becomes snakes, the sun is grey, the landscape is bleak.

We cannot see what is going on and have forgotten that there was another way of seeing. We go through life's journey without experiencing the sun in its full brightness.

Unbeknownst to us, there's a sudden turn in life's windy road and we crash the car. This is what it's like to be diagnosed with an illness. That crash can be the wake-up call we need to wash our damn windshield. Most times we're not going to wash the windshield unless we've already crashed the car, and even then we might not. Something has got to awaken a desire within us to see.

The untrained driver may question, "What is the point of continually washing my windshield? It seems like so much effort when it is just going to get dirty again."

Another kind of driver exclaims, "Oh my! My windshield has to be spotless, and if I see a speck of dirt, I am going to stop my car, clean it, and also freak out about it in the process." Neither is helpful. The first is avoiding; the second is obsessing and creating more anxiety for themselves. Both result in suffering.

The third person says, "I want to have a clear windshield so I can enjoy my journey. I know that dirt is inevitable. Even when the weather's perfect, I know that stuff will show up, so I will be prepared. I am going to keep cleaning it regularly for the sake of doing it. I value everything that I do and will put the same worth into the mundane work of cleaning my windshield." This person may not be as fast as the first or as arduous as the second, but inside they are as free as the view outside. The only way to truly appreciate the effect of a clear view is to clean your windshield regularly. When the dirt comes back you can see it for what it is: just a film covering your view of your true path.

Washing the metaphorical windshield is a lot like the practice of yoga. The goal is to clean the residue covering the inherent light of the mind. The obstacles on the journey are many, and unless we are shown what a clear view is, it is hard to make out the sun and sky even if we get a glimpse of it. By developing our mind's perception, we improve the quality of our life. We act better, are conscious of our actions, make fewer mistakes because we are able to evaluate our decisions, stop doing what is not working, and add more of what is helpful.[1]

1 Desikachar, T. K. V., Skelton, M. L. and Carter, J. R. (1980) *Religiousness in Yoga: Lectures on Theory and Practice*. Washington DC: University Press of America. p.2.

The Causes of Suffering

According to yoga philosophy, the mind creates suffering.[2] It does this when it forgets that its purpose is to act as a conduit for us to experience the light of our true nature. The mind is an instrument to understand, learn, discern, and transform through direct knowledge and perception from consciousness. The mind is our windshield; it is how we experience the world. When the pathways are open, the mind is clear and we can hear our inner wisdom. When it is dirty, we cannot see and we forget what is behind the grime.

The windshield is like an impure mind, so we are always seeing things from a distorted point of view. The film on the windshield blinds the driver from experiencing the pure light of the sun and may cause them to veer off course. Yoga has a name for it; it is called avidyā, an absence of truth. Some say it is ignorance, and others say it is knowledge that is not the right knowledge.[3] We think that we are correct when we are wrong and think we are wrong when we are right.[4] Deep grooves of habituated belief and conditioned behavior set in and misguide our actions.

Avidyā's origin can stem from past lives like a factory tint on the windshield, always obscuring our view (vāsanā). It can also accumulate from our actions, like the grime accumulating from the journey (saṁskāra). We hardly recognize that we are the masters of our domain. We reach outside ourselves to answer the questions as if fate and destiny were in the hands of something other than ourselves.

The driver has to *identify* avidyā to clean it up. Because avidyā is so subtle, it is hard to see, especially when layers and layers of it have accumulated and it gets lost in the chaos. By cleaning your windshield regularly, you can see avidyā when it splatters in front of your face.

Once you have seen a miraculous view, you lose your tolerance for dirty windshields. Many consider it the duty of a yogi to reduce the film of avidyā so that their consciousness can shine through them, as love, kindness, and devotion. As avidyā is subtle, it can be hard to identify and eradicate.

---

2 Tigunait, P. R. (2014) *The Secret of the Yoga Sutra: Samadhi Pada*. Honesdale, PA: Himalayan Institute. p.331.

3 Desikachar, T. K. V., Skelton, M. L. and Carter, J. R. (1980) *Religiousness in Yoga: Lectures on Theory and Practice*. Washington DC: University Press of America. p.3.

4 Desikachar, T. K. V., Skelton, M. L. and Carter, J. R. (1980) *Religiousness in Yoga: Lectures on Theory and Practice*. Washington DC: University Press of America. p.2.

For instance, you may not see the film of avidyā on your windshield, but you feel the physical pain of crashing your car when you veer off the road.

Patañjali expounds in the Yoga Sūtra-s that we might not always be able to identify avidyā, but we can identify its "children," known as the *kleśa-s*. Here are some examples of how they could show up in diabetes:

Avidyā in Diabetes Experience

Asmitā: Often translated *ego*, it the sense of I-am-ness. It's the "I" and "ME" identification with the changing diabetes experience.

I am diabetes. I am sick. I am this insulin bill at the pharmacy. I am this broken insulin pump. I am the A1c. I am the healthcare system and a crappy doctor who does not get it. All that goes into diabetes care is directly linked to your self-worth. It is the failure to recognize that the changing nature of diabetes is not who you fundamentally are. It is the identification of the true self with this personality that is conditioned and formed by what others perceive it to be.

Practiced correctly, asmitā can also be a means of spiritual advancement, for instance the feeling of I-*am*-ness is the same feeling of *that*. I *am* not separate from *that*.

Rāga: This is the attachment to some aspect of diabetes as being the object of happiness. For instance, a blood sugar reading of 108 mg/dL (5.9 mmol/L) = happiness, versus a blood sugar reading of 300 mg/dL (16.7 mmol/L) = unhappiness. The individual lives in fear of keeping these numbers perfect, otherwise suffering the wrath of self-ridicule when the numbers are imperfect. Another example is being attached to a piece of diabetes technology like a CGM, insulin pump, or brand of insulin.

Dveṣa: This means unreasonable dislikes. People with diabetes learn at diagnosis that consistency is critical for success. On one level, consistency is helpful to predict the unpredictable, but on another, it creates inflexibility and hardening, deeper grooves of aversion, and resistance towards trying new things. The problem with this is that it closes off the possibility of trying something different that could be better. They may harbor fear about living by the "seat of their pants," arguably stifling their ability to live, love, and experience the spontaneity of life. We would rather stay in the discomfort of what is not working than work through the fear of something different or new.

Abhiniveśa: This means fear of death (fear in general). A diagnosis of any type of diabetes is an existential crisis, and even as a child, you may have to question your mortality, something most do not do until much later in life. On the one hand, reflecting on the temporal nature of life can be helpful for some to live their lives more intentionally; for some, it imbues a type of fear into all experiences. The fear of what if? What if I do not have all the supplies that I need and there is an apocalypse—how will I survive? What if I can never get my A1c below 7.0%, and how will this impact my longevity, life, and health? Another source of diabetes fear is hypoglycemia (see Chapter 9), which can be fatal. Whether it is about the short term or long term, the fear of death is part of all human conditions, but especially that of diabetes.

We might not see our role in the cycle of ego, attachment, aversion, and fear, but we can recognize pain. The word duḥkha is the experience of avidyā and the kleśa-s. It is a feeling experienced within the body and the mind. Directly translated as "bad space," it is a disturbance of the mind and a feeling of physical restriction in the body.[5] Sadness is duḥkha; fear is duḥkha; judgment is duḥkha; hyperglycemia and hypoglycemia are duḥkha; any action caused by avidyā results in duḥkha.

Duḥkha is experienced by our minds, and in order to understand it, we must also understand the three qualities of the mind detailed by yoga. The *guṇa-s* are the manifestations of *prakṛti*, the nature of the universe that is in constant flux, anything manifested and material. In the context of the mind, the guṇa-s relate to the movement of the mind as represented by its thoughts and emotions. The three qualities of the guṇa-s are *tamas*, *rajas*, and *sattva*. Tamas is the state of heaviness, mental inertia, and dullness in feeling and responses. Excessive mental tamas could be a tendency towards attachment, cloudiness, and even depression. In diabetes tamas can be seen during hyperglycemia when the mind and senses are dulled by excessive glucose. Rajas is constant mental movement and action, like a ping-pong ball bouncing back and forth. Excessive

5 Desikachar, T. K. V., Skelton, M. L. and Carter, J. R. (1980) *Religiousness in Yoga: Lectures on Theory and Practice*. Washington DC: University Press of America. pp.38–44.

rajas could be the inability to focus, anxiety, or distraction. In diabetes it is represented in hypoglycemia, diabetes distress, and fear. On a baseline level, many type 1 diabetics have a lot of mental rajas because of the requirements to manage their condition, i.e. being plugged in, injections, and highs and lows.

Sattva, the third guṇa, can only be described as the absence of tamas and rajas; it is clarity and discernment. Only sattva is impenetrable to duḥkha. It is our goal to try to create more sattvic qualities of the mind, but also to be less attached and affected by tamas and rajas.

The mind fluctuates constantly between the three guṇa-s of tamas, rajas, and sattva. Whichever mental guṇa predominates in an individual indicates how duḥkha could potentially manifest within them. The goal would be to practice to encourage sattva to reduce avidyā, duḥkha, and suffering.

Tradition says there are causes of suffering and we must be able to identify them if we are going to get rid of them. The main reason why we have duḥkha is that we have likes and dislikes, attractions and aversions. When we get what we want, there is no duḥkha, but when we cannot get what we want, we suffer. We once had a pleasant experience, but cannot recreate it; this is duḥkha. We have a habit or a routine that is disrupted and we feel uneasy; this is also duḥkha. Duḥkha is an opportunity to understand avidyā, become aware of the causes of suffering, and use self-awareness to transform ourselves and overcome challenges.

Self-awareness helps identify and stop avidyā. It is so important that it is the first step in all transformation. The aim of yoga, Buddhism, and Vedanta is to remove duḥkha to weaken the karmic bond of ignorance (avidyā) and transcend suffering (duḥkha).[6]

Change is Constant

Everything that we know to be in existence is in a constant state of flux. They say the only constant is change. At this moment, you are growing older, the world is turning, a star is dying, something is being born. Today diabetes is easy, tomorrow it is impossible. One minute there is joy, another there is sorrow. There is pleasure and pain, good and bad, health and disease. The list of opposites is infinite. The pendulum swings from one direction to another

6 Desikachar, T. K. V., Skelton, M. L. and Carter, J. R. (1980) *Religiousness in Yoga: Lectures on Theory and Practice*. Washington DC: University Press of America. pp.38–44.

in the face of our desire for the good, joyful, and pleasurable to always remain the same.

For some reason, despite our understanding that change is constant, we expect certain things to remain the same. The more we expect that all things will remain fixed, the more we suffer.

Change influences every aspect of our lives, including what we feel, think, and do. Its reach is subject to the cumulative effect of the past as habits, impulses, and perceptions. These are the *saṁskāra-s*, conditioned patterns that subconsciously influence our thoughts, emotions, and behaviors. Every relationship within us and outside of us is subject to change. Whether it is a personal object of attachment like your house or car, a loved one, your own body, or living with an illness, nothing escapes the law of nature.

Fortunately for us, if we are suffering, we know that it is temporary. Everything is impermanent; even change changes. Even better, if we do not agree with the direction it is going in, we can influence change's trajectory. The skill is to influence it for the better. We have been doing this since before we were bipeds—manipulating environments, creating tools, and transforming obstacles into pathways. It is part of our innate nature to find ways around and turn misfortunes into opportunities for discovery.

If our intentions are pure, the change will be made for the better. The more aware you become, the more skillful you are at it. You are able to see with clarity what is needed and apply appropriate effort. Even with a good intention, there is an attachment to an outcome. We put in effort, expect a result, and suffer when it does not come to fruition. We seek out gratifying experiences only to be disappointed when the result is different than the expectation. The more we place our self-worth into the law of change, the more we are likely to suffer.

You see this with diabetes. You put in all this effort to achieve a certain A1c, only to go to the doctor and find that it is not as good as you thought, or that they want it to be even lower. You do everything you can to maintain your numbers, but wake up at 300 mg/dL (16.7 mmol/L) after having a low-carb salad for dinner.

Change pertains not just to circumstances and conditions outside of us, but also, most importantly, to what goes on inside of us—the biological and psychological processes within that create our inner environment. In fact, all the change that occurs outside of our physical body can determine what goes on inside our body and mind. By witnessing the changes in the body, mind, digestion, and, as we will see, diabetes, we can start to understand just a little bit more about cause and effect, and therefore become greater commanders of change within our own worlds. As yogis we can influence change and study it. Through our appreciation for the cause of all creation we can access a part of ourselves that is beyond all change and circumstance.

Special Awareness

Behind the individual personality is a special awareness that exists unconditionally. This awareness has never experienced illness, suffering, or fear. It remains untouched by avidyā, diabetes, and the highs and lows, sadness, and grief. It is our true nature, the highest self, and everything else is subject to change. It goes by so many names, from the observer, to the witness, to the true self. We will call it puruṣa. In our car analogy, our puruṣa is like the inherent joy within the driver. The one who recognizes that it is experiencing itself when it sees the true light of the sun.

Most of us do not live in this realm of unsurpassed joy, and we identify with change. We spend our lives trying to recreate pleasurable experiences and avoiding unfavorable ones.

It is the goal of yoga to open the pathways of perception to continually access this special awareness, to abide by it during pleasure and pain. It holds us, keeps us safe, and reminds us that no matter what, we are always whole and always at peace.

According to tradition, the cause of suffering stems from the misidentification to and with change. We identify with the changing circumstances and conditions within us and all around us. Thoughts, emotions, and impulses perpetuate the false belief that we are the change when our essential nature remains untouched and pure. To forget this is **avidyā** and the root cause of all suffering.

Yoga asks us to look beyond the status quo and ask the proverbial questions "Who am I?" and "What is my purpose?" To know thyself is the goal of human existence—to understand who we are and what our life's purpose is. It is also essential for healing the relationship of an illness. Those who understand this and can access it experience greater joy, freedom, and health. It is the objective of yoga to help us figure out how to access this part of ourselves so that we can live in this world, but also live above it.

Except for a select few who are born with the ability to access it naturally, most cannot perceive their higher self without being shown it. The weight of experience, the chaos of the mind, and relentless identification with the external world block our ability to perceive a part of ourselves that remains untouched by cause and effect. Sometimes we have a glimmer of it. It is that gentle whisper that says "You've got this" and "I love you." But most of the time, this special awareness lays dormant throughout a person's whole life.

Diabetes is a disease that is seen by this perfect consciousness. Yet, due to the misunderstanding (avidyā) that the individual is the experience of diabetes (duḥkha) and not the observer of it, the individual suffers greatly. The identification with diabetes further perpetuates the original misunderstanding that the individual is inherently flawed; diagnosis is a sickness; sickness is a weakness. The individual becomes attached to and dominated by diabetes and the label of being sick.

Although puruṣa is omnipotent, it is incapacitated. It needs a vehicle to move through, otherwise it can only do half of its job. The mind is the windshield for puruṣa, and through the mind, consciousness can experience itself. Yet the mind is full of junk; thoughts, memories, streaming consciousness, and intellect all work together, or against one another.

Yoga is mind training, and we will soon learn about the methods to train the mind. The process of yoga uniformly organizes the mind's constant movement, and calms and stills its fluctuations, so that the wisest part of ourselves can listen to consciousness. Otherwise, the mind will flow in every direction it pleases, never allowing puruṣa to be known. This is important to note in the context of diabetes because puruṣa and health are intertwined.

The Yogic Concept of Health

In yoga, the concept of health relates to prāṇa, our life-force. Prāṇa abides everywhere—inside of us and outside of us. The more prāṇa is contained within the body, the greater the potency, vitality, and resolution to fulfill life's purpose (dharma). The definition of a yogi is one who contains prāṇa within the body. As yogis we are trying to influence prāṇa, so it concentrates and flows freely within us,[7] removing all types of obstacles that inhibit our health, happiness, and wellbeing. When our prāṇa is low, we do not feel well, we experience *duḥkha*. This is represented by the tightening and constriction

7 Desikachar, T. K. V. (1999) *The Heart of Yoga: Developing a Personal Practice* (Rev. ed.). Rochester, VT: Inner Traditions International. p.55.

often felt during moments of stress and sickness. Ancient texts say that when a person is unwell or disturbed, they have more prāṇa outside of the body than inside. It is our aim as practitioners to consciously direct prāṇa's flow inward for our longevity and health.

Tradition also says that prāṇa is low because it is leaked through our various orifices. We'll talk more about this in Chapter 6, but just to get an idea, improper digestion and physical exercise are examples of this. This is why we have the practices of bandha to contain and direct prāṇa intentionally within. Another way that prāṇa is leaked is through the various sensory organs: ears, eyes, nose, tongue, and skin, and their faculties of hearing, seeing, smelling, tasting, and feeling. Our senses are intended to help us relate to the world around us, to enjoy and experience life. They are also there to warn of danger. Our nose is the most potent of the sensory organs; smell only requires one neurotransmitter synapse to arrive at the amygdala in the brain. An example of prāṇa being lost through the sense of smell could be that you smell some food, which incites hunger by telling the brain to release insulin for food. This takes you away from your work, focus, or practice. Another example is a smell that triggers a subconscious memory, which triggers a stress response. Our eyes are another way for the prāṇa to flow outward. In most people, the eyes orient us to our surroundings and how we see ourselves in space and in time. In a world of excessive and overt stimulation, it can be nearly impossible at times to allow our eyes to close, internalize, and become still. They are constantly searching outward.

Prāṇa is also pushed out through the mind with our thoughts, worries, aversions, and attachments. The more our mind moves outward—hooked and bound by the identification with objects and change—the less prāṇa remains in the body. Recall the various diabetes stressors from the last chapter. These are also considerations in how prāṇa leaks outward through the senses, digestion, energy expenditure, and, of course, mind. When you have diabetes, especially with T1D, you are always on. The constant thinking, being plugged into a computer screen, dialing in numbers, fears about going low or high, and everything else that goes along with self-management depletes prāṇa. It is essential to be vigilant and present to diabetes, but also to recognize that there is a fine line between care and hypervigilance. People have a hard time "turning off" their minds, which also depletes prāṇa and vitality.

How do we contain prāṇa within our bodies when the nature of a disease like diabetes implores you to externalize to survive? It is through the mind that we access the potency of the mind. The mind is the filter through which we experience *puruṣa*, but an untrained mind will always revert to impulses over consciousness. The structure of the brain houses the physical mechanisms that represent what yoga is talking about. In sympathetic overdrive, the amygdala perceives a threat and will bypass the prefrontal cortex and immediately signal the hypothalamus to release stress hormones. This is an example of an automatic reaction. Part of containing prāṇa is choosing how and where to allocate our attention. If we are letting it fly this way and that for whatever perceived threat or whimsical distraction the brain improperly associates with, we lose personal power and vitality. The intention is to consciously influence prāṇa's flow to affect change on a systemic level via the ANS, its connection with the endocrine responses, and the mind.

In the last chapter, we learned that breathing practices are a pathway to deliberately influence the body's automatic responses towards down-regulation, increasing heart rate variability, vagal tone, and reducing stress. Regularly applying the breaks on automatic responses creates a pause between reactivity and conscious choice (Chapter 3). Yoga says the same thing. *When we influence prāṇa through the breath to be smooth and calm, the quality of our breath changes the quality of the mind. Conversely, the quality of the mind affects the quality of the breath. So, to change the mind, we must first change the way we are breathing.* Choppiness or tension in our breathing is indicative of the same conditions within the mind. By alleviating the strain in our breathing, we can help our minds become calm, still, and one-pointed. By practicing conscious breathing regularly, we train prāṇa to remain in the body, dominating the mind's roaming tendencies and containing our vital life-force within.

Practice trains us to remain in a place of calm, even during a stress response. Performance athletes in a flow state are no different than a diabetic treating hypoglycemia while staying completely peaceful. Remember, stress is not a bad thing, we just can't let it drive the chariot.

All of this remains a theory until it is put into practice. It takes time to develop the skills to tame the mind to naturally flow inward. In the Kaṭha Upaniṣad, a famous symbol system of the mind is represented by a horse, chariot, charioteer, and passenger. The horses symbolize the impulses driven by the sensory organs of perception. The reins represent the mind, and the charioteer is the intellect. The passenger is consciousness, the one who is always present and at peace, the "dweller within the city."

To control the horses, the charioteer needs skill and strength. Without both, the horses (or in our case, the senses) will always overpower the intellect. An untrained driver is likely to let the horses take over and, eventually, crash the cart, but a steady driver understands how to skillfully use the reins (mind) to their advantage.

The skillful manipulation of the reins by the charioteer is analogous to the skillful use of the breath to influence the mind's direction.

The goal of yoga is to gain dominion over the inherent biological impulses through the mind's skillful influence. Through the mind, we can drive our senses in the direction of choice and allow our higher intellect and consciousness to be in the driver's seat.

The conscious manipulation of the breath, prāṇāyāma, trains the ANS to move seamlessly from sympathetic to parasympathetic and protect its function. This helps down-regulate habituated stress responses and override the biological imperative for survival, which left to its own devices will always choose a fear response rather than a conscious deliberation. Remember, the horses are strong; you have to be more skillful than the horses. The mind is distinct from neuroanatomy because we cannot see it, but no matter the starting point for your focus, whether it is physiology or yoga, it all goes back to the place in between reaction and response.

It is in our interest to examine the mind, as it is the filter of perception and choice. By clearing the mind of avidyā, as we have seen represented by the kleśa-s, our true nature can experience itself. That can mean so many things, but in the context of diabetes, it is clear discernment and appropriate action to contain pranic vitality that is continually being challenged to remain within.

It is in our interest as yogis and therapists to examine the mind, as it is the filter through which we discern truth from falsehood, vidyā from avidyā. By clearing the mind of avidyā our true nature can experience itself.

Diabetes creates its own level of avidyā, in both the body and the mind. Every aspect of the disease and the experience of living with the illness depletes pranic vitality. For a person living with diabetes, one's ability to contain prāṇa within, rather than without, helps maintain physical and mental wellbeing. This is valid for all humans, but especially so with a chronic disease.

Consciousness needs a medium through which it can be accessed; that medium is our mind. Through the mind, we experience the essence of mind—higher intelligence as a reflection of consciousness—but unless we know how to control the mind's movement, avidyā will continue to color our identifications, causing suffering on a multidimensional basis.

This is an important concept, as it applies to all humans, but especially in our conversation about overcoming the suffering of diabetes. Its influence extends intimately into the body and mind, reflected as an illness and the chaos of taking care of an illness. The mind of a person with diabetes can be cluttered. This is called *saṁkīrṇa*. The mind is mixed up. There is no clarity, only chaos, and when there is chaos individuals get caught up in the experience of suffering, subject to the will of their urges, fears, and impulses. This creates a context for acute and chronic diabetes stressors to deplete prāṇa, and when that occurs, people have less vitality and are more sensitive to future challenges.

The purpose of practice is to get the mind to experience itself by calming its movement through various practices and allowing it to become established in its true nature. When it is there, it can hear, perceive, and listen to the wisdom of puruṣa. It is not about getting the mind to be absolutely still, but *rather learning how to go deeper than the chaos*. By going deeper than the experience, one can avoid the consciousness crossing paths with the chemical and electrical messages of the mind that tell you that you should identify with the experience of diabetes.[8] This way you can abide in pure consciousness, unpenetrated by the suffering of disease. It is the power to be aware of opposites and yet remain in the heart space.

When this happens, the attitude towards diabetes undergoes a change. With practice, the individual is able to hold this space consistently and during intense moments, remaining unaffected by change. This is contentment. The more prāṇa that a person has inside, the better they feel and the more content they are. Contentment is not about always being happy. It is the ability to be even minded in pleasure and pain.[9] Just because your pancreas is broken does not mean that you are essentially flawed. In the moment of a hypoglycemia episode, it is helpful to reflect on how the rest of your body is fine! Yes, the low blood sugar is uncomfortable, but it is temporary. What about all the faculties of your body that work, and do it well? How about your liver—your miraculous liver that is working so much harder to make up for the pancreas? That is working well. Or your lungs breathing every day. Work with what is working for you. Link with that. Let the rest go.

By resorting to the interior strategies of dropping deeper, one can witness

8 Bharati, S. V. (2001) "Illness and Meditation." *Ahymsin*. Accessed on 01/07/20 at: https://ahymsin.org/main/swami-veda-bharati/illness-and-meditation.html.

9 *The Bhagavad Gita* II.14–II.15.

the chaos but remain *unaffected* by it. This is how illness becomes an opportunity for empowered resilience. One can be in the moment and remain unaffected by it. Through this regular practice, one can transform the experience of diabetes into the opportunity for a much more profound understanding of the body, health, and "Who am I?"

A New Relationship

A relationship is a fluid connection between two objects, a give and take, a co-existing mutual exchange. The relationships that last are adaptive, and the best ones teach us about what is important. Even the ones that end, or are ill-fated, can be opportunities to learn about what you want and don't want in life.

Relationships act like mirrors of ourselves. We may not like everything that we see, but what surfaces can teach us about who we are, what is meaningful, what to do away with, and what to add more of.

Yoga cultivates a relationship between your true self and the idea of who you think you are, or who you could potentially be. Yoga aims to support the process of transforming all of our relationships into mirrors for deeper understanding and sovereignty of choice. The clearer the reflection, the more accurate the perception, the more skillful the action. When established in accurate perception, so says tradition, there is only freedom. Freedom is not just an idea, it is a way of being. It is our power to live in this world, yet also rise above it.

Living with diabetes is another type of relationship. It can also serve as a mirror to strengthen the bond within ourselves. But unless we can look at the experience of disease objectively, the ego will identify with the pain of illness and the label of sickness. The feeling is so real at times that it is difficult to separate from it. Unless we have help along the way, the relationship between self and illness imprisons us rather than liberates us.

Part of the confusion is the misunderstanding that we are what we feel, think, see, and do. All of these perceptions are influenced by conditioned patterns and beliefs. Unless we find a way to study them, they will always be the driver of our chariot. We have to be able to feel the fear but not let it drive the horses.

There is a saying in the diabetes community that "I am greater than the sum of the highs and lows," which is very appropriate for this conversation. The feeling of low BG, for instance, is so intense and debilitating, it is hard *not* to identify with it. But the ability to observe the low objectively, from the standpoint of an observer witnessing the chaos from a distance, makes all the difference when it comes to living with a complicated relationship. This does not mean that one ignores their condition, but rather can attend to it without the influence of conditioned impulses. The highs and lows change, the illness persists, the observer remains unfazed. This is self-mastery.

"I am high, I am low, I am diabetes" is the identification, and any change that occurs within the invisible parameters of 80–180 mg/dL (4.4–10.0 mmol/L), good and bad, healthy and sick, informs the sense of I-*am* and, in turn, all action. The cumulative burden of displaced identification weighs heavily on the body, mind, and senses, depleting vitality and resilience. *The very act of taking care of diabetes aggravates the same factors that are necessary to take care of diabetes.*

A simple shift, a brief self-reflective pause in the cycle, can make all the difference. This is what yoga practice does. This is the breath pause we experienced in the last chapter.

With the nervous system in balance and the mind at bay, the individual perceives more clearly. They can begin to notice that there is a feeling associated with their blood sugars, a quality of emotion—there is a correlation between a number, their thoughts, and their actions. When they see the link, they can actively choose how to respond, or not respond. The relationship between the self and the experience of diabetes suddenly has much more space. This is the freedom to rise above one's condition. To be above the wave of highs and lows, and to de-link with the identification of "I am diabetes."

Diabetes is an Opportunity

It sometimes takes something cataclysmic to wake up consciousness. You hear about people who are changed by a near-death experience, a recovery from a terminal illness, and, yes, a diabetes diagnosis. Sometimes we need a hurdle to stir up something more inspired within us to say, "Hey, hello, are you living your potential? Are you fulfilling your greatness? Or are you just caught in the hamster wheel, getting by on the surface, unaware of the potential that life has to offer?"

Diabetes can be a blessing or a curse; it depends on the attitude. An attitude can lead to destruction or be that which inspires us towards greatness. It is both the wake-up call and the foremost obstacle in the way of improved health and personal transformation.

In Yoga Sūtra 1.30 Patañjali classifies disease as the first obstacle in the way of enlightenment. As a person who lives with T1D, an incurable disease, my ego gets a little jab when I hear this. It seems unfair that something I have not chosen could hinder my personal evolution.

The verbatim translation may imply that an incurable illness, like T1D, would hold me back from fully evolving as a spiritual being. But like all things, it is up to our own interpretation. Perhaps the reason why disease is listed as the first obstacle is that we can actually do something about it. That there is a *different* type of cure.

It's more plausible in the world in which we live to believe that the answer lies in a doctor's procedure or in a prescribed pill. We have been taught that we are not enough. I am fully aware that there is *no medical cure* for my condition and that I will always (at least for now) have to take insulin, but maybe this is not what Patañjali is alluding to (or at least my interpretation of it). Perhaps what he is saying is that I do have a choice, and there is a different type of remedy, one that exists within my own mind and heart.

Heyaṁ Duḥkham Anāgatam YS 2.16 states that all the suffering that is yet to come is avoidable, implying that there is some level of choice in our destiny. But to thwart the onset of pain, we must first cultivate the power to rise above it.

It is easier to fall down than it is to stand up. It is easier to lay idle than it is to apply effort towards achieving our goals. To avoid future suffering, we bring power to our choices and decisions. We cultivate this ability through yoga sadhana.

Upāya—the Means to Do It

My teachers stress that theory remains theory until it is directly experienced from within. The gift of the yoga practice is transforming ideas into fruition. The practice of yoga gives us an opportunity to realize the meaning of yoga in every moment of our lives. Whether that is during āsana, prāṇāyāma, meditation, reading texts, or through living with diabetes, it can be yoga if we are present.

The means by which we cultivate the power to remove the obstacles and awaken our potential is practice (sadhana). Remember that yoga is not passive;

it is active. It is to move from where you are to somewhere better. If the nature of the world and the mind is to move, we may as well influence its flow.

Yoga is a process that empowers a movement of change by building our internal fortitude, by refining self-awareness, and through the connection to something bigger, a source of inspiration. Patañjali outlines three main paths towards achieving this. Abhyāsa (practice) and vairāgya (non-attachment), kriyā yoga, and the yamas and niyamas. All are applicable paths, but for our conversation I will focus on the middle path: kriyā yoga, the yoga of action, because it is what was taught to me. 'Kr' of kriyā is to do. Kriyā yoga is the actual means by which we attain the promised result of yoga, whatever that is to the individual,[10] whether it lies within diabetes or it extends beyond it.

Kriyā yoga consists of three parts: tapas, svādhyāya, and īśvara praṇidhāna.

The first step of kriyā yoga is tapas. The traditional definition is to heat or to cleanse. By removing physical and mental impurities, one gains greater control over the regulatory systems of the body. Tapas, in our context, is to strengthen willpower to overcome the cause of avidyā and duḥkha. Another translation of tapas is austerity. I see the image of a long-haired, bearded fellow standing on one foot for 12 years. That is austerity, but it can mean something entirely different in the context of yoga, and in our conversation about diabetes. The Upanishads say that disease is the highest form of tapas—through which life can be revealed. In this frame of reference, a disease is the opportunity to know thyself.[11]

The second step is svādhyāya, the study of ourselves and the development of self-knowledge. It is not enough to keep the body fit, eat right, and take insulin. We have to understand what causes our pain and what inspires our purpose. Svadhyaya is to examine yourself, your mind, your condition, your breath. Classically, svādhyāya is the study of sacred texts that hold the abiding truths of the practice. Just as we would read a book and study its words, we do the same with ourselves.

It can also refer to the study of the mind, and, in our context, the study of diabetes. I paraphrase David Frawley when he says that life is learning and development of self-knowledge. That we should view disease in this

10 Desikachar, T. K. V., Skelton, M. L. and Carter, J. R. (1980) *Religiousness in Yoga: Lectures on Theory and Practice*. Washington DC: University Press of America. p.10.

11 Frawley, D. (2000) *Ayurvedic Healing: A Comprehensive Guide*. Second rev. and enl. edition. Twin Lakes, WI: Lotus Press. p.57.

light to understand it. Not just treating disease but also using it as a tool for understanding ourselves.[12]

How do you actively practice svādhyāya? The breath. By witnessing our breathing we become more acutely aware of our inner nature and how we can influence change within the regulatory systems of the body and, principally, the mind. But we do not have a mirror for our minds like we have a mirror for our bodies. We cannot see our minds like we can see our physical features. Does this mean that we do not have a mind? Of course not. No one negates the existence of their minds when they are perpetually talking to themselves all of the time. We do, however, rarely study what it is we are saying.

But one must also apply svādhyāya to their actions. Study your habits, look at the correlations between actions and negative results. If you continually wake up with BG at 300 mg/dL (16.7 mmol/L), do a svādhyāya on what the cause is. If you cannot figure that out, infer it and apply changes. If we notice that rajas is predominant, we are experiencing anxiety—inquire into that. What is it? Am I scared about something? Is it real and valid? Often, just recognizing it is enough to promote sattva and dissipate some of the duḥkha.

Lastly, īśvara praṇidhāna is a quality of action. It is the quality of intention that we put behind our efforts. It is often translated as surrender to a higher power, god, the universe, or anything meaningful to you. Īśvara praṇidhāna is active surrender. But it is also about doing for the love of doing, without attachment to a result. In the context of diabetes care, īśvara praṇidhāna teaches how to take care of diabetes without an attachment to the desired result. Yes, you can have goals. You can put all your tapas and svādhyāya into producing the best health and diabetes equilibrium possible, but there is always something that goes wrong. Īśvara praṇidhāna teaches us to let go of the tightened fist around what we believe we should be or what diabetes should look like and allows us to be more fluid in our efforts. This frees up space and teaches us how to forgive our mistakes and cultivate a positive attitude. Īśvara praṇidhāna is based in sattva, the purest form of the manifested material universe.

Desikachar says that rather than focusing on a specific goal, īśvara praṇidhāna teaches us to attend to a process. One that allows Īśvara to work through you. Do the work, see clearly, reduce suffering, and open the pathways

12 Frawley, D. (2000) *Ayurvedic Healing: A Comprehensive Guide*. Second rev. and enl. edition. Twin Lakes, WI: Lotus Press. p.57.

to enable consciousness to move through you to fulfill your destiny, achieve physical health, and radiate this onto others.

There is no specific goal other than to actualize our purpose, while never being fixed or sure about what that will bring. Inner harmony and joy can overcome all external difficulties.[13]

13 Frawley, D. (2000) *Ayurvedic Healing: A Comprehensive Guide*. Second rev. and enl. edition. Twin Lakes, WI: Lotus Press. p.57.

CHAPTER 5

Yoga Therapy Tools

Yoga is a spiritual path with an overarching goal of liberation from the ego and freedom from suffering. But to achieve the goal, good health is necessary. One must acquire the physical and mental stamina to make the long haul because our whole life is a practice and our life is a gift.

Although the original objective of yoga was (and remains) about enlightenment, health has always been at the forefront of the journey. Even Patañjali says the first obstacle on the path is disease. The ancients employed yogic tools to overcome health limitations so they could have a primed vessel for the real work of attaining self-liberation.

The tools of yoga therapy are the same as the tools of yoga, but the distinction is that we are using yoga therapy to address a specific condition within a unique person. While the long-term goal of yoga therapy may be the same as the goal of yoga, the route there is through the health condition or challenge. Friction creates the quest for self-knowledge and freedom.

This is why the practices should not stop at the condition. It is not about just diabetes; it is about learning how to practice self-care because of diabetes. Yoga is a self-care practice that teaches and empowers individuals to take an active role in their own health, happiness, and destiny with an illness and beyond that illness.

In this chapter I will walk you through the familiar terrain of yogic models and tools as they relate to yoga therapy for diabetes. It is true that the tools of yoga are beneficial to all people; the precise application of them for diabetes is what makes it such a detailed art and science.

What is Yoga Therapy?

The concept of yoga therapy stems from the yoga tradition of Patañjali and the Ayurvedic system of health.[1] Classically, yoga therapy was called yoga cikitsā, referencing the application of consciousness (or cit, the Sanskrit term for consciousness) or caring for one's health.[2] It is founded on the basis that everything we do, feel, and think, the relationships we have, and the way we live and connect with our environment are intimately connected to our wellbeing.[3] Āyurveda focuses on the health of the bodily systems and yoga on the transformation of suffering. Both serve the other in practice and in theory. The convergence of yoga and Āyurveda as yoga therapy is called *kaya kalpa*,[4] a term emanating from Āyurveda as a science of *immortality*.

Yoga Therapy is Individualized

Yoga therapy blends the knowledge and practices of yoga and Āyurveda into a complete health-providing tool to promote longevity. It is the ultimate self-care practice. In yoga therapy the traditional practices of āsana, prāṇāyāma, meditation, and so on are modified, adapted, and even simplified to suit individual needs.[5]

Yoga cikitsā recognizes that the experience of suffering is unique to the individual, and therefore the methods of practice should also be unique to the individual. One of the central models employed in yoga therapy assessment is the koshic model. I will not detail the koshas in this book, but the fundamental premise is that an individual is a complex layering of gross physical matter, subtle energy, mind, intellect, and higher consciousness. These layers are manifestations of matter that cover the true and essential nature. To treat a person holistically is to consider all of these sheaths.

1 Kraftsow, G. (1999) *Yoga for Wellness: Healing with the Timeless Teachings of Viniyoga*. New York: Penguin/Arkana. p.129.

2 Prabhu, U. M. (2020) "Yoga Therapy and Ayurveda: The Meaning of Chikitsa." *American Institute of Vedic Studies*. Accessed on 01/07/20 at: www.vedanet.com/yoga-therapy-and-ayurveda-the-meaning-of-chikitsa.

3 Kraftsow, G. (1999) *Yoga for Wellness: Healing with the Timeless Teachings of Viniyoga*. New York: Penguin/Arkana. p.129.

4 Kraftsow, G. (1999) *Yoga for Wellness: Healing with the Timeless Teachings of Viniyoga*. New York: Penguin/Arkana. p.130.

5 McCall, T., Satish, L. and Tiwari, S. (2016) "History, Philosophy, and Practice of Yoga Therapy." In S. B. S. Khalsa, L. Cohen, T. McCall and S. Telles (eds) *The Principles and Practice of Yoga in Healthcare*. Pencaitland: Handspring Publishing. p.44.

This consideration offers yoga therapists a unique vantage point in ameliorating the causes of individual suffering and the construction of health-providing practices that go much deeper than addressing just a condition. It is saying that health is about the whole being, not just one element. Diabetes is a metabolic condition, but if we just practice to treat the disease, we neglect the impact that the illness has on every layer of a person, just as every layer can impact one's own experience with a disease. Problems with anxiety, independent of a diabetes diagnosis, will influence the way a person copes with diabetes. By treating the whole person through complete practices that extend beyond the scope of an illness, we promote the objective of yoga therapy, which is the science of immortality. I see that as longevity, empowerment, and resilience.

It is common to hear "It depends" in the yoga therapy community because ultimately there is no such thing as a one-size-fits-all format in holistic health. We are all individual expressions of puruṣa, and upon diagnosis we arrive on the mat with different goals, physical constitutions, psychological proclivities, experiences, attitudes, and support systems.

Yoga is to move from where we are to somewhere better; perhaps a place we never thought possible. We achieve this with action and perception. Through yoga sadhana, we acquire the skills to produce beneficial results. In the therapeutic application of yoga there are two inherent elements of this process: to separate from what is not working, and to link with what is.

There are two fundamental components to the process of yoga cikitsā: *viyoga* and *saṁyoga*.

> *Duḥkha Saṁyoga Viyoga Yogaha* "Yoga is separating from identification with suffering." The Bhagavad Gita 6.20–6.23.

"Vi" means separation. It means to separate ourselves from whatever is undesirable in our lives.[6] In a way, the active practice of viyoga is to cultivate the discernment to see what is causing harm and apply methods to remove it. The awareness may start on a mat, but over time it is put into practice off of the mat. This occurs progressively and naturally as self-awareness improves.

"Saṁ" is to link with, denoting a connection between two things, but it is a little different than the "yoking" we commonly think of as being the definition of yoga. Saṁyoga is to link with what is most meaningful and constructive

6 Kraftsow, G. (1999) *Yoga for Wellness: Healing with the Timeless Teachings of Viniyoga*. New York: Penguin/Arkana. p.129.

in our lives.[7] Positive attributes like compassion, forgiveness, vulnerability, and love symbolically replace what is removed from viyoga. With time, the bond with positive associations becomes more significant than the bond with negative ones. This imbues positive virtues into actions, priorities, and even moments of difficulty. The work for the individual is to realize what is helpful and what is harmful so that they do not have to suffer.[8]

A lot of time, a person suffers but does not know why. How can a person see what is creating their suffering when they are caught up in it? The practice of self-care is no different than the practice of yoga sadhana. Taking care of oneself by attending to the elements of physical, mental, emotional, and energetic wellbeing as a sacred ritual awakens people to their potential for health and freedom.

Self-Care is Yoga

I think that in the Western world we want to be able to say "Do this one thing," and that one thing will create a specific result. People do it all the time in yoga. This posture does this, or they claim that it cures that. While it sounds incredible, these claims are unfounded. We are not always aware of what exact benefit the practice is having, just like we cannot always give exactly one formula for diabetes self-care that will improve a person's BG or quality of life. The impact is cumulative.

The recommended pillars of diabetes self-care are: *diet, exercise, behavioral adaptiveness, mental and emotional health, relationships support, energy management, rest, and sleep.*

Yoga therapy directly and indirectly helps with all of these pillars from a physiological, psychological, and behavioral standpoint.

In yoga therapy we are modifying, adapting, and even simplifying the traditional practices of yoga āsana, prāṇāyāma, and meditation to address the missing link in diabetes healthcare. Doctors recommend that individuals with diabetes add self-care practices into their daily routine to fulfill the requirements listed above, but there are no precise methods described other than exercise, eat right, take medicine, and watch your stress levels. The beauty of yoga therapy as self-care is that it empowers people to take charge of their own lives, but also that it extends well beyond the treatment of diabetes. It is

7 Kraftsow, G. (1999) *Yoga for Wellness: Healing with the Timeless Teachings of Viniyoga*. New York: Penguin/Arkana. p.130.

8 Kraftsow, G. (2014) Lecture at Mount Madonna Institute.

about maintaining good health, and if in the process a person understands themselves better, achieves greater freedom and joy, and can overcome negative behaviors and replace them with more positive ones, then we win.

Prāṇa—the Energetic Palette

We talked in the last chapter about how low prāṇa is a factor in disease and how containing prāṇa within the body is a method for increasing vitality and longevity for health. Yoga, as a practice of spiritual evolution, similarly uses the concept of prāṇa to accelerate development. Whether the goal is yoga or yoga therapy, we use prāṇa as the basis to achieve a beneficial result. We do this by influencing change's inevitability by altering the flow of the breath and the mind. This is part of the process of empowerment, the understanding that I can change the way I think, feel, and perceive through practice. It can be physiological, psychological, or behavioral. To influence prāṇa's flow, we employ breathing practices throughout all the tools of yoga from āsana, to prāṇāyāma, to meditation. An example of this would be encouraging a chest inhalation in a backbend to accentuate an extension, or a seated prāṇāyāma ratio to create a specific energetic effect, or to simply witness the breath in meditation as an anchor point for the mind to rest upon.

Prāṇa is divided into five directions within the body, known as the vāyus or the winds. Each has a specific movement, location, and function.

- **Prāṇ vāyu** (not to be mistaken for prāṇa; we will call it prāṇ, although in some contexts it is also called prāṇa)—Governs the inward movement of prāṇa, supporting intake of vitality. Associated with the chest and heart space.
- **Apāna vāyu**—Downward and outward, supporting elimination. Located from the navel down to the base of the spine.
- **Vyāna vāyu**—Abides everywhere, supporting the movement, cohesion of all the vāyus, and circulation.
- **Samāna vāyu**—Moves from the periphery to the center, supports assimilation and integration. Strong association with the navel region.
- **Udāna vāyu**—Located around the throat, an upward movement, inspires creativity and the ascension of consciousness.

Prāṇa exists everywhere, so it needs containment to potentiate it. It is stressed that we cannot increase prāṇa, we can just contain and direct it. Prāṇa can be more dominant in some regions of a person's body and lacking in others. This also creates a type of imbalance. Just to throw out a stereotype, a tall, lanky vāta type has a tendency to "live in the clouds" metaphorically speaking. The reference is to the amount of prāṇa, perhaps excessive, in their heads. It may be beneficial for them to focus on breathing into areas of their body, like the abdomen or the lower body, to encourage prāṇa to flow more evenly throughout their physical body, and promote balance.

An effect of hyperglycemia, for instance, is sluggish digestion. A potential tool would be to encourage the breath to move into the abdominal organs by focusing breath in the abdomen, relaxing abdominal musculature, lengthening the exhale, and suspending the breath. On a physical level, this will improve motility; on a more subtle physiological level, the abdominal focus on exhalation will stimulate the vagus nerve, which innervates the gut.

People with diabetes are at an increased risk of developing heart disease. Practices that encourage inhalation, open the thoracic cavity, improve circulation, and increase heart rate are potential methods to influence pranic movement for improved health.

You see, when considering prāṇa as a tool and encouraging its flow to move into areas in which it is lacking via the various methods outlined in yoga, we are teaching the individual to align with the elemental forces within them. These are concepts, qualities, and states of consciousness that are inexplicable by science but essential in the process of practicing yoga therapy as self-care. It is the framework for self-awareness and self-regulation.

The skillful and intentional use of prāṇa as an energetic palette for self-care is a starting point to begin sequencing. It helps us consider another dimension of yoga, the ultimate health-providing tool. If a practice offers up everything, it loses its potency. By homing in on how and why prāṇa moves, we become true designers of the art and science of self-empowerment.

The Tools

The main yoga and yoga therapy tools highlighted in this book are āsana, prāṇāyāma, chanting, guided relaxation (including Śavāsana and the preparation for yoga nidrā), and meditation.

Āsana

Āsana (physical yoga postures) develops interoceptive and proprioceptive awareness. Proprioceptive awareness is the awareness of the body, its muscles and structure, and how it moves with other parts of the body. Āsana helps to mobilize areas of tightness and strengthen areas of weakness. We learn in āsana how to identify and adjust harmful movement patterns and replace them with a more functional one. Interoceptive awareness is the ability to identify, access, understand, and respond appropriately to the patterns of internal signals—it provides a distinct advantage when engaging in life's challenges and ongoing adjustments.[9] This is especially interesting when we consider yoga therapy for diabetes as a strategy for improving self-care.

Āsana is divided into the five spinal directions (flexion, extension, lateral flexion, rotation, axial extension) and in orientation (supine, prone, kneeling, standing, balancing, and inversions). Each direction and orientation has an anatomical and physiological effect, supporting the movement of pranic influence within the body. At times, we are unaware of the impact that āsana has on the body's internal organs, supporting their redistribution and function.[10]

As you will see, all of the āsanas in the practices in this book are breath centric, meaning that they are not only sequenced with the breath, but also in service of a better breath. In the breath-centric tradition, we move in and out of postures synchronized with breath to increase the influence of prāṇa throughout the bodily systems. Repetition prepares the body to stay in a pose and builds physical and mental strength.

Moving in and out of postures with the breath focuses the mind, increases circulation, and naturally calms the mind's roaming tendencies. The postures also serve as tools to support the energetic condition, something we will address later in the chapter. As the practice evolves and the practitioner advances in their acuity of prāṇa, the postures become subtler. What may not look like much movement to an outside observer is quite exciting and potent. The reason you will not see advanced positions in this book is that they do not serve the general practitioner with diabetes, and ambitious postures can externalize and disrupt the meditative and therapeutic benefits of the practice. Compared with other exercises of equal metabolic intensity, walking for instance, yoga āsana

9 Price, C. J. and Hooven, C. (2018) "Interoceptive awareness skills for emotion regulation: theory and approach of mindful awareness in body-oriented therapy (MABT)." *Frontiers in Psychology* 9, 798.

10 Robertson, L. H. (2019) "Perspective: Srivatsa Ramaswami on the fundamental intentions of yoga." *Yoga Therapy Today*, Winter.

is found to be more advantageous to improving mood and reducing anxiety, supporting claims that the benefits of the physical portion of the practice extend beyond just a pose.[11]

Āsana directly serves the pillar of exercise, behavioral adaptiveness, and mental-emotional health. The most obvious benefit is that of exercise. Yoga āsana is a relatively safe, low-risk exercise compared with other forms of aerobic or strength training. Just about anyone can do it. It is a good starting point for exercise because the caloric and energetic expenditure is not as intense as running, for example. For people with T2D who are encouraged to exercise but may not feel confident in their fitness levels, yoga āsana is a great and effective way to get moving and help them feel successful without overworking. Yoga is modifiable to all bodies and can be practiced within the confines of one's home. Studies comparing yoga-based movement with conventional exercise have shown yoga to be just as if not more effective at improving energetic levels, reducing fatigue, and increasing self-esteem.[12] Āsana is also a safe and easy way to employ movement when there is concern for hypoglycemia. However, let it be known that yoga āsana is still a risk for hypoglycemia when there is too much insulin in relationship to the metabolic intensity of a practice. The intensity is easily modifiable and offers an intermediary physical exercise that increases circulation, heart rate, and physical fitness without the high energetic demand and recovery time of other exercise.

And while yoga may not meet all cardiovascular fitness needs, āsana provides a framework to adjust the duration and intensity of physical movement for people with diabetes, reintegrating physiological responses and mental focus. While feed-forward exercise activities can be performed without conscious awareness, yoga āsana is a feedback orientation where the individual is continuously assessing, feeling, and observing their body, mind, and breath. It can be as simple as noticing the foot, and paying attention to how it moves and the sensations present. For people with diabetic neuropathy, a risk factor is the lack of awareness in physical extremities. They run a higher risk of getting an infection in the foot, for example. It is proposed that coordinated

---

11 Schmalzl, L., Streeter, C. C. and Khalsa, S. B. S. (2016) "Research on the Psychophysiology of Yoga." In S. B. S. Khalsa, L. Cohen, T. McCall and S. Telles (eds) *The Principles and Practice of Yoga in Healthcare.* Pencaitland: Handspring Publishing. p.50.

12 Schmalzl, L., Streeter, C. C. and Khalsa, S. B. S. (2016) "Research on the Psychophysiology of Yoga." In S. B. S. Khalsa, L. Cohen, T. McCall and S. Telles (eds) *The Principles and Practice of Yoga in Healthcare.* Pencaitland: Handspring Publishing. p.50.

movement of moderate intensity is more likely to assist parasympathetic vagal tone than more vigorous exercise.[13] It has been shown that yoga āsana can affect neuroendocrine levels, risk propensity, and pain tolerance.[14] On a psychophysiological level, āsana teaches people how to remain in a pose, even when uncomfortable, and stay calm. They learn to observe and be less reactive to the sensations that surface in their bodies.

Prāṇāyāma

If you haven't realized it yet, prāṇāyāma is the most important tool in your toolkit for yoga and yoga therapy. Prāṇāyāma is the expansion, influence, and unobstructed life-force as it flows within the body.

It is much more than taking an inhale and exhale. Prāṇāyāma helps us improve blood circulation, the venous return of blood into the heart, and the exchange of gas and blood in the lungs, and reduces the strain on the heart.[15] The diaphragm is the engine of the breath.[16] The pericardium, the sack that surrounds the heart, is connected to the diaphragm. The regular practice of prāṇāyāma helps you work with and exercise the heart function. As we know, people with diabetes are at an increased risk for heart disease; working with the breath improves heart function.[17]

Prāṇāyāma is the bridge between the mind and the physical body and governs our energetic condition, which is related to our emotional state and perception of wellbeing. As we have learned, the ability to self-regulate and apply conscious choice to all decisions is empowerment.

The way we breathe constitutes the way we think. Prāṇāyāma removes the mental disturbances and focuses the mind for meditation.[18] We achieve this by

---

13 Schmalzl, L., Streeter, C. C. and Khalsa, S. B. S. (2016) "Research on the Psychophysiology of Yoga." In S. B. S. Khalsa, L. Cohen, T. McCall and S. Telles (eds) *The Principles and Practice of Yoga in Healthcare*. Pencaitland: Handspring Publishing. p.50.

14 Schmalzl, L., Streeter, C. C. and Khalsa, S. B. S. (2016) "Research on the Psychophysiology of Yoga." In S. B. S. Khalsa, L. Cohen, T. McCall and S. Telles (eds) *The Principles and Practice of Yoga in Healthcare*. Pencaitland: Handspring Publishing. p.51.

15 Robertson, L. H. (2019) "Perspective: Srivatsa Ramaswami on the fundamental intentions of yoga." *Yoga Therapy Today*, Winter.

16 Kaminoff, L. (2010) *How is your Diaphragm like the Engine in your Car?* Accessed on 01/07/20 at: www.youtube.com/watch?v=9UJIAiEThBw.

17 Robertson, L. H. (2019) "Perspective: Srivatsa Ramaswami on the fundamental intentions of yoga." *Yoga Therapy Today*, Winter.

18 The Yoga Sutra-s of Patanjali (2.52, 2.53).

making the breath long and smooth[19] and consciously changing our disturbed breathing patterns.[20] Disturbances of the body and mind alter our breathing patterns,[21] so influencing our mind's direction from tamas and rajas, towards sattva, and disease towards equilibrium, starts with the breath.

Prāṇāyāma is the main tool for bringing about change not only in our mind, but also in our physiology. Breath regulation can have a number of physiological effects depending on the type of breathing.[22] Our breath, the exhale specifically, is one of the only ways that we can self-regulate and activate the parasympathetic branch of the ANS, transforming the perception of threat and conserving the neuroendocrine responses for actual life-threatening situations.

There are four parts to the breath: inhale, retention, exhale, and suspension.

Exhale is produced by a progressive contraction of the abdominal musculature, supporting the relationship between the pelvis and the lumbar spine. Exhalation strengthens the abdominal muscles, tones the abdominal organs, and encourages *elimination* on all levels. According to Yoga Sūtra 1.34, exhale reduces the disturbances of the mind on a psychological level. Given its cooling orientation, the exhale activates the parasympathetic branch of the ANS, rendering it a vital method to calm, soothe, pacify, and reduce physical and mental instability. Another way to improve challenges with the inhalation is to work with the exhalation first. Exhale is the precursor to inhale; without it, the inhale has a tendency to be strained and choppy.

Inhale, like sustenance, is the nourishment that we take in on all levels. Like any food, it is essential to limit the amount to avoid aggravating the system.[23] Inhalation can be applied therapeutically. Its application benefits anatomical structure by opening the chest, ribcage, and upper back. Inhale activates the sympathetic branch of the ANS and is considered to be heating and stimulating.

Kumbhaka is the pause after inhale (retention) and exhale (suspension). Its use intensifies the energetic effect of the breath. It can be applied in āsana to fortify a posture, encourage a specific physiological focus, and prepare the mind for meditation.

19 The Yoga Sūtra-s of Patanjali (2.50).

20 The Yoga Sūtra-s of Patanjali (2.49).

21 The Yoga Sūtra-s of Patanjali (1.31).

22 Schmalzl, L., Streeter, C. C. and Khalsa, S. B. S. (2016) "Research on the Psychophysiology of Yoga." In S. B. S. Khalsa, L. Cohen, T. McCall and S. Telles (eds) *The Principles and Practice of Yoga in Healthcare*. Pencaitland: Handspring Publishing. p.52.

23 Mohan, A. G. and Mohan, I. (2004) *Yoga Therapy: A Guide to the Therapeutic Use of Yoga and Ayurveda for Health and Fitness*. Boulder, CA: Shambhala Publications. p.129.

Types of breath:

- Ujjāyī—Employed by constricting the back of the throat. This is the primary breath used in physical postures. Ujjāyī means *victorious breath*; the victory is over the mind's roaming tendencies. Ujjāyī breath with emphasis on inhale, exhale, and/or kumbhaka is a means to still the mind.
- Alternate nostril—There are several alternate nostril breaths, the classic being nāḍī śodhana. The purpose of alternate nostril breathing is to purify the energetic pathways as represented by the nāḍī-s.
- Bhastrikā and kapālabhātī—These are rapid, purifying breathing kriyās. The fast breath stimulates sympathetic activation and can be a means for promoting mental focus, memory, and sensory motor performance. They require a higher rate of breath coordination and respiratory muscle activity, which can help to strengthen the respiratory system.[24]

Mṛgī mudrā is the hand placement for any alternate nostril prāṇāyāma practice like nāḍī śodhana, candra and sūrya bhedana, and anuloma and viloma ujjāyī. In mṛgī mudrā, the index and middle finger are folded toward the palm of the hand, leaving the thumb, ring, and little finger. Its specialized use allows for greater control over breath rate due to a valve created by the fingers at the nose. In mṛgī mudrā one nostril is completely closed, and the other is partially closed or valved more or less where the bone and nasal cartilage meet. This is a crucial step that many practitioners miss (and many teachers neglect to teach), meaning they have less command over their breathing during alternate nostril breathing practices.

I'll explain how to use mṛgī mudrā in the context of nāḍī śodhana: Using the right-hand thumb, close the right nostril, and valve the left nostril with the ring finger where the bone and nasal cartilage meet. Inhale through the valved left nostril. You will feel a slight resistance at the nasal passageway, allowing you to slow down the rate at which you are inhaling. To exhale, slide the ring finger down to close the left nostril and the right thumb up to where the bone and cartilage meet and valve the right nostril. Exhale out of the right nostril.

24 Schmalzl, L., Streeter, C. C. and Khalsa, S. B. S. (2016) "Research on the Psychophysiology of Yoga." In S. B. S. Khalsa, L. Cohen, T. McCall and S. Telles (eds) *The Principles and Practice of Yoga in Healthcare*. Pencaitland: Handspring Publishing. p.55.

Repeat the inhale through the valved right nostril, switch the fingers, and exhale out of the valved left nostril.

Bandha

A bandha is a seal or a lock, implying the containment of prāṇa within the body. In esoteric terms, bandhas are a way to directly collect impurities that stagnate in the lower region of the abdomen and push them into the fire of agni (purification) at the navel. This is the spiritualization of the body—the removal of the obstacles so that prāṇa can flow freely in the central channel.

On a more practical level, uḍḍiyāna-bandha (abdominal lock) is a beneficial strategy to help tone the abdominal organs as an intervention and management strategy for people with diabetes. I recommend the practice of agni sara and treta bandha (all three locks) for some gastrointestinal issues due to conditions caused by hyperglycemia and autonomic neuropathy like gastroparesis.

Bandhas are not applicable for most students unless they can breathe without tension in āsana and practice a comfortable seated kumbhaka ratio. Without these prerequisites, bandhas can be injurious to a person's health, overstimulating them and creating unnecessary anxiety.

To keep everyone safe and utilize the benefit of bandha without aggravating anyone's system, you can instruct bandha-"like" action during āsana. For instance, lowering the chin (jālandhara-bandha-like) while transitioning through poses promotes the mind's internalization and encourages spinal length. Movement in and out of a forward bend on exhale suspension gives an uḍḍiyāna-bandha-like feel, intensifying a posture's energetic potency, and encouraging elimination (apāna vāyu) and parasympathetic activation. For the advanced practitioner with diabetes, a regular bandha practice, especially uḍḍiyāna-bandha, is recommended as a general maintenance strategy to tone the abdominal organs that are taxed by diabetes, so long as it does not create excessive stimulation or anxiousness.

Chanting

Chanting serves multiple benefits in the application of yoga and yoga therapy. I like to think of it as a cheater tool for dropping in. There is something that chanting does on a physiological level that is distinct from other tools of the practice.

The origins of yoga were passed down audibly through chanting. It was a means of focusing attention and retaining memory. Now, in a world where everything is at our fingertips, we have lost our patience and ability to listen. If we place chanting into practice, the student learns to focus their attention inwardly and intensify any posture or energetic condition. Krishnamacharya used chanting with children in āsana for mental focus,[25] and, in a therapeutic context, chanting in āsana is used to evoke a physiological response in the body.

First and foremost, chanting is prāṇāyāma, sound, and subtle meaning. I have included it as one of the main tools of practice because it works with the mind and physiology, and it inculcates a reverential quality of intention in practice. In yoga and yoga therapy, chanting is in Sanskrit; however, it does not have to be. It just has to be meaningful to the practitioner. In Sanskrit, each sound has a meaning beyond direct translation. The meaning of sound, known as pranava, is an eternal resonance. Chanting a mantra, a poem, or anything of inspiration infuses a subtle and spiritually potent significance into any practice that, without it, could be limited to physical mechanics. You can chant in āsana or seated prāṇāyāma, audibly (out loud), or mentally (silently from within), with the breath (as prāṇāyāma) or independent of the breath (as in some meditations).

As diabetes is aggravated by stress, chanting is a potent tool to help people relax and train their nervous systems to heal from overactive sympathetic responses. Chanting is another way of breathing and training the breath. Practiced out loud, chanting is a replacement for exhaling and teaches a person how to exhale without tension. High BG damages the vagus nerve, the prime regulator of the parasympathetic branch of the ANS. Exhale is a way to trigger a parasympathetic response, and for many who struggle to exhale, there is an underlying mental disturbance. Chanting is a way to resolve agitation in the breath and train the balance of sympathetic and parasympathetic activation. Chanting helps synchronize the left and right hemispheres of the brain, oxygenating the brain, improving heart rate variability, lowering blood pressure, and assisting in reducing brain wave activity.[26]

Perhaps more profound than the physical and mental benefit of chanting is

25 Gardner, P. (2010) "Sonia Nelson brings chant to life in practice." *Yoga Chicago*. Accessed on 01/07/20 at: www.yogachicago.com/jan10/sonianelson.shtml.

26 Dudeja, J. P. (2017) "Scientific analysis of mantra-based meditation and its beneficial effects: an overview." *International Journal of Advanced Scientific Technologies in Engineering and Management Sciences* 3, 21.

its meaning. Sonia Nelson, a student of both Desikachar and Krishnamacharya, and one of the foremost authorities on Vedic chanting, says that, "When we chant, we chant from our heart, and the chant is, therefore, received in the heart of the listener."[27] By chanting anything that is of significance, we imbue into our practice the deeper meaning behind our intention. This potentiates the method and helps a person embody the essence of the sound through direct experience.

Not everyone is comfortable with sound. It is best to educate new students on the importance of sound and its physiological healing potential. Yoga therapy and science are both revealing that a connection to faith, spirituality, and deeper meaning are important, if not essential, tools for managing chronic illness. Chanting is one way to access this potency without turning people away from something that may seem dogmatic.

Yoga Nidrā

This is a state of being; it is not something you do. Most people think they are practicing yoga nidrā when in fact they are doing the preparation for yoga nidrā, which is a progressive guided relaxation. Yoga nidrā is the fourth state of consciousness, *turīya*, a place beyond wakefulness, dream, and sleep.

Yoga nidrā can and should be utilized as a tool for all types of diabetes and related complications. First of all, everyone can do it. Second, it has an extraordinary nourishing effect on the body and mind, a profound way to manage energy, reduce fatigue, and dissolve unconscious habituated tension.

I honestly cannot say enough about its potential to heal, transform, and embody peace. The benefit is ubiquitous for all humans—surrender. It is especially beneficial in the context of diabetes, where we are chasing the highs and the lows and never fully given the opportunity to turn off and be. It is a method that benefits hypervigilant personalities and absentmindedness equally.

I practice it daily and use it as an intervention strategy to restore balance from every single physiological and psychological deficit. It can be a standalone practice, but it is even better when combined with other yogic tools like prāṇāyāma and meditation.

Research shows yoga nidrā's efficacy in treating anxiety and post-traumatic

27 Gardner, P. (2010) "Sonia Nelson brings chant to life in practice." *Yoga Chicago*. Accessed on 01/07/20 at: www.yogachicago.com/jan10/sonianelson.shtml.

stress disorder (PTSD), and it has also been shown to help individuals with T2D lower their A1c.[28] Although studies on guided relaxation and T1D are inconclusive,[29] I can confirm from direct experience that yoga nidrā is profound. I have seen clients with all types of saṁskāra-s resolved by resting and surrendering. A lot of the aggravation behind T1D and T2D is emotional and behavioral, so the art of surrender is quite profound. Ironically, in yoga nidrā people do not have to put in so much effort to achieve. It teaches you how to "just be" and witness what surfaces when you allow yourself to simply be. It teaches you how to loosen the grip and remain present without checking out, wandering off into inertia.

In the effortless space you find a wealth of information about your own habits, responses, and reactions. This is especially important for those who struggle with hypervigilance in their diabetes care and for those who are, conversely, resistant to self-care. Through direct experience of surrendering effort, people grant access to the subconscious underpinnings of their conditioned beliefs, reactivity, or aversion. It allows them to witness what surfaces as a thought, emotion, or sensation, and transform the contraction into an opportunity for release.

When people are exhausted, which is common with new students, they will fall asleep. This is not ideal, although I let it slide the first few times under the assumption that they probably need the rest, but I do communicate that the goal is to remain present. When people fall asleep during yoga nidrā, it represents their own habit of falling asleep in their waking life. Of course, if an individual drifts off to sleep here and there, it could mean that they are tired, but if they perpetually sleep without memory, despite your explanations as to the importance of remaining aware, it could represent deeper aversions and avoidance tendencies. Do what you can to help them remain aware. Useful strategies are propping their torso up with a bolster, having the head slightly above the heart, or keeping an arm up in an L-shape.

In a study[30] on the effects of yoga nidrā on hyperglycemia, researchers looked at 41 adults (35–65 years) with T2D on oral hypoglycemia medications.

---

28 Amita, S., Prabhakar, S., Manoj, I., Harminder, S. and Pavan, T. (2009) "Effect of yoga-nidra on blood glucose level in diabetic patients." *Indian Journal of Physiology and Pharmacology* 53, 1, 97–101.

29 Rubin, R. R. (2009) "Psychotherapy and Counselling in Diabetes Mellitus." In F. J. Snoek and C. T. J. Skinner (eds) *Psychology in Diabetes Care*. Chichester: Wiley & Sons Ltd. p.237.

30 Amita, S., Prabhakar, S., Manoj, I., Harminder, S. and Pavan, T. (2009) "Effect of yoga-nidra on blood glucose level in diabetic patients." *Indian Journal of Physiology and Pharmacology* 53, 1, 97–101.

The study defined yoga nidrā as "a state of relaxation and awareness on the border between sleep and wakefulness, allowing contact with the subconscious and conscious mind." Participants were divided into two groups: (a) 20 on oral hypoglycemics and yoga nidrā; (b) on oral hypoglycemics alone. Participants in control group (a) practiced yoga nidrā for 45 minutes a day for 90 days with reviews every 30 days. Results showed a reduction in diabetes-related symptoms (insomnia, distress, etc.), fasting BG, and postprandial BG (after meal) compared with oral hypoglycemics alone.

By learning how to relax while remaining aware, individuals with diabetes can also understand how to be more present with diabetes and awake in their lives. It is not uncommon to check out, turn away, and essentially fall asleep to diabetes care and all of our lives.

A big part of diabetes self-care is adaptability. Yoga nidrā teaches people how to remain aware and also relaxed at the same time. Unless we are awake to diabetes it is hard to be adaptive and present.

A.E. came to me in a dire state. A T1D for over 20 years, she was suffering from multiple diabetes-related complications and was on dialysis awaiting a kidney transplant. She wanted to build physical strength, but I knew that if we were to do anything too strenuous, it would actually deplete her rather than nourish her. In her fragile state, the method to strengthen physically was less about physical postures and more about helping her experience effortlessness through deep relaxation. This would not only support her compromised physical state but also attend to her worry as she awaited a transplant.

Together, we developed a yoga nidrā practice to help her build vitality, nourish her system, and calm her mind. The elements of this healing practice were inspired by my teacher Rod Stryker's work with specific healing.

What is significant about this style of yoga nidrā practice is establishing the witness—this is the part of every person that remains unaffected by change and disease. By abiding in this space of observation, one can impartially observe duality, promoting self-acceptance.

Over time, A.E. was more vibrant, her skin color returned to her face, and she would come to me less exhausted. We were able to use yoga nidrā as a tool to increase her stamina to withstand daily challenges until she could receive a transplant.

A Yoga Nidrā Practice for Diabetes

This is the basic outline for a yoga nidrā sequence for vitality and healing inspired by the work of my teacher Yogarupa Rod Stryker.

1. Preparation: Set up in a comfortable supine position, with support under the knees. Cover the body with a blanket and put a light cloth over the eyes.
2. Say to yourself, "Now begins the practice of yoga nidrā," and "I will remain open and aware." (Pause.)
3. Take ten to twenty conscious belly breaths, counting backward on exhalation. Relax the body on exhale into the earth. (Pause.) Inhale vitality, exhale let go.
4. Relax the breath.
5. Awareness of the body: The points of connection with the earth. Relax all holding and tension. Relinquish all effort, allow yourself to be open to experience. Every contraction of the body or engagement of the mind is an opportunity for release.
6. Awareness of sound: Allow sounds to enter and leave effortlessly.
7. Awareness of the part of you that endures, always at peace and at rest. (Brief pause.)
8. Awareness of the natural breath: Watch the rise and fall of the effortless breath. The exhale meets the inhale, the inhale meets the exhale.
9. The chest becomes still and the abdomen softens.
10. Recognize that you are not the breather. (Pause 1–2 minutes.)
11. Rotation of consciousness: 61 points with a blue star-like point of light.

    1) Eyebrow center
    2) Throat center
    3) Right shoulder
    4) Right elbow joint
    5) Right wrist joint
    6) Tip of the right thumb
    7) Tip of the right index finger
    8) Tip of the right middle finger

9) Tip of the right ring finger
10) Tip of the right little finger
11) Right wrist joint
12) Right elbow joint
13) Right shoulder joint
14) Throat center
15) Left shoulder joint
16) Left elbow joint
17) Left wrist joint
18) Tip of the left thumb
19) Tip of the left index finger
20) Tip of the left middle finger
21) Tip of the left ring finger
22) Tip of the left little finger
23) Left wrist joint
24) Left elbow joint
25) Left shoulder joint
26) Throat center
27) Heart center
28) Right chest
29) Heart center
30) Left chest
31) Heart center
32) Navel center
33) Pelvic center
34) Right hip joint
35) Right knee joint
36) Right ankle joint
37) Big toe of the right foot
38) Second toe
39) Third toe
40) Fourth toe
41) Right little toe
42) Right ankle joint
43) Right knee joint
44) Right hip joint
45) Pelvic center
46) Left hip joint
47) Left knee joint
48) Left ankle joint
49) Big toe of the left foot
50) Second toe
51) Third toe
52) Fourth toe
53) Left little toe
54) Left ankle joint
55) Left knee joint
56) Left hip joint
57) Pelvic center
58) Navel center

59) Heart center

60) Throat center

61) Eyebrow center

12. Observe the body as space and points of light. The breath moves through the space. (Pause 3–5 minutes.)
13. See or experience the body resting on a rose-colored cloud. Do not try to create it. Relax, and experience the body merging with a rose-colored cloud, healing the body and mind. (Pause 2–5 minutes.)
14. Resolve: "I am perfect health." Repeat mentally, three times, at the heart.
15. Awareness of breath. Deepen the inhale and lengthen the exhale. Return slowly. Roll to the side before sitting up.

Meditation

There are so many ways to meditate in yoga and yoga therapy that it can be rather daunting and overwhelming. How do you even start? My recommendation is to find a teacher from a reputable tradition that sources its information from sacred texts. Then, whenever you doubt the efficacy of what anyone is saying, there is a text to back it up. Some meditation traditions focus on something in particular; others are open and free-associative. Sometimes a meditation can be to self-reflect and question yourself, either with the hopes of finding an answer within or to remind yourself of what is meaningful. You can meditate on the breath, a symbol, a chakra, or a mantra. They are all means to arriving at one end; that is the true self.

Whereas yoga nidrā is about concentration, meditation is about cultivating your attention and sustaining that attention. This is helpful in our practice of diabetes self-care for a variety of reasons. It trains our attention. Increased mind wandering is associated with negative mood states.[31] We just talked about how āsana helps develop interoception; this is our awareness of emotion as bodily sensation. Meditation also helps to develop this skill in a different kind of way. It improves the ability to witness bodily signals (something as simple as feeling your BG level) or the sensations associated with emotional states like

31 Schmalzl, L., Streeter, C. C. and Khalsa, S. B. S. (2016) "Research on the Psychophysiology of Yoga." In S. B. S. Khalsa, L. Cohen, T. McCall and S. Telles (eds) *The Principles and Practice of Yoga in Healthcare.* Pencaitland: Handspring Publishing. p.54.

anxiety, and not get caught up in them.[32] In meditation we cannot run away (well, I guess we can get up and stop meditating or distract ourselves with something) but instead you are required to sit in it and be with it. Even if you find a way to distract yourself, in meditation you are given the opportunity to witness it and eventually change it. Although the disturbance may not be immediately resolved, over time and with consistent practice, meditation can dissolve the negative patterns and transform self-concept.

Success with diabetes is about being open to your potential as your caretaker and always discovering nuance in treatment strategies. Just when we've figured out the right way to manage our condition, it always throws in a new variable and we have to adapt. Meditation shows people how to cultivate an inner state of equanimity while in the midst of chaos. It helps us shift from this self-centered "Why is this happening to me?" attitude and be able to look at diabetes from a more objective vantage point. This is what we were talking about in the last chapter on witnessing the periphery but not getting caught up in the signals. All of diabetes, and life if you want to think of it like that, is a meditation.

Everyone knows that they "should" meditate but we do not always make time for it. No one can know the benefit it provides unless they commit to it and do it every single day. For me as a person with T1D, not only does meditation help me self-regulate, but also the self-awareness helps me to identify dysfunctional habits as they may or may not relate to diabetes care. It is in the quiet space where I recognize what I am not seeing clearly. What habits and tendencies do I consistently repeat or am I drawn to that are negatively impacting my BG? What thoughts and emotions continuously surface when diabetes throws me a curveball, and are those emotions necessary?

The mind is going to move; that is its nature. Meditation is not about controlling your mind, it is about witnessing it and then influencing its direction. That is self-mastery. We have learned that the breath is the vehicle for this. Without the breath, the mind will be unsteady and you will not receive all the potential benefits from your meditation practice. Studies show

32 Schmalzl, L., Streeter, C. C. and Khalsa, S. B. S. (2016) "Research on the Psychophysiology of Yoga." In S. B. S. Khalsa, L. Cohen, T. McCall and S. Telles (eds) *The Principles and Practice of Yoga in Healthcare*. Pencaitland: Handspring Publishing. p.54.

that a combination of movement and breath may provide a larger "array" of experience than a seated practice alone.[33]

STEPS TO MEDITATION

I was taught to prepare the body and mind for meditation with āsana and prāṇāyāma. You do not have to do much for it to be effective. It could be three to four dynamic postures linked with breath, for example Uttānāsana, cakravākāsana, Dvipāda Pītham, and Śavāsana, and then a brief prāṇāyāma (like nāḍī śodhana), before beginning the meditative process.

There are three main stages to meditation: dhāraṇā, dhyāna, and samadhi. My recommendation is to not worry about the second and third stages: they happen naturally with the right preparation. If we are too focused on the end result, these "higher" states will not occur.

The first stage of meditation is dhāraṇā, focused concentration. Concentration is not achieved with forceful will; it is an effortless effort. Our breath influences the mind, just as the mind influences the breath. In meditation we do not manipulate the breath; we watch its flow. Something happens when we do this; our brains become sensitized to prāṇa. Remember, prāṇa is not the breath; prāṇa rides along the breath. By watching the natural flow of the breath at the tip of the nose, the inhale entering and exhale leaving, the mind begins to "link" to the presence of prāṇa. It is a presence that is always there, but our minds are too outwardly oriented; we lack the awareness to perceive it. My magnificent teachers have stressed to me that this is the most important step in meditation. It is called *prāṇa dharana*. We want to use it to really condition the mind to be centered and prepared for the next stages of meditation. Once prāṇa is concentrated in the mid-brain, you can go on to the next step of meditation, like a mantra, chakra, or reflection.

Other traditions offer different focal points, but it seems that prāṇa dharana is pretty universal. Get the mind to rest on the natural presence of the breath, and then direct that energy into the next stage.

---

33 Schmalzl, L., Streeter, C. C. and Khalsa, S. B. S. (2016) "Research on the Psychophysiology of Yoga." In S. B. S. Khalsa, L. Cohen, T. McCall and S. Telles (eds) *The Principles and Practice of Yoga in Healthcare*. Pencaitland: Handspring Publishing. p.54.

PRĀṆA DHĀRAṆĀ MEDITATION

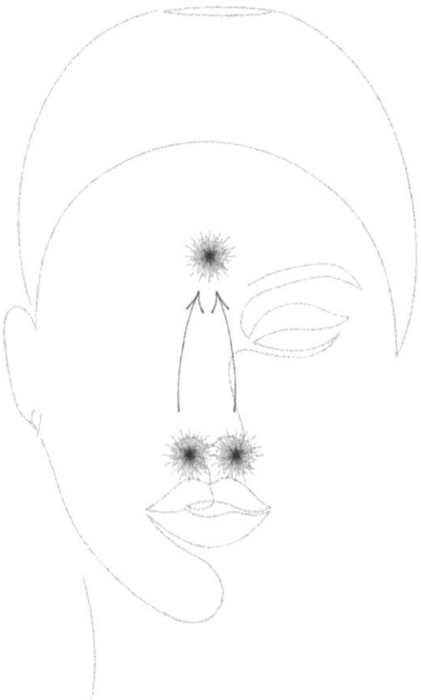

prāṇa dhāraṇā

FIGURE 5.1

1. Sit with the spine comfortably straight, either on a cushion or in a chair. Progressively lengthen and deepen your breath (ujjāyī prāṇāyāma). Spend the first several minutes checking in by deepening and lengthening your breath in a rhythm that is without tension or strain. On the inhale, follow the physical shape change of your breath in expanding the chest and ribcage, as well as down to the spine's base, relaxing the abdomen almost completely. On the exhale, contract the abdominal musculature; sense the exhale move up the spine from the bottom to the top and out as the lungs empty slowly. Maintain for about five minutes. Reflect on yourself, your day, what's going on for you currently—without getting lost in the story.
2. Relax your breathing completely. Be effortless.
3. Place attention just below the right and left nostril. Feel the breath moving in and up on inhale and down and out on exhale. Be effortless; just watch the breath and its sensations. Inhale is distinct from exhale; exhale unique from inhale.
4. Recognize that the feeling of the breath is the feeling of presence and

that presence is universal. You may sense the flow of the breath as a sensation—a river or channel of light, or even both.

5. Watch the sensation of the inhale rise from the nostrils up to the top of the inner nose. Note an expansion of sensation there. Spend some time here. Remind yourself to be effortless.

6. Allow the inhale to move up to the space between the eyebrows. Awareness expands between the eyebrows. Spend some time here. Remind yourself to be effortless.

7. Once awareness is concentrated between the eyebrows, now let it move back into the mid-brain. Inhale from the tip of the nose to the mid-brain; exhale from the mid-brain to the tip of the nose. Spend some time here. The more effortless you are, the more this presence will become magnified and the mind will rest in its effulgence.

8. Now relax your attention at the tip of the nose. Feel it completely contained inside the brain—like the presence expands from the center of the mid-brain on inhale and is absorbed from the periphery to the infinite center on exhale.

9. Rest in this space for some time. You can continue on to a mantra practice, or direct the presence you just cultivated to an area of the body like the navel or the heart for a specific healing effect.

The Energetic Condition

This is where all the information we have gathered comes together in one cohesive method for sequencing yoga therapy. In yoga and yoga therapy, the art of sequencing is vinyāsa krama. Vinyāsa means to place in a special way, and krama signifies steps. Vinyāsa krama are the intentional steps to move a person from where they are to somewhere better. That focus can be a pose, a physiological state, or preparation for a specific meditation. In yoga therapy, we use these principles to address a specific condition. The basic premise for all practice is to look at the subtle energetics, like prāṇa, to determine the "flavor" of the practice.

Our energetic condition is how we see ourselves in the present moment. It determines our sense of self, how we feel about our place in the world, and our subsequent actions. Throughout the day, our energy changes. There are moments when energy is low and we feel tired and need a boost. There are times when energy is high, we bounce off the walls, and we need to calm ourselves down. Our energetic condition is always changing, and its predominance influences our thoughts, emotions, and behaviors.

On a psychological level, humans identify with their energetic state, which determines their perception of vitality, attention, and conduct throughout the day. "I feel good or bad" is a general way of identifying our current feeling state with the ego. When the energetic condition shifts, so does the mind's perception. This understanding empowers self-care practices and dis-identification with changing circumstances and conditions.

By paying attention to the ebb and flow of the current energetic state, we can carefully design a yoga therapy practice to suit our needs and goals. There are times when it is beneficial to increase and times when we need to reduce or eliminate. A morning practice should serve the needs of the day to come, and an evening practice should prepare for sleep and processing the day. By and large, the way we feel determines our perception of vitality, self-efficacy, and focus. Depending upon a person's lifestyle and constitution, they may possess proclivities towards an energetic archetype. A type-A personality could be attracted to *stimulation* because they value productivity. A type-B personality is more laissez-faire in their attitudes and perhaps drawn to calm energy because they value being relaxed.

Nothing is wrong with either, but sometimes our energetic condition accumulates in one extreme more than another and turns into a chronic imbalance, which can result in disease. When this happens, it can be a precursor for disease or aggravate existing disease pathways. A baseline example of this is the overactivation of the HPA axis from the stress response and its correlation with depression and hyperglycemia.

Being in an aroused state all day is not only impossible, but it would burn out a person's energy. Being in a calm or even sedated state, although relaxing, would not help you accomplish goals. If we want to affect our energetic condition, it is first necessary to understand the goal (short and long term) and the starting point. Often the starting point is the current state. We cannot ask a type-A person to relax unless we first *pacify* mental hyperactivity, or a type-B person to awaken unless we first purify mental dullness and physical inertia.

Ultimately, we should seek balance, and recognize our likes and dislikes, aversions, and attachments, as these proclivities can cause the duḥkha we wish so desperately to remove. Practice serves the energetic needs throughout our day and over the extent of our lives. If we never consider the energetic condition, we are more susceptible to imbalances and reliant upon external sources to enhance or decrease our energy.

The Bṛṁhaṇa/Laṅghana Paradigm of Energetics

All forms of yoga therapy can be classified under two general categories: **bṛṁhaṇa** and **laṅghana**. You can cultivate bṛṁhaṇa and/or laṅghana by adapting physical postures and breathing practices to suit a specific energetic orientation.

Bṛṁhaṇa is for deficiency at any level, and results in the qualities of strength and nourishment. It has a "brightening effect" and helps to increase self-confidence. Not to be mistaken for stimulation, bṛṁhaṇa is nourishing to the body and mind. You can make any āsana bṛṁhaṇa, but generally it is a backbend orientation with some lateral flexion. Standing poses and longer holds in challenging postures increase bṛṁhaṇa. Bṛṁhaṇa is encouraged through the conscious lengthening of inhalation and the pause (retention) after the inhale. Inhalation activates the sympathetic branch of the ANS, which in excess can trigger anxiety; however, bṛṁhaṇa can be a strategy to reduce anxiety when followed by laṅghana.

Laṅghana is for excess at any level. It means "light," weightlessness, in Sanskrit. Laṅghana reduces, supports elimination, slows down the heart rate, and is generally a parasympathetic orientation. Typical āsanas that create a laṅghana effect are forward bends and some twisting. Supine and restorative supportive poses with a longer, restful stay increase laṅghana's calming quality. Laṅghana is encouraged by consciously lengthening the exhalation and a short pause (suspension) after the exhale.

Paradoxically, a laṅghana practice may have an overall effect of bṛṁhaṇa. For instance, reduction eliminates toxins, calms the nervous system, and restores balance. The overall quality may be bṛṁhaṇa because it ends up tonifying and building energetic strength.

A bṛṁhaṇa practice can also have a laṅghana effect. For instance, a person who exhibits physical and mental arousal (sympathetic and rajasic) may experience relaxation after a bṛṁhaṇa practice, and the cumulative result is calming. You cannot ask a hyper-aroused person to relax, although it is what they need. Giving them bṛṁhaṇa first and then moving towards laṅghana will result in laṅghana, but you used bṛṁhaṇa to get there.

I know this is confusing, and everyone admits that it is. It is best not to hold these paradigms in strict categories. My recommendation is to practice and feel the shift yourself before you apply it to others.

All of the complete yoga therapy practices in this book are modeled after the bṛṁhaṇa/laṅghana paradigm. There are more paradigms of the energetic condition: balancing (samāna), purification/stimulation (śodhana), pacification (śamana), heat (sūrya), and cooling (candra).

Although I will reference some of these qualities in our practices, they are not the main focus of this book. I mention them to show the reader that there are infinite options. This is a science and an art.

As long as you have a reason and can back it up with a rationale, it is valid.

Bṛṁhaṇa/Laṅghana in the Disease Process

Disease is the product of energetic imbalances, and illness is the experience of it. People suffer from a disease because of the effects of underlying energetic imbalances—either deficiency or excess. When I say energetics, I am talking about our neuroendocrine responses and psychological state. You can reference any model you like—from the ANS/HPA axis, to the guṇa-s, to the doṣa-s—that makes sense to you.

A depressed state, for instance, is a hypo condition. An anxious state is a hyper condition. By understanding the qualitative forces behind them, we can use prāṇa to move energy intentionally, attenuating the causes of suffering and restoring balance.

By consciously altering our energetic state with the methods of yoga and yoga therapy, we can also change the way we feel on both a short- and long-term basis. Every practice has an immediate energetic effect as well as a post-digestive one that lasts throughout the day. A consistent daily practice has a longer-term, cumulative benefit, promoting homeostasis on both a physiological and psychological level and increased resilience. A short-term gain may have a completely different effect than a long-term one. For example, a practice for anxiety may be calming and soothing initially, but its long-term cumulative result is nourishing and strengthening.

The result is especially impressive when we consider yoga therapy's role in diabetes management. It is challenging to discern what many people with diabetes are feeling: are they tired, or is it a product of blood sugar changes? Are they hungry or is it hypoglycemia? BG alters the energetic condition in a way that is different from anything else. The cumulative effect of BG swings and daily diabetes management requirements (stress) creates energetic deficits. For example, hyperglycemia is excessive glucose in the bloodstream, and creates a sluggish effect in the body (increasing insulin resistance) and mental inertia. Hypoglycemia (low BG) is a sympathetic fight-or-flight state exhibited by a deficiency of glucose in cells and the brain. Depending upon its severity, hypos deplete the nervous system's important stress responses, and the post-hypoglycemia effect feels draining.

This is why it is helpful for both therapists and individuals with diabetes to meditate on what type of energetic effect is created by their diabetes challenges. Hyper and hypoglycemia have distinct qualities both in the short and long term, and everyone is different. The experience of a persistent hyperglycemia is similar physiologically to the after-effect of a severe hypoglycemia episode.

We can apply these strategies for immediate situational triage and long-term sustainability. Throughout each chapter, we will dive deeper into the physiology and psychology of the leading diabetes challenges as they relate to T1D and T2D, and allow you to inform your practice.

Let's say you are working with a person with T2D, insulin resistance, and obesity. If they can manage it, I would recommend an active āsana practice with a focus on lengthening exhale. Why? Exercise will support the uptake of glucose from the bloodstream, and the exhale will help to reduce the underlying cause of insulin resistance and obesity, which is chronic activation of sympathetic activation. We want to activate sympathetically to spark the uptake of insulin and also eliminate through the lengthening of exhalation. What are we removing? The very mechanisms that cause insulin resistance in the first place.

Let's say you are working with a person who recently experienced a severe hypoglycemia episode. After the blood sugar has normalized, there is still a residual effect from the low. Since lows are a fight-or-flight response of the sympathetic branch, the result is depleting, and they need nourishment. But because the person's starting point is such a vulnerable state, you cannot ask them to build their strength before they first calm their system. What looks like a laṅghana practice has an overall bṛṁhaṇa effect in the long term.

I offer these strategies as a template for you to understand the mechanics behind our yoga therapy practices. By considering the energetic condition, the starting point, and the result—the short- and long-term goals—you can create simple practices with transformative outcomes.

Examples of Breathing for Bṛṁhaṇa and Laṅghana

Bṛṁhaṇa

- Ratios that will increase inhale and inhale retention: inhale is never longer than exhale; 1:1, or 1:2 with a longer inhale retention such as 1:1:2:0 or 1:2:2:0.
- Anuloma krama.
- Viloma ujjāyī.
- Sūrya bhedana (inhale right, exhale left).
- Chest inhale, belly exhale, hold the belly in as you begin the inhale to encourage the chest inhale.

Laṅghana

- Ratios increasing exhale, and exhale suspension: such as 1:0:2:0 or 1:0:2:1.
- Viloma krama (two- or three-step exhale).
- Anuloma ujjāyī (alternate nostril exhale, ujjāyī inhale).
- Candra bhedana (inhale left, exhale right).
- Chanting on exhale.
- Belly inhale, belly exhale.

CHAPTER 6

Āyurveda and Diabetes

Āyurveda does not live in books; it lives in the world.[1] It is a science of relating to the manifested universe, a part of nature inside of you, and in everything. It is a way for us to understand how nature forms and develops into individual personalities, constitutions, and even diseases. It shows us, through its complex and yet incredibly simple view, how the immutable laws of nature can be manipulated to create harmony in every aspect of our lives; this is the science of immortality. Essentially, Āyurveda is a life science—the science of health and wellbeing, a way of living, and a way of understanding the world, health, and nature. *Āyur* translates as life and *veda* as science, and she is the sister science to yoga. It is one of the oldest living health sciences, whose origins can be traced back at least 5000 years.[2]

To become mastered in Āyurveda requires a lifetime of practice and study, but every yoga therapist should have a firm understanding of Āyurveda, just as Ayurvedic specialists benefit from possessing experiential knowledge of yoga therapy. There is a tendency to be better versed in one than the other, which can cause confusion and misinformation. But you cannot really have yoga therapy without Āyurveda and Āyurveda without yoga therapy. They are meant to co-exist and to support the other in view and practice. Āyurveda empowers diabetics by teaching how to have a vested interest and joy in self-care.

One of the biggest challenges that people with diabetes face is upholding self-care and disease-management practices. The problem is the lack of proper methods and enthusiasm for doing the work. It is not the fault of the person: if diabetes were as simple as eating right, exercising, and administering insulin, there would be no need for this book, nor would so many people be struggling

1 Clarke, J. (2020) Personal communication. March 16.

2 National Ayurvedic Medical Association (n.d.) *History of Ayurveda*. Accessed on 06/07/20 at: www.ayurvedanama.org/history-of-ayurveda.

every day. The challenges that people with diabetes face are represented not only in the illness pathology and symptomatology, but also in the attitudes that they hold about taking care of themselves. Management is seen as a burden and many cannot uphold the recommendations of doctors. Not only that, but the self-imposed judgment when a person fails to uphold the metrics for a "good" diabetic is just as damaging as high or low BG.

Just as Āyurveda views the body to be a microcosm of the universal macrocosm, we can use diabetes to be a more subtle example of that microcosm. The practice and wisdom inform health on a broader level, empowering the individual to understand what throws them out of balance, makes them feel unwell, and makes them feel better. By understanding diabetes as a disease and how that disease manifests in the individual in body, mind, and spirit, we can learn so much about life. Now that might be hard to absorb in the midst of diabetes turmoil, but this is the consistent message that Āyurveda and yoga aim to inspire on an individual level.

Both Āyurveda and yoga therapy address the individual. T1D looks different in me than it does in another person. There are many profiles of T2D; nothing can be brought down to a stereotype. I have dedicated an entire chapter to Āyurveda because it informs so much of what otherwise is rather inexplicable in the laws of nature. It brings the formless to life and helps all of us in this technology-saturated reality to take a step back into the wisdom of nature.

If you have done any reading on Āyurveda, you'll have seen that it is a vast and intricate system. In this chapter I hope to simplify, but not diminish, Ayurveda's perspective on diabetes to provide a practical approach to support our work with diabetes. As such, please remember that although Āyurveda is a science of health, it holds a unique perspective on health, which is not the same as that of Western medicine. If you try to correlate everything that Āyurveda says with a Western viewpoint you will become increasingly frustrated and may even throw away its gifts, as they could seem impractical. But let me also remind you that Āyurveda is one of the oldest health systems in use today. Āyurveda was one of the first systems to recognize what we know of as diabetes and recognize a distinction between T1D and T2D. Just like yoga, Āyurveda was transmitted orally before it was ever written down. The dates are shaky but the first classical texts go back as far as 1000 BC.

I invite you to see Ayurveda as a complementary science to yoga and modern medicine's recommendation for diabetes care. Its wisdom is ancient and, like anything very old, it holds abiding truths about life, health, and the cause of disease processes. Āyurveda is not the answer, but it is part of the equation. The goal of Āyurveda is to remove the contributing factors for disease, create balance on both physical and psychological levels, and increase longevity by empowering the person to take care of themselves. When disease cannot be removed, in the case of T1D and long-duration T2D, the goal is to reduce suffering by working with systemic imbalances that aggravate existing disease. Many of these "factors" are related to our behavior and lifestyle proclivities.

The missing link in diabetes management is transforming behavior and attitudes about self-management from being a chore to a curious exploration of one's own potential when harmony is created inside the body and mind. The root of all suffering is improper perception. Yoga therapy informed by Āyurveda helps support the progressive purification of the mind, awakening the individual's innate intelligence and vested interest in their own health and wellbeing. Before we dive much deeper into Āyurveda for diabetes, it is important to review Āyurveda to provide a context and palette to work from.

Our Constitution

Āyurveda, just like yoga, is informed by Sāṁkhya philosophy. According to Sāṁkhya, the cause of all of the manifested universe is *prakṛti*.[3] Beginning and endless, prakṛti is the primordial cause of all creation and destruction. All gross physical matter when refined down to the smallest atom is still a refinement of prakṛti's effect. Prakṛti is not consciousness (puruṣa); it is primordial (unmanifested) potential. Yoga and Āyurveda fine-tune the effect of prakṛti to align it with the perfect reflection of consciousness. On one level this is health; on another level it is transcendence. Prakṛti possesses the three guṇa-s—sattva, rajas, and tamas—which are the inherent nature of prakṛti. Another translation for the guṇa-s is ropes; like ropes, the guṇa-s are braided together and their union is prakṛti. The only way we can understand prakṛti is through the combination of all three guṇa-s.

Sāṁkhya says that the guṇa-s are the cause from which the entire universe is created.[4] The unique combination of the guṇa-s creates all physical matter in the form of the five elements (mahābhūta-s) of earth, water, fire, air, and ether.

3 Tigunait, P. R. (1983) *Seven Systems of Indian Philosophy*. Honesdale, PA: Himalayan International Institute of Yoga Science and Philosophy of the USA. p.125.

4 Tigunait, P. R. (1983) *Seven Systems of Indian Philosophy*. Honesdale, PA: Himalayan International Institute of Yoga Science and Philosophy of the USA. p.126.

The specific combination of the five elements form the living force of the doṣa-s, which create individual personality and constitution.

The Defects

The doṣa-s represent the physiological, biological, and psychological processes that govern all creation and destruction within the body. They are the systems of *vāta*, *pitta*, and *kapha*, catabolism, metabolism, and anabolism activities, respectively.[5] The term doṣa means "defect" or "that which causes things to decay." Once their nature is disturbed, our systems are thrown off balance.[6] Popular belief is that the doṣa-s represent a physical constitution; this is true but the knowledge of the doṣa-s extends well beyond a type. Understanding our doshic constitution is a way to understand what is balance and imbalance, what is disease and health, and how to avoid falling into poor health and disease.[7] One of Ayurveda's most beautiful parts, and why yoga therapists should learn from its wisdom, is that it acts as a model to help identify and understand a person's proclivities, personality, and imbalances. However unique an individual is, they will still fall into classifiable and anticipatory patterns that mirror nature's forces represented by the doṣa-s.[8]

Essentially, when looking at the doṣa-s to inform health, Ayurveda's goal is to align the doṣa-s with the birth constitution, deter the disease process, and maximize longevity. Many readers will have taken a doṣa quiz to determine whether they are vāta, pitta, and/or kapha predominant. But these quizzes rarely address the fact that there are two doshic constitutions: *vikruti* (current state) and *prakruti* (birth constitution). What we think we "are" might not necessarily be what we *need* or vice versa. When in doubt, it is best to treat what is out of balance.

It is incorrect to assume that if a person is obese, they have a kapha imbalance; in fact, many obese people actually have a vāta imbalance. But seeing the doṣa-s as symptoms provides us with an extra layer of subtle nuance in constructing a self-care practice. An individual with T2D who wants to

---

5 Tigunait, P. R. (2014) *The Secret of the Yoga Sutra: Samadhi Pada*. Honesdale, PA: Himalayan Institute. p.146.

6 Tigunait, P. R. (2014) *The Secret of the Yoga Sutra: Samadhi Pada*. Honesdale, PA: Himalayan Institute. p.331.

7 Frawley, D. (1997) *Ayurveda and the Mind: The Healing of Consciousness*. First edition. Twin Lakes, WI: Lotus Press. p.12.

8 Frawley, D. (1997) *Ayurveda and the Mind: The Healing of Consciousness*. First edition. Twin Lakes, WI: Lotus Press. p.12.

lose weight but is vāta vitiated would not fare well with vigorous exercise; it would aggravate their system. Slower, gentle practices will be more beneficial for this person.[9]

Remember, the doṣa-s are the defects—what goes out of balance and causes decay. Therefore it is in the interest of the observer to reflect on their own imbalances to help achieve harmony. Classical wisdom informs that there are many levels of doshic influence—including the environment (seasons), time of day, stage of life, and types of food. By understanding how the doṣa-s are at play in every area of life, and how they influence our inner state, we acquire a greater understanding of ourselves, mother nature, and the laws of cause and effect. The interesting thing is that the doṣa-s are easy to impact through diet, lifestyle modifications, and practice. The annoying thing is that you have to follow through for the changes to work. The frustrating thing for many people of our modern era is that they want automatic results. Āyurveda and yoga are about adjusting your lifestyle to promote circumstances that create harmony and prevent disease.

The Disease Process

The current state is never set in stone and is always in flux. However, a lifetime of ingrained habitual patterns and environmental stressors will heighten specific imbalances, dampen the digestive fire, and accumulate toxins, and, according to Āyurveda, this is where disease sets in. All disease is viewed as an imbalance of the doṣa-s, which often originates within our digestion.

To understand diabetes within Āyurveda, we must also look at Ayurveda's perspective on health and disease. Disease is disorder and health is harmony. Health in Āyurveda is described as balance or equilibrium between the digestive fire (agni), the seven tissues (dhātu-s), the bodily humors (vāta-pitta-kapha), the three waste products (urine, feces, and sweat), and the senses, body, mind, and spirit working together in harmony.[10] Disease is the disorder of any one or many of these factors. When in harmony, the body is set up to fulfill its purpose. When out of harmony, vitality is disrupted and disease manifests.

9 Yang, K. and Rioux, J. (2015) "Yoga Therapy for Metabolic Syndrome and Weight Control." In S. B. S. Khalsa, L. Cohen, T. McCall and S. Telles (eds) *The Principles and Practice of Yoga in Healthcare.* Pencaitland: Handspring Publishing. p.273.

10 Lad, V. (2002) *Ayurveda: The Science of Self-Healing. A Practical Guide.* Delhi: Motilal Banarsidass. p.37.

The use of the doshic model to understand the complexities of the body and the mind is an indispensable tool for yoga therapists and for people with diabetes who want to understand their own imbalances. Next, we will go through all of the doṣa-s or "defects" to illumine their qualities, function, and imbalances, and how all of this relates to diabetes.

Vāta Doṣa

Vāta is the maha (great) doṣa, which regulates the other two doṣa-s and all physical processes.[11] Vāta governs the biological activity of catabolism, that which breaks down cells and reduces. It comprises the elemental forces of air contained in ether. In the body, vāta resides in the empty spaces and subtle channels. Its qualities are dry, cold, light, and aggravated. Its nature is movement.

Vāta is linked with rajo-guṇa and the vital essence of prāṇa. Vāta is formed by the five prāṇas of pran, udana, vyana, samāna, and apana. Its primary site is the colon, and it governs the breath, lungs, circulation, and sensation.[12] Vāta doṣa regulates catabolic processes, the breakdown of cells to release energy and remove waste.[13] When in balance, vāta is the source of creativity and inspiration. When out of balance, vāta creates chaos exhibited by mental and physical instability. Vāta types are generally very sensitive to the external stimuli and quick to get upset or have their feelings hurt. They are equally as quick to let go of anger.

Vāta Vitiation

Given vāta's mobile nature, it is the easiest doṣa to influence and also the most susceptible to vitiation (excessive imbalance). While vāta people are more likely to be vāta vitiated, anyone can experience it. In fact, it is so commonplace because of modern-life stress and overstimulation that whenever I teach a general class or a beginner student I am always addressing vāta imbalances. Vāta imbalances are prone to constipation, gas, and bloating. Vāta vitiation

11 Frawley, D. (2000) *Ayurvedic Healing: A Comprehensive Guide*. Second rev. and enl. edition. Twin Lakes, WI: Lotus Press. p.11.

12 Frawley, D. (2000) *Ayurvedic Healing: A Comprehensive Guide*. Second rev. and enl. edition. Twin Lakes, WI: Lotus Press. p.12.

13 Lad, U. and Lad, V. (2007) *Ayurvedic Cooking for Self-Healing*. Delhi: Motilal Banarsidass.

is reflected in the skin (dry), nails (brittle), and digestion (gas, bloating, and constipation).

That being said, it is interesting how many vāta types are attracted to vāta-vitiating qualities, such as raw food, drying food, and drying climates (has anyone ever tried driving in Santa Fe, NM?).

When vāta is excessive, prāṇa and the mind lose connection with the body, resulting in decay of the bodily tissues and physical coordination.[14] The movement of the mind towards an outward plane is exhibited in the body, represented by a lack of physical stability and stamina in postures. High vāta types may find it challenging to remain still, exhibit involuntary movement in their fingers and eyes, and sometimes seem as if their body vibrates. They may live with their "head in the clouds," closer to the causal plane. Emotionally, excessive vāta elicits fear, nervousness, and anxiety. Vāta-type anger arises just as quickly as it dissipates. Over time, too much vāta depletes vitality and increases vulnerability on both a physical (disease) and mental (oversensitivity) level. When in balance, vāta is the source of higher creativity and inspiration, but when out of balance, ideas lack action and continuity to bring their concepts into fruition. There is too much air and not enough fire.

Pathogenesis of Vāta Disease

As vāta is the primary doṣa, it rules over the other two and is broadly responsible for all the physical processes in the body. Vāta is viewed as being a major factor in the disease process.[15] *Vāta diseases are associated with the nervous system, arthritis, and hyperactivity. As vāta regulates all catabolic (breaking down) activity, vāta disorders are associated with dryness and cold, as well as the wasting of the bodily tissues.*[16] Āyurveda holds that all vāta diseases start in the small intestine.

If we look at the qualities of vāta, we can understand its function in relationship to the body. Related to prāṇa, vāta is the mover. Its action is to push. It pushes accumulated āma (toxins) from the gastrointestinal (GI) tract into cellular membranes. This coating of toxins around the cell membrane challenges

14 Frawley, D. (2000) *Ayurvedic Healing: A Comprehensive Guide*. Second rev. and enl. edition. Twin Lakes, WI: Lotus Press. p.12.

15 McCall, T., Satish, L. and Tiwari, S. (2016) "History, Philosophy, and Practice of Yoga Therapy." In S. B. S. Khalsa, L. Cohen, T. McCall and S. Telles (eds) *The Principles and Practice of Yoga in Healthcare*. Pencaitland: Handspring Publishing. p.43.

16 Frawley, D. (2000) *Ayurvedic Healing: A Comprehensive Guide*. Second rev. and enl. edition. Twin Lakes, WI: Lotus Press. p.43.

the uptake of nutrition into the cells. Cellular receptor sites are covered with metabolic toxic debris, creating depleted tissues due to lack of nutrition.

Vāta in Diabetes

All types of diabetes can develop a vāta vitiation, but it is most commonly connected to the autoimmune varieties of diabetes. Just as the human constitution falls into general patterns, these patterns also show up in the cause (etiology), development (pathogenesis), and result (pathophysiology) of diabetes. High vāta causes decay, emaciation, and hyperactivity at the expense of the vital fluids and the physical body begins to waste away.[17] This sounds eerily like the pathogenesis for type 1 and LADA.

Vāta is classically associated with the profile of what Āyurveda calls inherited diabetes, not caused by behavioral factors. We'll learn more about this later on in this chapter, but just know that vāta is most associated with the development of T1D and is the main aggravator of existing T1D. T1D is by its nature vāta aggravating. Represented by volatile BG extremes, relentless self-management requirements, sensory overstimulation from diabetes devices, and the psychological burden of living with chronic illness, many people with T1D suffer from vāta imbalances even if their constitution is not vāta.

Hypoglycemia is a perfect example of this: symptoms of aggravated vāta in disease are dizziness, disorientation, incoherent speech, and confusion. The same symptoms are represented by hypoglycemia.

People with T2D are also prone to vāta vitiation. A vāta-vitiated T2D profile could be represented by high levels of stress and anxiety.

Treatment

It is important for vāta types and those with vāta imbalances to work on containing, calming, and internalizing their prāṇa (attention). Vāta imbalances are treated by moving vāta towards kapha (grounding) and principally building the vital essence of *ojas*. Practices that are too vigorous and externalizing, with a lot of dynamic and strenuous movement, can aggravate vāta. Elements of a practice could focus on forward bends, jālandhara-bandha-like movements to help the mind settle in from the eyes into the body, and longer sustained holds in poses to promote physical and mental stability. The senses are part

17 Frawley, D. (2000) *Ayurvedic Healing: A Comprehensive Guide*. Second rev. and enl. edition. Twin Lakes, WI: Lotus Press. p.12.

of vāta's domain. By practicing sense withdrawal (pratyāhāra), internalizing the organs of perception, one is able to contain prāṇa and direct it inwardly. Prāṇāyāma is beneficial for all types, but excessive prāṇāyāma can also aggravate vāta.

F.K. was recently diagnosed with LADA, latent autoimmune diabetes in adults. She is in her early 50s and very active. For many years her LADA went by unnoticed, because of her athleticism. When she is not taking part in a sport, she is very busy with a full-time job that requires a lot of travel and her family—a husband, two kids, and a few dogs. She came to me complaining of weight gain and stress. Her digestion is variable and physically her constitution is pitta/kapha. As diabetes is relatively new to her, she is still struggling to figure out management and is having trouble sleeping because of the continuous alarms set by her CGM.

In the physical portion of the practice, although she is very muscular, F.K. lacked the mental stability to hold a pose and not freak out. When the sensation became too challenging, she would explode with anger (vāta pushing pitta). Together, we developed a daily routine so she could practice calming her vāta imbalance and, secondarily, stretch her hypertonic muscles. It was a challenge to get F.K. to prioritize her yoga therapy practice because of the deep *saṁskāra* to move vigorously. I asked if she would at least give it a month to see if there was a measurable difference.

I also recommended that she make a few behavioral adjustments:

1. Take two days off from exercise and limit her activity to walking the dogs instead of running up the mountain.
2. Eat one meal a day in silence with no distractions.
3. Prepare for bed an hour before by turning off electronics.
4. Put a night setting on her CGM to reduce the alarms (only allowing the necessary ones).

I run into F.K. several months later. She reports that although she has not upheld her daily practice, she has learned the benefit of not pushing her body so hard and is seeing a benefit from it. She has replaced the daily uphill burn with stretching and less intense exercise on two days of the week. Her weight has gone down some, but she feels lighter in her body and in her mind.

Pitta Doṣa

Pitta doṣa regulates all light and warmth in the body. It is the subtle fire that governs our metabolism, digestion, heat, and visual perception. Pitta manages our hunger, thirst, complexion, courage, and intelligence. Comprised of the element of fire, pitta doṣa exists in the body as water or "oil." Its qualities are oily, sharp, hot, light, and moist. On a spiritual level, pitta is the divine fire of transformation, that which yearns for the understanding of higher understanding and dharma.

In the body, pitta exists predominantly in the small intestine and coordinates with the liver, gallbladder, glands, lymph, and the organ of vision (eyes). Pitta doṣa is closely related to the overarching theme of agni, the subtle digestive fire that metabolizes the food that we eat and assimilates experience. Strong agni is a signifying factor for vigor and good health; low agni is a precursor to disease.

Pitta Vitiation

High pitta accumulates and results in excessive heat, inflammation, acid reflux, fever, and infections. We begin to burn ourselves up.[18] The word bile is another way of translating pitta doṣa.[19] When you look up bile in the dictionary there are two definitions: one relates to a bitter greenish brown liquid that aids in digestion and the other relates to the emotional qualities of anger, irritability, and vitriol.[20] Both descriptions uniquely describe aggravated pitta. As fire cannot exist in the body as fire, it exists as acid. The acidity of pitta is the bile that digests things from fat, eliminating worn-out blood cells and toxins from the body.[21] Emotional bile is angry, self-righteous, and sharp.

Pitta of the Mind

Pitta types are bright and vibrant, with a sharp intellect, purpose, and enthusiasm for doing things. Pitta types emulate the quality of tejas, the subtle essence of light. Pitta is the typical type A, doer personality. They are inspired by goals and tasks. Give the pitta the vāta's ideas and then it will actually get done!

---

18 Frawley, D. (2000) *Ayurvedic Healing: A Comprehensive Guide*. Second rev. and enl. edition. Twin Lakes, WI: Lotus Press. p.12.

19 Frawley, D. (2000) *Ayurvedic Healing: A Comprehensive Guide*. Second rev. and enl. edition. Twin Lakes, WI: Lotus Press. p.9.

20 Merriam Webster (2020) *Bile*. Accessed on 01/07/20 at: www.merriam-webster.com/dictionary/bile.

21 Mayo Clinic (2018) *Bile Reflux*. Accessed on 01/07/20 at: www.mayoclinic.org/diseases-conditions/bile-reflux/symptoms-causes/syc-20370115.

Pitta types have a tendency to be exceedingly self-righteous (it takes one to know one!). When they are angry, they know they are right, and there is very little you can say or do to change their minds. It is helpful when working with a pitta type to diffuse their intensity with space. Think vāta to meet pitta. Not too much vāta, otherwise you will push a pitta to explode. Excessive pitta over time burns up all vigor and strength, accelerating the aging process associated with vāta doṣa.

Treatment

Depending upon whether the pitta imbalance is physical, mental, or both, there are some different protocols for balancing excessive pitta doṣa. Moving pitta towards vāta is helpful, but too much vāta can make pitta explosive. Prāṇāyāma is helpful for pittas as it cools their heated nature and intensity. Giving pittas enough of a challenge so that their mind can relax will "trick" the pitta into balance. Depending upon the physical condition, it can be helpful to remember that, in general, excessive pitta is overheating, burning, and has liquidity. Food and diet should be regulated and sour and spicy flavors should be avoided. Diffuse pitta with a cooling bitter like aloe and cooling and mild spices like turmeric, cumin, coriander, and mint.

The pitta type would do well to avoid excessive heat-provoking situations, such as exercising in the heat of the sun or going to predominantly hot yoga practices. Cooling prāṇāyāmas like shitali, shitali with alternate nostril exhale, and candra bhedana are recommended.[22] Meditations focusing on the light of self-knowledge and self-reflection (vicāra) on emotions like anger and criticism can help quell the fire of pitta. Focus on creating space and the light of self-knowledge established in Īśvara.

Pitta in Diabetes

Pitta can be a causal factor for all types of diabetes, including T1D, although it is less common than vāta and kapha. According to Āyurveda, the liquidity of pitta originating in the large intestine lodges itself in the liver and the pancreas. It messes with the specific agni of the pancreas, burning out its function.[23] Pitta vitiation is exhibited in many effects of long-duration hyperglycemia like

22 Frawley, D. (2000) *Ayurvedic Healing: A Comprehensive Guide*. Second rev. and enl. edition. Twin Lakes, WI: Lotus Press. p.74.

23 Frawley, D. (2000) *Ayurvedic Healing: A Comprehensive Guide*. Second rev. and enl. edition. Twin Lakes, WI: Lotus Press. p.236.

hunger and thirst, burning sensations in the limbs (neuropathy), inflammation, and infections.

Kapha Doṣa

Kapha doṣa is like the mother who holds the whole family together. Comprising the elemental forces of water contained within earth, she is that which binds and supports the other two doṣa-s, upholding physical matter and bodily tissues. Kapha translates in Sanskrit as phlegm. Not the most lovely picture in your mind, but if you consider the quality of phlegm, as a thick and viscous substance, it helps to understand kapha's nature. Kapha governs the biological activity of anabolism, that which takes cells and builds them into larger cells.

The body consists predominantly of water. This water is contained within the confines of the skin and mucous membranes. Its qualities are cold, moist, heavy, dull, sticky, and firm. To the uninformed, kapha seems like an undesirable trait. However, kapha types have the most love, stability, and vigor of all the constitutions. Kapha provides physical and psychological stability, strength, patience, and love. A kapha type has the resilience to withstand long journeys and is rarely depleted like vāta or overheated like pitta. Kapha is associated with the vital essence of ojas, resistance against the excessive appearance of vāta and pitta doṣa-s.

Kapha Vitiation

High kapha increases its innate qualities as the building, stabilizing, protective force. It creates lethargy, resistance, laziness, and melancholy. There is an inherent heaviness that dampens all internal drive and the digestive fire of agni. Overtly kaphic individuals tend to hold on to weight and gain weight even with lack of appetite. They may exhibit hypoactivity, difficulty breathing, and depression.

Kapha of the Mind

The sweetness of kapha types is represented by their natural disposition towards love, patience, and compassion. They can be slower to learn but retain the knowledge forever. Negative aspects of kapha are greed, possessiveness,[24]

24 Frawley, D. (2006) *Ayurveda and the Mind: The Healing of Consciousness*. Delhi: Motilal Banarsidass. p.21.

and an inability to forgive. Kapha is associated with the mental guṇa of tamas. Tamas, inertia, blankets the light of perception, dulling the senses from awareness and putting the person to sleep in their life. When angry, a kapha type will hold on to their anger, internalize it, and never let it go. Their energy and emotion can be stagnant and repressed. They have poor self-care habits and are challenged to make changes.

Pathogenesis of Kapha as Disease

The main seat of kapha is in the stomach but it also resides in the lungs and throat. Kapha disease is characterized by phlegm, loss of appetite, heaviness, and excessive sleeping. The outcome is obesity and depression, and it also is linked with prediabetes and T2D.

Kapha in Diabetes

T2D is most strongly associated with a kapha disorder that is aggravated by excessive consumption of sweet kaphogenic foods, sedentary lifestyle, and excessive sleep. As kapha governs anabolism, the building of cells, high kapha accumulates weight and gravity in the body, causing hypoactivity and excessive tissue accumulation.[25] There is a clear correlation between both hyperinsulimia (excessive production of insulin) and insulin resistance (weakened insulin potency entering the cells), and obesity. Medical treatment for T2D is a kapha-reducing regimen: abstaining from heavy, sugary food to promote balance in the stomach. Exercise helps to reduce kapha doṣa and balance its stable, stagnant, and heavy nature.

When aggravated, kapha produces effects similar to *hyperglycemia*: nausea, lethargy, sluggish digestion, and heaviness.

Treatment

Given the nature of kapha, which is heavy, dull, moist, and stable, kapha types need to get things moving. The amazing thing about kapha is its longevity and resilience. In order to harness this potential, kapha types need to move their bodies regularly and they fare well with vigorous exercise. An overtly obese

25 Frawley, D. (2000) *Ayurvedic Healing: A Comprehensive Guide*. Second rev. and enl. edition. Twin Lakes, WI: Lotus Press. p.12.

individual (from kapha) would need to work progressively towards stronger movements and not harm their bones and joints.[26]

A strong, heating practice is best for a kapha type. Āsanas that focus on larger-class muscles that require more energy and oxygen are useful. Solar practices like Sūrya Namaskār-s (should they be suited to the person), inversions, and a focus on inhale with inhale retention are advised. Postures that open the chest, expand the lungs, and exercise the heart are useful. Prāṇāyāmas like sūrya bhedana, kapālabhātī, bhastrikā, and other stimulating and activating breathing practices are recommended.

Given kapha's emotional grip, incorporating active renunciation (tyaga) is a beautiful way of cultivating non-attachment and non-possessiveness. Try giving up something simple for one month. You can start small with something easy, like a type of food you like but are not attached to. See that you can live without it. Then try it with something that you have more attachment to, like chocolate or coffee (these are my vices!).

Generally, kapha types should avoid heavy, cold, and oily food. They do best when their food is light, warm, and dry. Warming spices should be applied to all food to spark their digestive fire. Kapha types should not eat frequently and should eat their largest meal during the middle of the day when digestion is the strongest.[27] Walking after eating will be helpful to reduce lethargy and promote strong digestion.

Table 6.1 Balancing doṣa vitiation

Balance K→P
Balance P→V
Balance V→K

K: Kapha
P: Pitta
V: Vāta

26 Please note, not all obesity is caused by kapha. Yang, K. and Rioux, J. (2015) "Yoga Therapy for Metabolic Syndrome and Weight Control." In S. B. S. Khalsa, L. Cohen, T. McCall and S. Telles (eds) *The Principles and Practice of Yoga in Healthcare*. Pencaitland: Handspring Publishing. p.273.

27 Frawley, D. (2000) *Ayurvedic Healing: A Comprehensive Guide*. Second rev. and enl. edition. Twin Lakes, WI: Lotus Press. p.95.

Longevity

From the moment we are born, we are aging. Aging is the breaking down of tissues and organs at a cellular level, causing deterioration and degeneration of the cells we need for rejuvenation and vitality. In Āyurveda, aging and disease are viewed in a similar fashion. It is the drying up of the prime vigor. To reduce the aging process, and in effect the disease process, Ayurvedic practices and lifestyle considerations are aimed at promoting longevity. According to Āyurveda, longevity is created through proper diet, exercise, and behaviors. Disease susceptibility is related to longevity. Initial imbalances may be miniscule, so subtle and imperceptible that they will go unnoticed until disease has set in. On a biological level, longevity is what counteracts the breakdown of cells, even the telomeres on the ends of our DNA, which hold our genetic makeup together to ward off the development of disease processes. To fight this breakdown it is essential to create protective mechanisms from our diet, lifestyle, relationship to nature's rhythm, and yoga sadhana.

To understand this concept of longevity, let's take the example of a brand-new baby in the kapha stage of life. She has rolls of fat, a lustrous glimmer in her eyes, and her laughter is pure joy. She represents the essential energy of ojas, the prime vigor. Compare her image with an elderly person. Their body is breaking down and losing muscle tone, their strength is weakening off, and they have arthritis of the bones. This is represented by a lack of ojas.

Āyurveda as the practice of kaya kalpa, the science of immortality, helps a person retain, maintain, and build that vital essence represented in the archetype of the baby. The more ojas we have, the greater the protection we also have against the effects of aging and disease; in fact, in Āyurveda aging and disease are synonymous.[28]

Vulnerability is the opposite of longevity. It is the cause of doshic imbalances and is created from improper diet, mental attributes, and behavior. By looking at the doṣa-s, and the more subtle qualities of them, we can begin to rewire the aging process and reduce our susceptibility towards disease. In the case of diabetes, an already existing condition, these processes support maintenance and health.

To achieve this, we have to look at the subtle essences, primarily ojas, the vital energy. The doṣa-s are influenced on a deeper level by the subtle essences

28 Devi, D., Srivastava, R. and Dwivedi, B. K. (2010) "A critical review of concept of aging in Ayurveda." *Ayu 31*, 4, 516–519.

of prāṇa, tejas, and ojas. The subtle essences are the master forms of the doṣa-s and they are key in achieving and maintaining health and higher evolutionary potential (should that be a goal).[29]

The subtle essence of prāṇa is associated with vāta doṣa, tejas with pitta doṣa, and ojas with kapha doṣa.

Prāṇa, associated with the life prāṇa (yes there are so many!), governs all life function. Tejas is linked with pitta doṣa and governs our digestion and nutrition. Tejas is the essence of the subtle fire, governing metabolism and agni. When tejas is deranged, it burns up ojas, compromising immunity and aggravating prāṇa. Ojas is the essence of kapha, the seven tissues (dhātu-s), and is the vital energy that presides over all bodily function with the support of prāṇa.[30] Ojas, in the Ayurvedic model of health, maintains our immunity.[31]

Longevity in Āyurveda is best conceived through the vital essence of ojas. Ojas is the quality of protection. Although ojas contains all of the elemental forces,[32] it is most associated with kapha doṣa and the elements of earth and water. With prāṇa's help, ojas regulates hormones and all life function. It governs the autoimmune system (lymphatic), reproductive fluid, and mental intelligence.[33] Ojas protects the body against the breakdown of age, and builds resilience against unforeseen risk and the toll that all catabolic processes have on the longevity of the system. It is the moisture that locks prāṇa (life-force) into the body, rather than letting it escape and continue to "dry up" the system.

Ojas, being the most positive essence of kapha, holds the body together and ensures that prāṇa is not wasted. Ojas is the essential energy of the body and means "vigor."[34] Of all the subtle essences, ojas is the most important to maintain as low ojas is associated with vāta vitiation and the acceleration of the disease process. As kapha and ojas have a unique partnership, one may assume

29 Frawley, D. (2006) *Ayurveda and the Mind: The Healing of Consciousness*. Delhi: Motilal Banarsidass. p.25.

30 Lad, V. (2002) *Ayurveda: The Science of Self-Healing. A Practical Guide*. Delhi: Motilal Banarsidass. p.110.

31 Maharishi Ayurveda (2017) *Restoring Depleted Ojas: Miscellaneous Articles*. Accessed on 06/07/20 at: www.mapi.com/ayurvedic-knowledge/miscellaneous-ayurvedic-articles/use-ayurveda-to-restore-ojas.html.

32 Lad, V. (2002) *Ayurveda: The Science of Self-Healing. A Practical Guide*. Delhi: Motilal Banarsidass. p.110.

33 Lad, V. (2002) *Ayurveda: The Science of Self-Healing. A Practical Guide*. Delhi: Motilal Banarsidass. p.110.

34 Frawley, D. (2000) *Ayurvedic Healing: A Comprehensive Guide*. Second rev. and enl. edition. Twin Lakes, WI: Lotus Press. p.48.

that high kapha would mean high ojas, but what Āyurveda says is that kapha vitiation can disrupt ojas by displacing it,[35] meaning it is not properly stored and impairing its function at all levels. An example of this is T2D, both a kapha and displaced ojas disturbance.

Dr. Lad, who is the foremost authority on Āyurveda in America, if not the world, says that a major cause of depleted ojas is "saying no to what is."[36] Practicing surrender is a key component in both yoga (īśvara praṇidhāna) and Āyurveda. Just as trees say yes to every season, we must also accept the nature of change. By practicing dinacaryā (is a self-care routine in alignment with the cycles of nature for optimal health and wellbeing), our self-care becomes a ritual of self-love and radical enthusiasm for health. When our bodies and minds are healthy, we are suited to fulfilling life purpose and accessing a higher development of spiritual realization.

Ojas can also be depleted as it is in the case of vāta vitiation. A key strategy for vāta imbalances is building ojas and, as vāta is present in most disease processes, increasing and redirecting ojas is important for all people with diabetes. T1D is caused by and aggravated by vāta vitiation. Low ojas shows up as fear, physical weakness, fatigue, and inability to perceive clearly, and eventually results in death.

In summary, people with T2D *generally* have displaced ojas—they have a lot of it, but it is not being properly directed and utilized. By helping to redirect ojas, and in turn balance the doṣa-s, people with T2D can improve their insulin sensitivity.

People with T1D tend to have low ojas. The treatment of T1D and the disease itself increases vāta and decreases ojas. Taking time to dedicate part of self-care to the building and cultivation of ojas promotes resilience against T1D risk and helps individuals recover faster from dramatic BG fluctuations. By focusing on ojas as the protector of all metabolic processes, people with T1D will build strength and immunity, and perhaps reduce the hyper-reactive nature of their BG in response to food, as well as the mind in response to stressors.

By recognizing these simple predispositions with the Ayurvedic model, people with diabetes can understand what aggravates them (body and mind)

---

35 Lad, V. (2002) *Ayurveda: The Science of Self-Healing. A Practical Guide.* Delhi: Motilal Banarsidass. p.110.

36 Svastha Ayurveda (n.d.) *11 Ways to Increase Healthy Ojas.* Accessed on 06/07/20 at: https://svasthaayurveda.com/11-ways-to-increase-healthy-ojas.

more subtly. Science is delving into these concepts more and more. *Resilience* and *longevity* are buzzworthy topics in the diabetes field and anyone in the know recognizes their importance. Āyurveda has known all of this for 5000 years. The concept of promoting longevity is old and can be applied to all diseases and all humans. Those who recognize their own proclivities towards imbalances can set about a path of intentionally reestablishing order to maintain balance and health.

However, disease is intricate and subtle. Often, we are unaware of imbalances until disease has already set in. Then we try to do everything we can to overcome it or we take a pill and avoid the cause of the disease, essentially masking it. Ignorance is what causes us to look outwardly for the answers to our ailments rather than looking within ourselves. For example, metformin is commonly prescribed for many people with T2D to promote insulin sensitivity. But if an individual does not address why they have insulin resistance in the first place, because of improper diet and lack of exercise, the medicine may lower the blood sugar but it will not address the origin of the problem. Those who dramatically change the way they eat and the lifestyle they lead, like engaging in regular exercise and reducing stress, have even been known to reverse their T2D.

Dinacaryā is the practice of being in balance with the laws of nature. Vāta, pitta, and kapha not only govern our metabolic processes and biological humors, but also fluctuate from season, time of day, and time of life. By following a dinacaryā routine, we create a sattvic or balanced lifestyle in alignment with the ebb and flow of prakṛti's changes. The goal of dinacaryā is to achieve optimal balance within the doṣa-s and especially maintain ojas. Problems on any level of the dhātu-s (seven tissues) from improper diet, lifestyle, and behavior in accordance with the laws of nature set the path for vulnerability and disease.

Practical Ways to Build Ojas When it is Depleted (T1D)

- Choose nourishing foods that are cooked and warm and have a balanced taste.
- Reduce physical exertion, visual stimulation, and sexual intercourse (reproductive fluid is considered to be vital for health).

- Āsana practice: Consider laṅghana or laṅghana toward a bṛṁhaṇa orientation with an emphasis on calm and stability.
- Prāṇāyāma (in moderation to avoid vāta derangement): Nāḍī śodhana and ujjāyī emphasizing lengthening exhale, slight pause after exhaling (suspension).
- Meditation: Pratyāhāra (withdrawal of the senses), mānasa pūjā to purify the mind, draw in compassion and love.
- Yoga nidrā: Less on expanding awareness, more on concentrated attention within the physical body's confines as a method for healing.
- Dinacaryā: Abhyaṅga oil massage.

Practical Ways to Redistribute Ojas When it is Displaced

- Diet: Avoid heavy, dense, and oily foods. Food should be easy to digest.
- Stoke the fire of agni with ginger and heating spices.
- Āsana practice: Consider bṛṁhaṇa orientation with standing āsanas, and emphasis on large-class muscles and the quality of building.
- Prāṇāyāma: Kriyās like kaphalabhati, bhastrikā to stimulate and activate the ANS. Central channel breathing with ujjāyī ratio emphasizing an equal inhale/exhale and equal retention/suspension.
- Meditation: Vicāra meditation (self-inquiry), niṣṭhā dhāraṇā meditation on the navel, any of the prāṇa vāyus.
- Yoga nidrā: Emphasis on transformation, saṁkalpa (intention), and fire of true perception.

The Digestive Fire of Health

Agni is the digestive fire, *the* biological energy of all metabolic processes. We learned about agni briefly when looking at pitta doṣa. They are related—agni is subsumed into pitta—but they are distinct. Whereas pitta is the system, agni is the enzyme that digests the food. It helps the body digest nutrients from food and eliminate what is non-essential. It is the internal flame that provides the vital essence of ojas and preserves prāṇa, and is the glow of optimal health in the body.[37] Strong agni promotes a long and healthy life. When agni is out of whack, the metabolism is greatly affected, food is improperly digested, toxins build up in the body, and resilience and immunity are impaired. On a psychological level, agni helps to digest memory and experience. Unprocessed negative experiences cultivate lasting impressions that color the clear lens of perception. These undigested experiences accumulate as mental contaminants like fear, anxiety, and depression. Āyurveda and yoga co-exist as health-providing tools to balance agni as the main source of nourishment.

If we are going to get technical, there are 13 different agnis, but the central agni that governs all is jathara agni and it abides in the stomach. Therefore, at least in an Ayurvedic view, all disease, all imbalance, originates in the stomach and all healing, all curative capacity, also resides in the stomach. Lifestyle habits, diet, food combining, and repressed emotions aggravate the doṣa-s, and aggravated doṣa-s disturb agni. Hypoactive agni slows digestion, leading to slow metabolism. We see this with kapha imbalances. This may lead to obesity, hypotension, and T2D. When agni is hyperactive, the digestive balance is burned up and the individual does not absorb nutrients. Think of emaciation, autoimmune disease (yes, T1D), and hyperthyroidism. These can be related to vāta (wasting) and pitta (burning up). The elemental forces of the doṣa-s help us to systematize the qualities of imbalance and balance to help us understand in a less cognitive and more experiential way how to promote homeostasis.

When agni is disturbed, physical and mental toxins accumulate and a person feels unwell.[38] These toxins are known as *āma*. Āma is a sticky, putrid-like substance that blocks prāṇa's ability to flow. It inhibits the biological function of vāta, pitta, and kapha and lodges itself in vulnerable areas of the body. Think of āma as being like unprocessed nutrients; undigested, improperly combined food creates āma. Signs of āma are fatigue, heaviness, constipation,

---

37 Lad, U. and Lad, V. (2007) *Ayurvedic Cooking for Self-Healing.* Delhi: Motilal Banarsidass. p.40.

38 Lad, U. and Lad, V. (2007) *Ayurvedic Cooking for Self-Healing.* Delhi: Motilal Banarsidass. p.39.

gas, indigestion, and diarrhea. Bad breath, mental confusion, physical aches, and stiffness can also be symptoms of āma. Even our food cravings are linked with āma, possessing you to eat foods that perpetuate your own imbalances. Āma is attracted to āma. Āma accumulates āma. The only way to stop it is to cultivate the opposite and move towards sattva.

It is Ayurveda's belief that all curative abilities also begin in the digestive system.[39] This is why diet is such a huge component of self-care. Digestion requires a lot of energy, and if we are eating too much food or improper food, too much of our agni goes towards digestion and it fizzles out. Āyurveda says that to reduce the impact of āma and increase agni, the stomach should always be partly empty.

Food should be nutritious and limited in quantity and in alignment with the seasons, time of day, and doṣa-s. One third of the stomach is for food, one third is for water, and one third is empty. Small amounts of nutrient-dense food are best for the reduction of āma. Āyurveda cautions against leftovers and constant snacking, as these are seen as contributing factors in the development of āma. Lifestyle factors like inactivity, overstimulation, and improper sleep patterns like sleeping late or during the day can all contribute to the buildup of āma. The individual's constitution and propensity will determine their weaknesses and how āma may influence disease process.

For people with diabetes, food can be a source of contention between impulses and willpower. For many with T2D, their relationship with food can be a contributing factor in the development of disease (although this is not always the case) and a source of emotional distress. Food causes stress in a person with T1D, as they have to think about what they are eating, how much insulin to take, and subsequently what they are doing after they eat and how the food will impact their blood sugar. There is a lot of emotion wrapped up in both experiences. People with diabetes have a tendency to overeat, either for emotional reasons, like night binging, or to treat hypoglycemia. One of the most common symptoms of hypoglycemia is extreme hunger, where all reason is overridden by the instinctive impulse to eat.

Hyperglycemia can also cause false hunger pangs, signifying a disruption of agni. All hyperglycemia challenges digestion, as excess glucose can cause GI distress, candida (a yeast overgrowth), and sluggish digestion. A common

39 Carter, K. (2017) "Diabetes: An Ayurvedic Perspective." *California College of Ayurveda.* Accessed on 06/07/20 at: www.ayurvedacollege.com/blog/diabetes-anayurvedicperspective.

effect of the long duration of diabetes combined with a history of high glucose levels is gastroparesis, a type of autonomic neuropathy in the stomach (more on this in Chapter 10). With gastroparesis, the stomach releases food very slowly, making it difficult to discern how and when to administer insulin, and it is physically uncomfortable. Nausea, bloating, and abdominal pain can accompany gastroparesis. These effects hamper the agni and increase āma, aggravating diabetic weaknesses. For some, a day or two of hyperglycemia and/or hypoglycemia episodes, although treated, retards the digestive fire that is so necessary for proper elimination.

If we look deeper at the motivations behind eating, for people with diabetes, the very act is embroiled in stigma. Knowledge of right from wrong does not take away underlying desires and cravings rooted in emotion. The act of eating and our choices of what we eat become a contentious source of fear, embarrassment, and protection. From the moment of diagnosis, we are told what we should eat and what is right and wrong to eat. And everyone else has an opinion about it. What we put into our bodies is viewed by others, and by ourselves, as the cause of our very dysfunction. Judgment and fear pervade a person's experience. Food is no longer considered to be nourishment or something to be enjoyed, but instead is viewed as a mechanical, survival-based action. We have to hold back, avert our choices from others, and hide from others to avoid their criticism.

This can create secrets and obsessive control surrounding food and body image. People with diabetes can become compulsive night eaters who do not eat in the day and overeat at night. People with T1D are also at higher risk for developing an eating disorder.

I struggled for most of my adolescence with food and still find myself asking, "Am I really hungry, or is this my blood sugar talking?" Yoga and the practices of prāṇāyāma and meditation provide me with the clarity to know the difference, support my willpower, and improve my choices.

Next, we will look at the Ayurvedic view of diabetes, its causes, and how Āyurveda and Ayurvedic lifestyle practices can support a person living with diabetes.

Ayurvedic View on Diabetes: *Pramēha* and Mādumēha

Āyurveda is one of the earliest recorded sciences to recognize what we consider to be diabetes as a major disease, using the term *pramēha*. The concept of *pramēha* first appeared in the ancient texts of Ṛg Veda and Atharva Veda as far back as 1900 BCE.[40] Over a long period of time, Āyurveda evolved within two main source texts: the *Suśruta-saṃhitā*, dating back as far as 1000 BCE, and the *Cakāra Samāhita*, dating back as far as 400 BCE.[41]

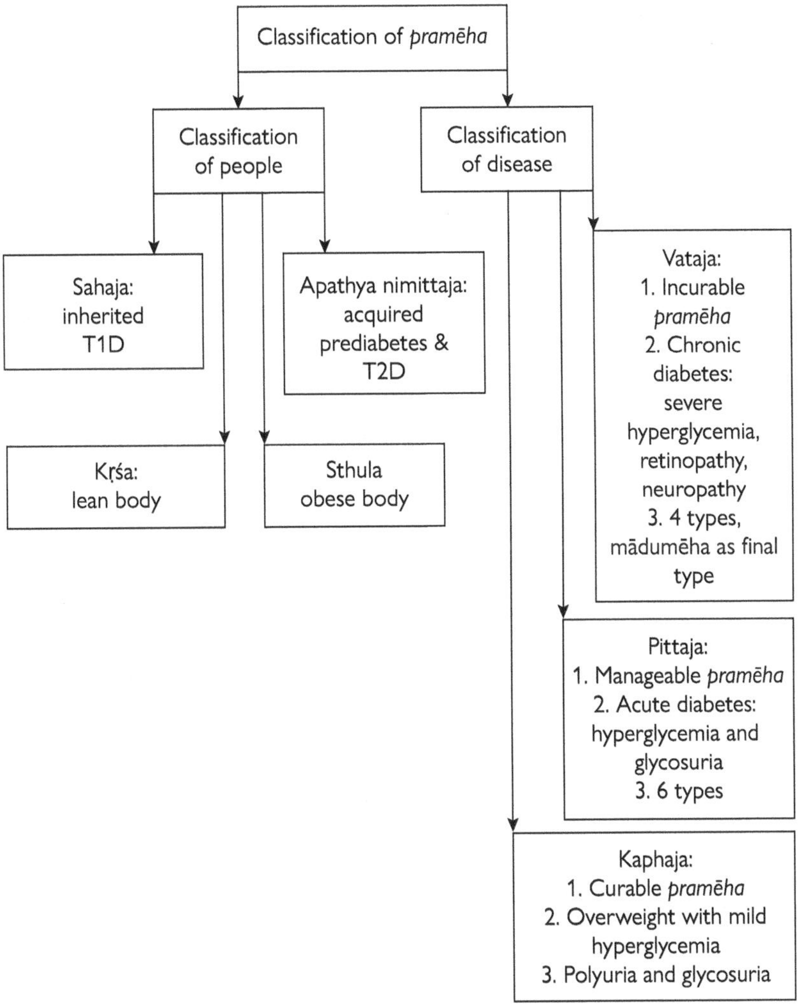

FIGURE 6.1[42]

40 Wikipedia (2020) *Vedas*. Accessed on 06/07/20 at: https://en.wikipedia.org/w/index.php?title=Vedas&oldid=959891235.

41 Wikipedia (2020) *Charaka Samhita*. Accessed on 06/07/20 at: https://en.wikipedia.org/w/index.php?title=Charaka_Samhita&oldid=958640559.

42 Sayyad, M. G. *et al.* (2011) "Computer Simulation Modelling for the Prevention of Diabetes Mellitus (Prameha)." *Journal of Applied Sciences 11*, 15, 2670–2679. doi:10.3923/jas.2011.2670.2679; Murthy, A. R. and Singh, R. H. (1989) "Concept of prameha/madhumeha (contradictions and compromises)." *Ancient Science of Life* 9, 2, 71–79.

Pramēha is a disease of profuse urination in Āyurveda, described mainly as a water metabolism imbalance.[43] Pra means abundant, and meha means "passing of large quantities of urine." Incidentally, the term "diabetes" is derived from the Greek term "Diabainein," meaning the continuous free flow of water. Therefore the terms "*pramēha*" and "diabetes" have similar meanings.[44]

There are 20 different gradations of *pramēha*, classified by the three doṣa-s. Of the 20 types, not all will land us in what we view as prediabetes or diabetes. What is important is Ayurveda's view of the disease process. When we understand the cause of imbalance, we can treat the imbalance.

Ten of the *pramēhas* are *kapha disorders*. This is interesting when we look at the origin of T2D. Kapha vitiation in *pramēha* is represented by adipose tissue, muscle tissue, and an increase of the waters of the body. Kapha is the bodily humor responsible for anabolism, the building of cells, and kapha vitiation of *pramēha* is represented by a similar profile.

Six *pramēhas* are pitta. Pitta-type *pramēha* is represented by a vitiation of pitta, muscle tissue, and an increase in urine and sweat. Pittas have high agni, which can burn out the pancreas.[45]

The final four *pramēhas* are vāta, and they are considered to be the final and most severe stage of *pramēha*. Vāta is responsible for all catabolic processes that break down cells for energy. Vāta *pramēha* is the vitiation of vāta doṣa, represented by a depletion of connective tissue and tissues of the nervous system, and it can infiltrate into other spaces.[46]

Of the four vāta *pramēhas*, the final is known as mādumēha. It is the closest to what we know of *diabetes* today. Mādumēha is the most advanced and final progression of *pramēha* and is considered to be incurable.

It is one of the eight major diseases of Āyurveda, demonstrating the significance of the disorder in populations before the advent of modern diseases. Interestingly enough, the word madu is analogous to "mellitus," both meaning honey.[47] Thus the terms mādumēha and diabetes mean the passing

43 Frawley, D. (2006) *Ayurveda and the Mind: The Healing of Consciousness*. Delhi: Motilal Banarsidass. p.235.

44 Murthy, A. R. and Singh, R. H. (1989) "Concept of prameha/madhumeha (contradictions and compromises)." *Ancient Science of Life* 9, 2, 71–79.

45 Murthy, A. R. and Singh, R. H. (1989) "Concept of prameha/madhumeha (contradictions and compromises)." *Ancient Science of Life* 9, 2, 71–79.

46 Aubin, K. (2020) Personal communication. March 15.

47 Murthy, A. R. and Singh, R. H. (1989) "Concept of prameha/madhumeha (contradictions and compromises)." *Ancient Science of Life* 9, 2, 71–79.

of large amounts of sweet urine. The 20 types of *pramēha* may refer to polyuria (excessive volume and frequency of urination), whereas mādumēha refers to sweet urine—what we know as diabetes. As we will see, the etiology, pathology, and physical manifestation of each type subsumed into the term mādumēha is distinct.

You might be wondering why I am spending so much time on this. Please, just wait. By looking at the Ayurvedic view of what we know as diabetes, we can see how it differs from the Western medical perspective, which is usually focused more on treatment than prevention. Ayurvedic wisdom holistically attends to diabetes in a way that Western science is only just beginning to value and attend to.

Etiology

Āyurveda sees diverse causes for the development of *pramēha* and there are some correlations with Western models of T1D and T2D. It classifies the disease as either inherited (sahaja) or acquired (apathya nimittaja). And although Western models would agree that both types of diabetes can have a genetic origin and also an environmental component, T1D is generally classified as *inherited* while T2D is *acquired.*

Under the acquired classification, we see 19 subtypes of *pramēha*. The 20th subtype, mādumēha, is the final stage of acquired *pramēha* and is also the direct progression of *inherited pramēha*. Therefore, Āyurveda implies that acquired *pramēha* is avoidable, whereas inherited is unavoidable. Interestingly, the causes of acquired *pramēha* like over nutrition, sedentary habits, and obesity aggravate the management of inherited *pramēha*.

Inherited *pramēha* (sahaja—etiological factor) lands a person directly into mādumēha, the final stage of vataja *pramēha* (disease classification). In this classification of *pramēha*, the patient can exhibit weakness and extreme fatigue, and be afflicted by excessive thirst, loss of appetite, and a need to be treated with a nourishing diet.[48] They tend to have a smaller build and be emaciated and thin.

48 Chandola, H. M. (n.d.) *Prameha in Terms of Diabetes Mellitus, Metabolic Syndrome and Obesity with Recent Advances in its Management.* Jamnagar: Institute for Post Graduate Teaching and Research in Ayurveda, Gujarat Ayurved University. p.9. Accessed on 26/08/20 at: www.ayurvedinstitute.com/Presenations/ChandolaSir.pdf.

Acquired *pramēha* develops slowly and, unless treated, moves from kapha, through pitta, and progressively into vāta.

The constitution of acquired *pramēha* resembles a kaphic profile. These people typically have a larger body mass, a tendency to gain and retain weight, and obesity is listed as one classifier. The classic view is that all untreated acquired *pramēha* will develop into the final, terminal stage of mādumēha (diabetes); however, not all Ayurvedic practitioners hold this view. Some will say that just two *pramēhas* actually relate to the development of T2D, and the rest can be classified as urinary disorders[49] and metabolic disorders like obesity and metabolic syndrome.

Of the two kaphaja classifications as T2D, iksu meha is the most relevant. Iksu meha is one of the ten kapha disorders. It is a buildup of āma at the receptor sites (see the disease pathology of kapha doṣa in Chapter 6). This buildup of āma occludes metabolic action,[50] possibly leading to what we know of as insulin resistance.

In summary, the diagnosis of any type of *pramēha* is an indicator of diabetes susceptibility but is not analogous with diabetes per se. There is a strong correlation between *pramēha* with obesity, insulin resistance, and metabolic syndrome too. It might not look like diabetes or even prediabetes in a Western sense, but recognizing it is an early detection strategy that can reduce the potential development of diabetes as mādumēha.

According to Āyurveda, if caught early on, acquired *pramēha* in a kaphaja and even pittaja stage can be managed, attenuated, and even eradicated by following Ayurvedic protocols. Once the disease has progressed to the vataja stage of mādumēha, it is impossible to treat with Āyurveda alone.

The Stages of *Pramēha*

- **Kaphaja *pramēha***: Early stage with ten subtypes. Considered to be curable with lifestyle and diet changes.

49 Chandola, H. M. (n.d.) *Prameha in Terms of Diabetes Mellitus, Metabolic Syndrome and Obesity with Recent Advances in its Management.* Jamnagar: Institute for Post Graduate Teaching and Research in Ayurveda, Gujarat Ayurved University. p.9. Accessed on 26/08/20 at: www.ayurvedinstitute.com/Presenations/ChandolaSir.pdf.

50 Aubin, K. (2020) Personal communication. March 15.

- **Pittaja *pramēha*:** Intermediate stage with six subtypes. More challenging to treat than kaphaja but not totally incurable.
- **Vataja *pramēha*:** Advanced stage with four subtypes, the final of which is mādumēha. Complicated, incurable, and terminal.

Causes and Potential Treatment

From an Ayurvedic view, all types of *pramēha*, including mādumēha, stem from a single cause: metabolic derangement.[51] Agni is at the core of metabolism, so it is part of the cause as well as the treatment. Insufficient agni leads to increased sugar in circulation. Too much agni can burn out the system—think hyperinsulimia and insulin resistance. When we look at the potential causes of metabolic dysregulation, Āyurveda recognizes that all acquired *pramēha* is a result of behavior.

Behavior is further classified into *diet* (*āhār*) and *lifestyle* (*vihār*) proclivities. What we put into our bodies, how we eat food, when we eat food, our daily rhythm of activity and sleep, and the level of stress we experience all contribute to the development of disease and to existing disease aggravation. Certain foods challenge agni's function, dampening its ability to metabolize, and increasing āma. Food should be well balanced, nutrient dense, and easy to digest; not too heavy, sweet, or spicy. Imbalances in food, i.e. types of food that require a lot of agni to digest, will progressively fizzle out a person's digestive flame.

Certain lifestyle habits like "idle" sitting, excessive sleep, and lack of exercise also contribute. Mental habits like excessive worry, thoughtlessness, anger, interrupted sleep, and sorrow all derange and accelerate the disease process. No matter the type of diabetes, when considering prevention and treatment, we are always looking at how to build a person's agni, reduce āma, and create balance within all systems, including the mind. Unprocessed negative thoughts are just as harmful and destructive as not exercising and eating well.

51 Murthy, A. R. and Singh, R. H. (1989) "Concept of prameha/madhumeha (contradictions and compromises)." *Ancient Science of Life* 9, 2, 71–79.

T1D

It should be clear by now that Āyurveda views T1D as being inherited more than acquired. And although it is unclear whether Āyurveda also sees T1D as being acquired from behavior, it is certain that behavior (diet and lifestyle) is a contributing factor to diabetes management and the progression of long-term associated co-morbidities.

It is widely accepted in Āyurveda that there is not a reliable cure for T1D, and treatment should be a combination of insulin injections and Ayurvedic lifestyle protocols. T1D is viewed predominantly as a vāta condition; the recommendation is a vāta pacification protocol.

The very nature of managing T1D is aggravating to vāta. Constant testing, alarms, and dramatic BG fluctuations are a recipe for crazy. People with T1D are already in an energetic deficit due to the vāta and should therefore focus their self-care efforts on building and nourishing their system and reducing the cause of vāta vitiation, which is largely stress related.

People with T1D should prioritize practices that calm and pacify the mind, build vitality, and connect regularly with spirit. Attending to vāta, pacifying the body with balanced nutrition, and the mind by reducing mental rajas, will help a person with T1D maintain their vitality and nourish their whole body from the inside out. These lifestyle practices reduce the sharp BG swings associated with stress, overwhelm, and overstimulation. Diet and exercise are also important behaviors to focus on in treatment. Both should be sattvic in nature, meaning well balanced. Exercise is important, but vigorous exercise without adequate self-care will derange vāta and deplete ojas.

T2D

It is the classical view that the progression of acquired mādumēha starts in kapha, moves to pitta, and eventually arrives in vāta. This is why you may see early-stage T2D as a kapha imbalance (prediabetes) and, over the duration of the disease, the person moves to vāta (insulin dependent). This could also be age related, as the later stage of life is a vāta stage. Either way, there is a movement from kapha to vāta. When vāta is predominant, there is a weakening of the systems and nourishment is essential.

For our purposes, let's look at the stage of kapha where the progression of the disease is the most manageable. The earlier stages of the disease progression are kapha vitiation. It is common to see kapha vitiation co-occurring with tamas.

Excessive kapha increases body mass and decreases metabolic function (low agni), and high toxins (āma), coupled with psychological tamo-guṇa predominance (dull, heavy, depressive mind), block the fire of willpower, determination, and transformation. From a yoga therapy perspective, T2D treatment is one that stimulates agni, and increases insulin sensitivity (or reduces insulin resistance), weight loss, and stress reduction (a contributing factor in depression and insulin resistance). The general Ayurvedic protocol for reducing kapha uses diet and exercise. This is to remove the accumulation of āma that is a result of lowered agni from poor lifestyle choices. Essentially, the goal is to balance the guṇa-s, but tamas has to move through rajas to arrive at sattva. Creating physical heat will stimulate mental rajas and awaken the mind, perception, and intellect towards individual responsibility. Āyurveda often prescribes a regimen of panchakarma (Ayurveda's purification and detoxification treatment) to remove excess āma, accelerate the weight loss, and promote insulin sensitivity by removing āma.[52]

It is absolutely clear that Āyurveda cannot replace allopathic medicine in T1D and T2D. Insulin is necessary for T1D and certain forms of T2D. Āyurveda has an important contribution to the prevention of T2D, as well as the reduction of diabetes complications in both types of diabetes. Although the view in Āyurveda is that T1D is genetic, this does not mean that the disease process cannot be influenced by Ayurvedic practices, including yoga therapy. The application is multifactorial. On one level, Āyurveda reduces the disease process of T2D, perhaps avoiding the diagnosis of diabetes all together. On another level, Ayurvedic practices help mitigate the complications of both T1D and T2D with āhāra/vihār and dinacaryā. It provides a framework of understanding the contributing factors to disease progression and what an individual can *personally* do to avoid risk while building resilience against future risk.

Practical Approach

Here's the gist: let's wrap this chapter up with a summarized digestive enzyme. Upon designing a yoga therapy practice informed by Āyurveda, consider what is out of balance constitutionally through the doṣa-s. Essentially, the movement

52 Carter, K. (2017) "Diabetes: An Ayurvedic Perspective." *California College of Ayurveda.* Accessed on 06/07/20 at: www.ayurvedacollege.com/blog/diabetes-anayurvedicperspective.

is from imbalance to balance. Balance is the essence of health in Āyurveda. Every type of imbalance can be traced back to the doṣa-s and the guṇa-s. By understanding the models of Āyurveda, we can begin to see similarities in what goes out of balance with diabetes. Every chapter in this book relates to a specific diabetes challenge that can be traced back to Āyurveda and treated with both Āyurveda and yoga therapy practices. By merging the wisdom of Āyurveda with yoga therapy, we can look at diabetes treatment with new eyes. This depth of awareness affords all yoga therapists, as well as people with diabetes, the chance to identify and treat diabetes from a more holistic perspective, addressing the person as a whole, and not just diabetes. The experience of diabetes will differ dramatically from person to person.

Just as yoga has rules of inner and outward practices known as the yamas and niyamas, Āyurveda holds a similar approach with the āhāra rasāyana-s, which promote a sattvic, or balanced, lifestyle. These steps help to preserve ojas and reduce the qualities of tamas and rajas that inherently make up the doshic imbalances. As Āyurveda views all disease as having its origin in digestion, these practices support agni's function and balance appropriate ojas. In the case of T1D, we are working with building vitality and reducing depletion. With type 2, in general, the work is on redistributing ojas and reducing kapha imbalances to promote effective energy metabolism.

Khecharī Recipe Adaptations for Diabetes

Khecharī is a healthy and soothing dish frequently prescribed by Ayurvedic specialists to help restore digestion and increase agni. However, khecharī can be challenging for diabetics to digest because of its high carbohydrate density and the fact that it is made in large batches, making it more difficult to dose appropriately with insulin in the case of T1D. I love khecharī and believe in its medicinal qualities. It as a reset for my gut or when I am needing nourishment.

I have come up with two adaptations for people with diabetes of a classic khecharī recipe. The first is for people who are carbohydrate friendly and the second for those who wish to limit their carbohydrate intake. The second one can present some challenges if a person is eating khecharī to reduce gas and bloating, as it contains cauliflower. The recipes are adapted from Vasant and Usha Lad's *Ayurvedic Cooking for Self-Healing.*[53]

RECIPE 1: KHECHARĪ

This is a classic recipe for khecharī. The adaptation is to cook the dal and the grain separately. This way you can measure the carbohydrates for your meal with greater ease and flexibility. I choose to use quinoa, as it is a complex carbohydrate.

Dal

- ½ cup yellow split mung dal
- 3 tbsp ghee or high-quality oil (not coconut, as it increases vāta)
- 1 tsp cumin seeds
- 1 tsp black mustard seeds
- Pinch of hing
- ½ tsp turmeric
- 4 cup water
- ½ tsp salt
- Cilantro as desired

Quinoa

- 1 cup white quinoa
- 1 ¾ cup water

Rinse the quinoa and mung dal. If there is time, soak the mung dal for an hour to help digestion.

In a small pot, heat up the oil on medium, and toss in the cumin, mustard seeds, and hing. When they start to pop, add in the dal and turmeric, and stir. Add the 4 cups of water, bring to a boil for 5 minutes,

53 Lad, U. and Lad, V. (2007) *Ayurvedic Cooking for Self-Healing.* Delhi: Motilal Banarsidass.

and then cover slightly and reduce to simmer for about 20 minutes. Keep an eye out that the dal does not dry out. Add salt and cilantro at the end.

Place the water and quinoa in another pot. Bring it to a boil and then cover and simmer for 15 minutes. I personally like to use a ratio of grain to water of less than 1:2. Try it out.

RECIPE 2: CAULIFLOWER KHECHARĪ

Follow the same steps and ingredients for the dal in recipe 1. In the last ten minutes of cooking, add about 2–3 cups of cauliflower rice and another cup of water if it looks dry.

CHAPTER 7

The Role of a Yoga Therapist in Diabetes Care

The role of a yoga therapist is to empower individuals to take responsibility for their health, happiness, and wellbeing through the use of yoga teachings and practices. Empowerment is one part education and one part experiential. Facts only go as far as a person understands them to be real within their own experience. If we are truly to help people transform their health, we also need to know how to transmit the tools in a way that means they can be "directly" experienced. This means the experience never leaves the person because it has awakened a part of them.

In this chapter, we will run through the scope of practice for yoga therapists in diabetes care: what you can do, my main assessment tools and strategies, and I'll also give you some words of advice that no one outside of the diabetes community will tell you.

Yoga therapy sees each person as a multidimensional system consisting of the body, breath, mind (emotions and intellect), and their mutual interaction.[1] The yoga therapist carefully assesses each person within this framework and maps out a path that will serve the individual's unique needs and goals. It is the role of the yoga therapist to help the practitioner awaken to their sense of personal power, transforming conditioned patterns, and encouraging them to become an equal contributor to their wellbeing. A skilled yoga therapist can see how to create an environment for the inner wisdom to awaken naturally, inspiring patient empowerment and responsibility for the long term.

---

1 International Association of Yoga Therapists (IAYT) (n.d.) *Introduction to the IAYT Scope of Practice*. Accessed on 07/07/20 at: www.iayt.org/general/custom.asp?page=IntroScope.

Working with Diabetes

If you are going to work with someone who has diabetes, it is essential that you first and foremost understand what diabetes is and how it impacts a person on a multidimensional level. Diabetes is tricky to work with because there is not a specific practice for diabetes. Diabetes is invisible for the most part, and even the person in front of you may not be aware of the degree to which they are negatively affected by diabetes. A person may come to you for a diabetes-specific goal or something else, like stress reduction or weight loss. It is good to have a goal but also to know that everything is interconnected. Just keep in mind that, no matter your goal, if diabetes is present, it is always part of your consideration.

If they come to you to manage stress, you know that stress impacts diabetes and diabetes impacts stress. If they come to you to help them reduce their A1c, managing stress may also be a strategy to help lower A1c, but so is self-awareness.

Yoga therapy is not about fixing diabetes; it is about facilitating a space for a person to get in rhythm with self-care so improved health can occur naturally. With an understanding of how diabetes is always part of the bigger picture of health, you will be able to skillfully assess and implement practices that will positively influence change in their lives. Whether or not this has a direct impact on their diabetes care is not definable in the immediate scope of the practice. All we can do as yoga therapists is create a safe space for the individual to move energy, process emotions, and, ultimately, feel more competent and confident within themselves.

First, create the parameters of a balanced practice informed by your client assessment. Teach the person who is in front of you. Ask whatever your connection is to a higher power that the practice be of benefit, and trust the process that you know to be meaningful and beneficial to you in your life. Trust that the work you have done on yourself will support the work you are helping to facilitate in the other. This is all you can ask. Then empty yourself of all of yourself, your biases, story, and preconceptions, to be a vessel for the work to be done through you.

Your ability to create a safe container for a person to be heard and met with your compassion is part of the healing process. For people with diabetes, it is less important to find a cure; we have come to terms with the fact that there is not a cure. What we want is to be heard, be understood, and have our feelings validated. We may not want an answer but rather a space to be safe where we can just be and maybe have a glimpse of feeling like we have some influence and control in our lives. The compassion you offer in your yoga therapy space will inspire compassion within the person in front of you. When people sense that their fears, struggles, and challenges are not only real but also reasonable, it helps them to let go of the anger and open to a more significant potential within themselves, one of loving-kindness and hope.

It is not the scope of a yoga therapist to advertise himself or herself as a licensed healthcare practitioner unless they are a licensed healthcare practitioner as well as a yoga therapist.[2] You are not a diabetes educator, and it is not your role to advise on diabetes management beyond the scope of yoga therapy unless you are certified to do so. It is your job to demonstrate, encourage, and support your client's needs and goals. Through this process, it is hoped that the person can improve their relationship with diabetes and, on a broader level, with themselves.

Diabetes is a self-care practice, and an important reason why people are unsuccessful at adhering to diabetes parameters set by healthcare practitioners is a lack of self-care tools and methods. One of the biggest frustrations for healthcare providers is figuring out a way to transform patient behavior outside of the office. The problem is that unless a person is developing self-awareness, looking at their deeper conditioned patterns and reconstructing them into more positive ones, and supported by a method, they will probably not change their behaviors. Education is not enough; it has to be inspired from within.

According to *Psychology in Diabetes Care*,[3] the main pillars of diabetes health are diet, exercise, self-management of diabetes such as insulin administration and calculating carbohydrates, emotional health, relationships, and energy management such as rest and sleep. In the overall picture of diabetes education and support systems, there is more support for diet, exercise, and self-management, but most people are falling short in the mental, emotional, relationship, and rest categories.

Although it is not the scope of yoga therapy to address the aspects of diabetes management like insulin administration, these are improved as a person develops self-awareness through yoga therapy. They are more likely to see the patterns in their habits, recognize when to stop and start implementing

---

2 International Association of Yoga Therapists (IAYT) (n.d.) *Introduction to the IAYT Scope of Practice*. Accessed on 07/07/20 at: www.iayt.org/general/custom.asp?page=IntroScope.

3 Snoek, F. J. and Skinner, C. T. J. (eds) (2009) *Psychology in Diabetes Care*. Chichester: Wiley & Sons Ltd.

new strategies, and seek out the help of healthcare specialists when they need extra support. The most important sectors of your work with the inner pillars of diabetes care are energy management, mental and emotional health, and relationship support.

The inner pillars, as I like to call them, are not measurable or tangible. They do not cater to the ego's limited view of self, i.e. our body, image, or a number on a glucometer. There is no metric for the inner pillars other than a feeling of wellbeing. We will typically put rest, relaxation, and mental and emotional health last on our to-do list and continue to rationalize why we do not have time to practice self-care. But we as yoga therapists, medical communities, and even people with diabetes know the importance of the self-care pillars; they just do not know how to do it.

I always ask people how they practice rest, and most look at me like I am crazy. They say, "What rest?" They may say that they nap, but the majority tell me that they rest when they sleep, and many do not sleep well. A personal practice addresses these often-overlooked pillars, which can make or break a person's resilience to diabetes risks. Consistent practice will benefit all components of care. You often hear about people trying really hard to achieve a physical goal of losing those last ten pounds. They strive so hard, and, in the process, end up gaining weight. Little do they realize that it is due to stress. Then they go on vacation for two weeks, eat and drink, break all their "rules," and end up losing weight. Why? They are relaxed.

This is where yoga therapy becomes a tremendous asset to every person with diabetes as a way to achieve their health goals and an adjunct for diabetes care specialists who are frustrated with low patient adherence. The yoga therapist narrows the gap between the individual, their condition, and personal responsibility. Understanding the importance of self-care in diabetes is the cornerstone of all improved action.[4] When people fully cognize their role and responsibility in their health, it inspires improved action. Studies show that scare tactics do not encourage diabetes self-care, it has to be awakened within the individual.[5]

Diet could be subsumed into Āyurveda, but unless you are qualified to

4 Anderson, R., Funnell, M., Carlson, A., Saleh-Statin, N., *et al.* (2005) "Facilitating Self-Care Through Empowerment." In F. J. Snoek and C. T. J. Skinner (eds) *Psychology in Diabetes Care*. Second edition. Chichester: Wiley & Sons Ltd. p.71.

5 Snoek, F. J. and Skinner, C. T. J. (eds) (2009) *Psychology in Diabetes Care*. Chichester: Wiley & Sons Ltd. pp.27–35.

address diet, it does not fit within the scope of practice. Your assessment strategy can ask about nutrition, to get a sense of likes and dislikes. People are not honest about what they eat. It is more beneficial to ask questions like: What is your guilty pleasure food? If there were no rules, what would you want to eat? Are you a snacker? When is your first meal of the day? What time is your last bite of food? And so on. These paint a better picture of the role of diet and nutrition in a person's health.

> D.Z., 54, with LADA, complains of high BG numbers in the morning. She reports eating her main meal late at night because her husband works late. Instead of making a dietary recommendation that is beyond the realm of yoga therapy, you could educate her about the role of agni in metabolism and how Āyurveda suggests that the main meal should be eaten during the pitta time of day. This way, you let D.Z. come to a conclusion on her own without telling her how to do it. By eating a more substantial meal in the daytime, she will be less hungry at night and will exchange her heavy evening meal for a lighter one, potentially avoiding the morning high BG.

There are so many intelligent ways to exercise these days; yoga is one of them. I do believe that it is within your scope as a yoga therapist to encourage people to move. Still, the specifics of exercise are beyond the scope of yoga therapy and better suited to an exercise specialist. In my work in the Rocky Mountains, many of my clients with diabetes are not the stereotypical high BMI, sedentary, kapha types. The majority are more likely to be over-exercisers than under-exercisers and need yoga as the counter pose that balances their hyperactivity.

Yoga āsana can be considered light exercise, and it may be enough exercise for some, especially for those who are just starting an exercise routine. However, the moment we think of yoga as exercise, it changes the psychological intention behind what would otherwise be therapeutic. It is my recommendation to consider some qualities of yoga therapy as "exercise like," as they build physical strength and increase stimulation on a physiological and mental level. These qualities are helpful in your construction of practices for diabetes energetics.

You have to know the population that you work with and assess how to appropriately present yoga as an exercise intervention or suggest other modalities for people to look into in addition to their yoga therapy practice. Gentle āsana may be a lot for some populations, and you will have to help them modify and adapt, so that they do not aggravate their system.

The Attributes of Empowered Yoga Therapy for Diabetes

- Awaken purpose and desire to be better.
- Identify obstacles to diabetes care and refine diabetes goals.
- Understand what is out of balance and what to do to restore balance.
- Encourage self-administered practice—the individual can influence change.
- Upgrade perception of self-efficacy.
- Build resilience against diabetes risks by increasing physical and mental vitality.
- Cultivate the witness, the one who is beyond diabetes.
- Transform perception of self-care from chore/work into an appreciation for the gift of life.

Client Responsibility

Diabetes belongs to the individual, and there is nothing that you can say or do that will deflect that responsibility onto anything other than the individual.[6] They must do the work themselves. This is why empowerment is an essential element of yoga therapy for diabetes. We want people to not only feel better because of their practice, but also be more capable of handling any challenge that diabetes throws at them. Please be mindful not to be attached to your efforts in helping your clients transform. All you can do is lay out the methods, carefully assess how to offer it to them, and encourage people to do the work. If they do it, and believe in it, with your support, they can really improve their lives.

6 Anderson, R., Funnell, M., Carlson, A., Saleh-Statin, N., *et al.* (2005) "Facilitating Self-Care Through Empowerment." In F. J. Snoek and C. T. J. Skinner (eds) *Psychology in Diabetes Care*. Second edition. Chichester: Wiley & Sons Ltd. p.71.

Assessment Tools and Strategies

The process by which we take on a client—from initial intake and assessment, to the co-authored construction of a yoga therapy practice—increases the effectiveness of the practice. I begin my assessment process at the moment I receive an inquiry. It is best to assess people when they do not realize that they are being watched. There is a lot that we can learn from a person before we ever meet them in person. I am listening in on every interaction, including the way they inquire about yoga therapy, and their questions, timeliness in response, availability, punctuality, etc. You can tell about a person's health just by observing them. When you greet them at the door, watch their movement as they walk down the hall or up the stairs. Observe the color in their face, clarity in their eyes, and how much or how little they talk—these things all inform the way you curate their experience. Uncontrolled diabetes has a look and a feel to it. Their skin is grey, eyes are dull, and vitality is low. They may not be engaged or present with you. Their attention span and memory retention will be low to moderate at best.

I want to know right away who I am working with, and what their risks, interests, and goals are, so I can be prepared. That way, we do not waste any time in our first session, or later on when they tell me about their herniated lumbar disc and we have been focusing on forward bends and twists for their anxiety for the last several weeks. A comprehensive intake questionnaire takes the doubt out of the assessment process; however, nothing compares to skilled observation. For all of my yoga therapy clients, I have a specialized intake form that I send to them before our first session. I have modeled this after the International Association of Yoga Therapists' (IAYT) suggested intake form and have added diabetes-specific questions below.

General Intake Questionnaire

- Why are you seeking yoga therapy? What do you hope to achieve? Do you have any specific goals?
- Have you practiced yoga before? If so, what is your previous yoga experience?
- Are you interested in a home practice? If so, how much time do you have to practice? Do you have a space to practice? What time

of day would be best for you? For example, for 30 minutes, on five days a week, in the mornings.

- List current and previous health conditions. Include medical diagnoses, surgeries, accidents, and injuries with approximate dates. What treatments have you had for these conditions?
- What do you consider to be your strengths in terms of current health and wellness?
- Please describe your typical eating patterns. How many meals a day? What time is your main meal? Do you like to snack? If you could have one food for the rest of your life, what would that be?
- Do you have an exercise routine? How many days a week do you exercise? Describe the duration and intensity.
- What kind of movement and activities do you enjoy?
- How is your energy level? Does it fluctuate or stay constant? When do you feel the most energized? And the least energized?
- How well do you sleep, on a scale of 1 (terrible) to 10 (perfect)?
- Do you feel rested in the morning?
- Do you nap in the daytime?
- How would you rate your digestion? How often do you have a bowel movement? Do you experience stomach aches, bloating, or gas after meals?
- How much water do you drink a day?
- What is your support system like? Are you married or single, and do you live alone? Do you have family close by?
- How do you rest and relax?
- What types of medication are you on?
- Do you have physical tension? If so, where do you generally hold your tension?

- Do you experience physical pain or discomfort? If so, where? What makes it worse and better?
- Do you experience sadness, anxiety, depression, or worry? If so, how often?
- What is your perceived level of stress, on a scale of 1 to 5?
- What is your definition of optimal health?
- If you could change a habit, what would you choose to change?
- Do you consider yourself a spiritual person?
- Do you seek more meaning and purpose in life?
- Are you interested in meditation?
- What aspects of your life bring you the most joy and pleasure?
- Yoga methods include postures, breathing practice, meditation, visualization, and chanting. Are there any aspects of a yoga practice that you are not comfortable with?

When a person seeks me out specifically for diabetes, I add to the initial questionnaire. You can edit it as you see fit. I want to get a sense of the relationship that a person has with diabetes and isolate any potential red flags. Do they exhibit any mental or emotional problems associated with diabetes care? I also want to know how a person feels about diabetes as a disease. How much is it consuming their thoughts, defining their actions, and impacting their life?

Diabetes-Related Questions

- What type of diabetes do you have?
- What was the date of your diagnosis?
- Have you had any complications from diabetes? For example, retinopathy in the feet.

- Have you had any hospitalizations for diabetes?
- Would you like to share the last A1c?
- What types of insulin are you on (if applicable) and what are your methods of administration (pump versus MDI or oral medications)?
- If you are on insulin, what is your average daily dose of insulin? Please include short- and long-acting insulin.
- How often do you experience hyperglycemia or hypoglycemia? For example, lows twice a week, highs once a day.
- Is there a pattern to your highs or lows? For example, highs after lunch, lows in the afternoon.
- Do you worry about lows?
- Can you feel your lows coming on?
- How do you treat your lows? Juice, glucose tabs, or something else?
- Please describe in your words what it feels like (symptoms, sensations, thoughts, emotions) when your BG is high.
- Please describe in your words what it feels like (symptoms, sensations, thoughts, emotions) when your BG is low (if applicable).
- Please describe your diabetes self-care routine. For example, balanced diet, low carb, low fat at night, exercise 30 minutes a day.
- Does diabetes wake you up at night?
- What is your biggest challenge with diabetes management?
- When you make a mistake with diabetes management, are you more likely to feel angry, guilty, worried, overwhelmed, or avoidant? Please choose one to two of these.
- How much do you feel your family support you with your diabetes, on a scale of 1 to 5?

- How much do you feel your healthcare providers support you with your diabetes, on a scale of 1 to 5?
- How confident do you feel about your ability to manage diabetes, on a scale of 1 to 5?
- How often do you think about diabetes, on a scale of 1 (not at all) to 5 (every 15 minutes)?
- How burned out do you feel by all the work that goes into diabetes management, on a scale of 1 to 5?
- If there were a cure tomorrow, how would that change your life?
- What do you think are your strengths with diabetes care?
- What are your weaknesses?
- How would you define optimal diabetes health?

Daily Questions

- What is the biggest challenge today?
- What is working well?
- What is your BG at this moment?
- How much active insulin do you have on-board?
- How is your energy level?
- What would you like to achieve today? How can I be of service?

Everyone is Individual

Some people need space; others require you to hold their hands. Some need auxiliary resources to explain why they are doing everything; others just want to do it without explanation. Some people need to be pushed; others need to be cared for. The skill of a yoga therapist is to understand how to meet each person in front of them.

Whenever I am with a client, I try to empty myself of myself, so as not to project my opinions about what they need onto the experience. Despite our efforts to understand diabetes and cultivate compassion for our clients, we can come into our sessions with biases, judgments, and opinions. There is a difference between what you think a person should do versus what they actually need. Watch out for if and when this is surfacing and continue to tune into your inner guide.

I rely upon a keen sense of listening to the presence of the person in front of me. I often begin sessions in silence, just bringing our attention to the breath, so I can drop in to where they are at energetically. This information overrides everything I receive in a questionnaire.

Assessment Tools

There are infinite assessment tools to choose from; it depends on what resonates with you and what works for the person in front of you. I generally rely to an extent on Ayurvedic models, although I am not a trained Ayurvedic specialist. The models of the doṣa-s and mental guṇa-s are invaluable to my assessment process. I am looking for imbalances just as much as strengths. This way, I can form a plan to meet the person where they are at and influence a direction of change that will support their constitution.

Breathing Assessment

One of the first assessment tools that I rely upon is a breath analysis, as it provides invaluable information about the state of a person's mind and resilience of their nervous system. Even if someone has prior yoga experience, in all probability they have not been taught how to breathe or to pay attention to the movement of breath in the body. Asking a person to pay attention to their breath reveals qualities of their mind often unobservable in a questionnaire and initial assessment. Just as everyone has a physical threshold in a pose, they also have a mental limit for maintaining a smooth and deep breath. For instance, how long can they pay attention to their breath without stopping? Do they fall asleep? Does the rhythm of their breath become shallow or intermittent?

Diabetes adds an intriguing layer of analysis to a yoga therapy assessment. Some, but not all, people's experiences with diabetes will have primed them to be more sensitized to the healing force of prāṇa and interoceptive awareness; this is the refined ability to sense presence within the body. Given that there is no advanced neuropathy stunting sensitivity, I find that many clients with diabetes have a "leg up" in the self-awareness category compared with non-diabetics, just by living with diabetes. Many are natural breathers and feelers. The concept of breath as shape change does not seem as strange as it can for some, and the conscious movement of breath in different body areas—like chest breathing versus belly breathing—is quite accessible. This is not always the case and should be adjusted on an individual basis.

Ultimately we want to help people improve the quality of their breath to enhance self-awareness and teach self-regulation of the ANS. Breath analysis in a supine position is a useful assessment strategy to understand what may be out of balance on a subtle level.

I generally begin all sessions in a supine position and invite the patient to direct their breath in various ways within the body. It helps them focus their mind and reveals subtle tension. Remember, the breath is to the mind as the mind is to the breath.

You can ask a person to breathe just into their belly, chest, or mid-body, providing cues to resolve tension and facilitate efficiency within their breathing. Then ask them to tie all the focal points together into a cohesive breath. This can be done from the top down on the inhale, and the bottom up on the exhale. It can also be applied from the bottom up on the inhale, and the top down on the exhale. Ultimately it is about breathing with ease, although what comes naturally to an individual is not always an ideal breath. A chest inhale may occur more readily than a belly inhale, but when they inhale into the chest, they over utilize the neck and shoulder muscles, creating more tension. For some, inhaling into the abdomen is more natural than inhaling into the chest, but they may exhibit tightness in their chest and ribcage and benefit from a chest inhale.

For our work with the energetic condition, inhaling into the chest is more energizing and nourishing, while an abdominal inhale will be more pacifying and relaxing. Ideally, we would like to be able to breathe in various ways, supporting personal adaptability and variability within a practice. It is natural for a person to struggle with part of their breathing, whether inhale, exhale, or both.

If a person struggles with inhalation, it could represent underlying anxiety, an ineffective exhale, or general tightness in the chest. Why there is tension is not as important as how to resolve said tension. When you help a person breathe comfortably in a new way and into areas of their body that they do not readily access, emotions can surface. If this happens, give them space, and encourage them to come back to their breath when they are ready. Do not be afraid to change your route for practice if you notice that a person is struggling to breathe and that it creates tension. If this occurs, I may not focus on breathing at all and will adapt the method to the body first, as in the Iyengar tradition, hoping that continued practice will improve the self-awareness, mental focus, and interest in breathing.

Breath Assessment Practice

This breath analysis is written for the therapist, but one can self-evaluate through the same process.

Start with the person lying in a supine position and place a folded blanket lengthwise under their mid-back, resting the bottom of the blanket just below the scapula in the mid-body. Fold the excess part of the blanket from behind the head under the neck should additional cervical support be necessary. This slight elevation of the torso helps to open the ribcage and facilitate the breath; however, it should not accentuate the cervical or lumbar curves. Straighten the legs, or place a bolster under the knees.

Some individuals may need more or less prop support depending upon their height, weight, pre-existing heart conditions, etc. The idea is that they can remain in this position for some time without effort but not be so relaxed that they fall asleep. When they are set up and comfortable, go through the exercise below.

There are three central locations for breathing: the chest, mid-body, and abdomen. The torso is divided into two cavities: the thoracic cavity above the diaphragm and the abdominal cavity below the diaphragm. The diaphragm, nestled below the lungs, is what Leslie Kaminoff dubs the "engine of the breath."[7]

"Pay attention to the breath and breathe normally. Notice the feeling of inhale and exhale."

Watch what comes up with their natural pattern of breath.

"Progressively deepen the inhale and lengthen the exhale by way of the throat."

Explain ujjāyī prāṇāyāma, the valving of the glottis in the throat, if necessary.

"Watch the flow of the breath and resolve any tension in your breathing. Tension is represented by strain, choppiness, or tightness."

---

7 Kaminoff, L. (2010) *How is your Diaphragm like the Engine in your Car?* Accessed on 07/07/20 at: www.youtube.com/watch?v=9UJIAiEThBw&t=12s.

Observe how a person breathes with ujjāyī. If ujjāyī is a struggle, you may need to apply further relaxation strategies before continuing.

Next, progress with localized breathing in specific sections of the torso including the abdomen, mid-torso, and collarbone. Limit the shape change to each area (i.e. if breathing into the belly, the chest should not move).

"Inhale into the abdomen, exhale from the abdomen. Sense the origin of the inhalation deep in the pelvic floor at the base of the spine. Relax the inhale entirely at the end of the breath. To exhale, squeeze the abdomen progressively but not strenuously, inwardly and upwardly."

"Inhale into the mid-ribs and sternum. Feel like the breath expands three-dimensionally—up, down, forward, and back. Limit the movement of inhale into the abdominal cavity by keeping the abdomen firm."

"Inhale into the chest and collarbone. Allow the breath to be shallow and sense the collarbone rising while keeping the neck and shoulder muscles relaxed. Limit the movement of inhale into the abdominal cavity by maintaining the abdomen firm."

Lastly, bring all three sections together into one cohesive breath. Generally, I teach this from the inhale chest to the abdomen and exhale abdomen to the chest, but you can do it in any way that facilitates a better breath.

"Inhale from the collarbone, chest, mid-body, and then belly, relaxing the abdomen almost completely. Exhale from the abdomen, feel the sternum lower and then the chest."

Spend several minutes on each section. Observe their mechanics and the patterns of how they breathe, and offer cues to help their breath flow freely. If you notice that an area is unavailable to them, for instance they are chronic chest inhalers and cannot breathe into their abdomen, perhaps work on belly breathing before you introduce chest breathing.

Often, when people are challenged with inhale, they are not exhaling correctly. There is a reverse breath that some people have where they push their belly out on the exhale, contracting their ribs to exhale. For these individuals, the work is first to improve the exhale by teaching them to exhale from an abdominal contraction versus the ribs.

Sometimes, these individuals need tactile awareness. You can place a sandbag on the abdomen or have them lie on their belly with a rubber exercise ball nestled into the abdominal cavity.

A Few Words of Advice

It was emphasized in my yoga therapy training that the most important aspect of yoga therapy is the relationship between therapist and student. Trust is part of what encourages student empowerment and adherence when they doubt themselves and the efficacy of their practice. When you are working with people with diabetes, there is an unspoken etiquette that no one outside of the diabetes community really talks about. I feel a responsibility as a person living with diabetes and a yoga therapist to impart this knowledge to you.

First of all, if you live with diabetes, you are sick of people telling you what to do or how to manage diabetes. We have heard it all, especially unsolicited advice from people who mean well but have no business advising on diabetes. Unfortunately, the holistic healthcare community is one of the worst demographics for this. Personally, I have been told how to manage my diabetes by yoga teachers, therapists, massage therapists, holistic healers, acupuncturists, teachers... the list goes on and on. For the most part, these people have no idea what they are talking about, and this is mainly because of the ignorance and misinformation about the types of diabetes.

I have been told everything from stop eating ketchup, to only eat egg whites, and that a special honey or cinnamon will "cure" me. The moment a person makes such a suggestion, it is basically over for me, and I will immediately discredit everything they say. Perhaps this is my own personal hang up, but I know that others feel the same way. I do not want this to happen to you or the person who you may help.

People with diabetes are generally wary of advice, even from accredited medical professionals. It is not our fault; even doctors do not fully understand diabetes. I have had doctors tell me all kinds of things, and because they are not endocrinologists, their understanding is limited. Even endocrinologists who are not diabetes specialized may not fully understand the self-care requirements for diabetes.

In general, we feel like unless you are living with it, you can never "fully understand." We may listen to what you have to say, but, at the end of the day, we are going to do what we feel is best. So please keep this in mind in your work with others.

Take your time to build a relationship with your client, and, as you get to know each other more, offer tidbits of advice as they pertain to practice for diabetes. For example, let's say a person comes to you complaining of fatigue from hypoglycemia. You can say, "This is a practice to help you nourish your system and recover after a hypoglycemia episode." If they are more science minded you could say, "This practice will help to down-regulate sympathetic overdrive and encourage parasympathetic activation to promote hormonal balance and reduce allostatic load." But you probably won't say that.

Do not risk being one of the many who make the mistake of assuming what is best or claiming cures. Let us figure out what is right within the trusting mutual framework you create. Asking questions like "What's the hardest thing for you right now with diabetes?"[8] will give you a better chance at getting them to open up about their experience than "What's your A1c?" We want to get a broader picture of what it is like for them to live with diabetes.

Another thing to keep in mind is that if a person takes insulin, anytime they move their body this potentiates insulin in the body, and blood sugar can drop dangerously low. It is the responsibility of the individual to be prepared for hypoglycemia episodes. However, as you will learn in Chapter 9, not all people can sense their lows. Many people have preventative diabetes technology like a CGM to detect the onset of hypoglycemia. But if you are to work with this population, you need to know the warning signs of hypoglycemia. Please review Chapter 9.

You need to understand the risks of hypoglycemia when working with an insulin-dependent population. The timing between a meal with insulin and exercise adds one extra layer of complication for blood sugar management. The closer to a meal a practice is, the higher the likelihood of hypoglycemia because there is active insulin on-board. Fast-acting insulin lasts in the system for three to four hours. An easy way to mitigate hypoglycemia from occurring during a session is to recommend, as you would for all clients, to refrain from eating a large meal within three hours of a yoga therapy session. This way, they will not have active insulin on-board, which decreases the risk of hypoglycemia. Please note that some people will still need to have a light snack and/or reduce their insulin rates before practice.

If a person's levels are consistently falling low and they are unable to make appropriate modifications for their yoga therapy practice, you have some leeway in your suggestions. You could suggest a different time of day for their session, like mid-morning or afternoon when there is less risk of complicating

8 Rubin, R. R. (2009) "Psychotherapy and Counselling in Diabetes Mellitus." In F. J. Snoek and C. T. J. Skinner (eds) *Psychology in Diabetes Care*. Chichester: Wiley & Sons Ltd. p.240.

movement with extra insulin in the system. Ultimately, it is their responsibility. Please just keep it in mind.

We practice yoga sadhana to influence change and shape what is real for us, and this shift is cumulative and gradual.[9] In a world where we expect instant results, it can be easy to fall off the path of practice when avidyā and duḥkha keep popping up. One day, practice may help automatically lower BG, and another day, it has no effect. Today, the anxiety is decreased; tomorrow, it seems stronger than ever. People get disheartened and stop believing in their own power to self-heal. It is plausible that if someone is seeking you out for help with their diabetes, they have tried many things, exhausted their resources, and harbor suspicion when it comes to receiving advice, even if they are coming to you. It is your responsibility as a yoga therapist to educate your client about what you can realistically provide for them if they follow your guidance and how they are ultimately responsible for the benefit that they receive from the practice. I will often tell my clients things like "It works only if you do it," or "Yoga is progressive, not automatic. Be patient."

Sometimes, people want to learn yoga therapy but also take part in various other types of holistic practice. They often have a hard time separating these practices from yoga therapy. To these clients, I suggest that if they want to get the most out of yoga therapy and know if it works for them, they abstain from other methods for at least three months. Three months is an adequate time frame to assess the efficacy of their practice.

If you decide to work with diabetes in yoga therapy, know that there are many elements and there is no such thing as a prescription. Your assessment intake and organization of a personal practice is carefully designed for each individual person, their unique goals, and their constitution. The scope of a yoga therapist is not to diagnose or advise beyond their skillset of yoga therapy. What we can and should focus on are the strengths of yoga therapy in the pillars of diabetes care: energy management, relationships (principally with the self), and emotional health. These are the areas where people receive the least amount of support and where yoga therapy can fill a huge void in their lives. Your role as a yoga therapist is to be an open, compassionate support system so that a person can shine through the conditionality of diabetes. This can be achieved by the invaluable skills of listening, appropriately assessing,

9 Desikachar, T. K. V., Skelton, M. L. and Carter, J. R. (1980) *Religiousness in Yoga: Lectures on Theory and Practice*. Washington DC: University Press of America. p.9.

and providing space for a person to move, breathe, and process without trying to fix anything. Encourage them to trust in their own ability to practice and to use their practice as a way to return hope to a real, lasting support system that is always present within.

CHAPTER 8

Hyperglycemia

Upon the sixth, and I swear the last, time I hit the snooze button, I muster the willpower to pull myself out of bed. Why does it feel like I've been hit by a truck? Glancing at my insulin pump, I see my BG reading is 400 mg/dL (22.2 mmol/L). *Oh, yeah, that's why.*

My mind spins, "What did I do wrong? How could a salad for dinner cause such destruction?" I muddily attempt to retrace my steps from the previous day, to deduce the cause of this unmerited effect, but my mind is cloudy. Plus, there is no time. I've got to get my BG down as soon as possible. I have a life, a job, and responsibilities, after all.

Diabetics like to tell themselves a story, and with good reason—it's happened before. Mine goes like this: "Evan Soroka, yoga therapist and T1D since 1998, has no idea about how to manage diabetes!"

If it's not the story, it's feeling like I am defined by diabetes and always complaining. I've learned that wallowing in guilt will not get you anywhere, but when you're high, emotions also run high.

Holding back tears, I trudge to the kitchen.

Coffee. Black. Dear old, reliable friend. You will stimulate my brain to work again.

But first, I've got to tackle this number.

Over the last 20-odd years of living with T1D, I've learned a thing or two about correcting a long night of hyperglycemia.

Sometimes it works, sometimes it doesn't. But *mostly it* works.

Here's my list.

- Rip out my insulin pump set—perhaps it is not absorbing correctly.
- Take an insulin correction—get it in now!

- Put in a new set.
- Wait and try not to stare at my CGM every minute for the number to budge.
- Abstain from taking more insulin.
- Try not to get low.
- Have that cup of joe. I don't care if it makes my BG spike, I need it.

That's a pretty good list, but it is doing one thing: treating the number. What about me? That number is affecting *me*. The way I feel, the way I think, my sense of wellbeing.

I have a choice. I choose to practice. Almost every part of me says, "No," but there is one part of me, who says, "YES."

After years of work, this voice is louder than the rest. It is just as much a part of me as diabetes. It knows that I always feel better if I only practice.

First, figure out a goal.

BG 400 mg/dL, (22.2 mmol/L) for 6+ hours, no ketones present.

Time available: 30 minutes.

Short-term goal: Increase insulin sensitivity, lower BG level, increase mental clarity, and reduce physical heaviness.

Long-term effect: Sympathetic/parasympathetic balance. I feel better for the rest of my day with increased energy and vigor. Anything else I learn or achieve, like awareness of why I woke up high, is an added bonus.

You'll soon learn about the methods.

What is Hyperglycemia?

The ADA recommends a BG target range for people with diabetes of between 80 and 130 mg/dL (4.4 and 7.2 mmol/L) before meals and less than 180 mg/dL (10.0 mmol/L) two hours after meals.

If you live with diabetes, you'll know how ridiculous that sounds, but, despite your feelings, it is true. Keeping your BG within that range will reduce your risk of complications and help you feel better every day. Staying within the lines is attainable, just not all the time. It's not so much about staying within the lines; it's more about what you do when you are outside of them.

Hyperglycemia is a hyper condition of glucose (sugar) in the bloodstream. Glucose is the primary fuel for our body and especially the brain. Everything we eat turns into glucose—not just sugar and carbohydrates, but also protein and fat. Whenever we eat something, glucose from those nutrients enters the bloodstream and is eventually metabolized. Unless glucose has a guide to transport it, it remains in the bloodstream, damaging the blood vessels and not fulfilling its dharma of providing fast-acting energy. This is where insulin gets involved. Insulin is a hormone produced by the beta cells of the pancreas, guiding glucose to its home—in the cells, the brain, or even the liver for storage. Without insulin, glucose stays in the bloodstream, and the body cannot use it for energy.

In normal non-diabetic physiology, the pancreas is always making a small amount of insulin to maintain glycemic levels. When a person eats, the pancreas releases even more insulin, and it knows how much to dose to cover the amount of glucose or energy in the food. The pancreas also knows when to turn off insulin production when BG levels drop too low, something you'll learn more about in Chapter 9. These mechanisms work synergistically to maintain glucose homeostasis.

Everyone can experience high blood sugars, even without diabetes. BG levels rise after a large meal and under times of prolonged stress. They just don't rise too high and don't stay high for too long. When they do, this is an indicator of prediabetes.

Diabetes is the inability to use insulin effectively, the result being hyperglycemia. Without sufficient insulin, produced by the beta cells of the pancreas, glucose has nowhere to go. It stays in the bloodstream and eventually damages the blood vessels. This is why diabetes affects so many organ systems of the body, causes other illnesses like retinopathy and cardiovascular disease, and will ultimately kill you. The reasons behind hyperglycemia in T1D versus T2D are the very distinctions between the disorders. T1D is the relative absence of insulin. People with this condition produce very little, if any, insulin and are required to inject it. T2D is both insufficient insulin production and insulin resistance. Some people with T2D can manage diabetes with just diet and exercise adjustments; others need to take some form of medication to help their bodies use insulin better.

The Many Faces of Hyperglycemia

Insulin Resistance

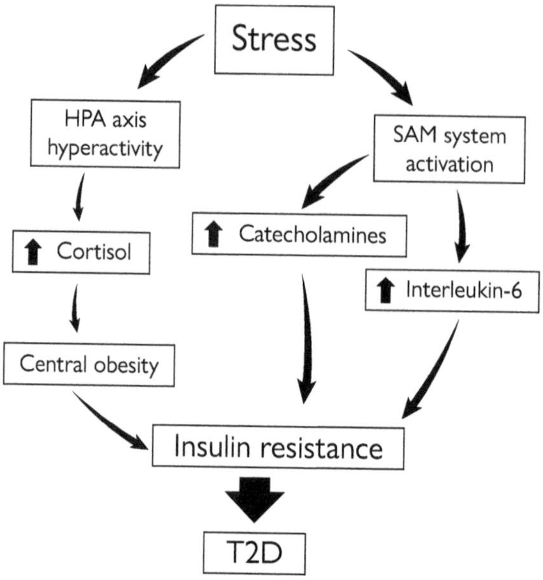

FIGURE 8.1

We need insulin to survive. Every creature on earth produces insulin, and without it you will die within a few months. Whether we are producing insulin on our own or injecting it, we need our insulin to work effectively. But sometimes it doesn't, and this is a big problem in managing diabetes, especially when we are looking at reducing hyperglycemia. To limit hyperglycemia, we need to first address insulin resistance, as it is a critical factor in why people with diabetes and prediabetes have high blood sugars.

When there is insulin resistance, there is hyperglycemia. When there is hyperglycemia, there is insulin resistance.

Insulin resistance occurs when insulin's effectiveness is reduced, meaning more and more insulin is required to transport glucose from the blood into the liver, muscle fat, and other cells.[1] Think of it like this: your cells want to absorb glucose from the bloodstream for energy but, for whatever reason, they cannot utilize insulin properly. Despite the presence of insulin, the body's cells fail to recognize it, glucose remains in the bloodstream, and you need more and more insulin to do the job.

---

1 Bernstein, R. K. (2011) *Dr. Bernstein's Diabetes Solution: The Complete Guide to Achieving Normal Blood Sugars*. Fourth edition. Boston, MA: Little Brown Publishers. p.100.

The cause of insulin resistance is multifactorial and complex. Still, the basic premise is that quality of food, amount of food, energy expenditure, and stress levels all play a role in how well your body can use insulin. Think of it like this: the more you ask your body to digest without giving it any help like eating less food or exercising, the higher the metabolic demand. Over time, that digestive fire we spoke of, *agni*, fizzles out. The body never gets a break from all the energy it is putting into just keeping you in balance; it produces more insulin (or you inject more of it if you have T1D). The glucose remains in the bloodstream, damaging your blood vessels and setting you up for the effects of uncontrolled diabetes.

There are a few ways to reduce insulin resistance and increase insulin sensitivity: eat less, move more, and manage stress levels.

When there is less pressure on the body to metabolize food, the insulin, either produced or injected, works better and faster, and you need less of it. This makes metabolic control easier, there are fewer blood sugar swings, and digestion is better. Taking less insulin and potentiating the existing insulin helps take out additional variables in maintaining glycemic control.

T2D is a disease of insulin resistance. People with T2D have a tired pancreas and not enough insulin to cover energetic demand. BG rises due to increased metabolic demand, the pancreas produces more insulin, and the increased insulin in circulation is blocked because of insulin resistance. A goal for people with T2D is to eat less and exercise more—give their pancreas a chance to rest and catch up. Improving insulin sensitivity by reducing insulin resistance will help to lower BG levels and potentiate the insulin that their body already produces.

Whether the cause is behavioral (lifestyle and diet), genetic, or both, a person becomes susceptible to prediabetes and T2D when their fasting blood sugar is higher than 126 mg/dL (7.0 mmol/L) on average.[2] Higher blood sugar levels increase the demand and production of insulin production. Cells get used to having so much insulin around that they need more and more of it to absorb glucose. The cells resist the insulin, blood sugars stay higher, more insulin is required to lower blood sugar, and the pancreas exhausts its insulin production.

The treatment of T2D involves reducing the demand for insulin production and increasing insulin sensitivity so that the insulin produced by the pancreas is utilized efficiently. Sometimes, adjusting diet and increasing exercise is

2 Mayo Clinic (2020) "Prediabetes." *Mayo Clinic*. Accessed on 10/11/20 at: https://www.mayoclinic.org/diseases-conditions/prediabetes/diagnosis-treatment/drc-20355284.

not sufficient. People need to take medications to help them reduce insulin resistance. Some people with longer-duration T2D need to take insulin as well.

T1D is not caused by insulin resistance, but people with this can also experience insulin resistance. It is kind of like a double whammy. You can't make insulin, and the insulin you inject is not properly utilized. It makes the management of T1D extra complicated. The less insulin that someone with T1D needs to correct a high BG reading or to cover a meal, the better. This does not mean that insulin is the enemy, just that we want to potentiate its effect. When we can achieve this, there is less variability in BG swings.

Similar to T2D, insulin resistance in T1D is caused by high blood sugars. *The longer the duration of prolonged hyperglycemia, the higher the insulin resistance.* A person who has been running 300 mg/dL (16.7 mmol/L) all night will need much more insulin to bring their BG down than someone with a reading of 300 mg/dL (16.7 mmol/L) after a meal or intense exercise. When you are insulin resistant with T1D and correct with an injection, it is essential to exercise patience and caution.

Postprandial Hyperglycemia

Keeping BG under tight control is important in the short term to help the person feel better and the long term to avoid the complications from a lifetime of hyperglycemia. Both T1D and T2D cause postprandial spikes, but T1D requires quite a bit of extra math and timing. An area where most people with diabetes can make an improvement is by reducing the post-meal (postprandial) BG spike. This is the rate of BG deviation after a meal. According to the ADA, postprandial hyperglycemia is the main unmet need in both T1D and T2D, and it becomes more difficult to control over time.[3] Without diabetes, a postprandial number should go no higher than 140 mg/dL (7.8 mmol/L), two hours after a meal; anything higher than that may indicate prediabetes.[4] With both T1D and T2D, the ADA recommends a postprandial number (up to two hours after a meal) no higher than 180 mg/dL (10 mmol/L) to avoid long-term diabetes complications.

Even when a person achieves optimal A1c numbers on paper (under 7.0%),

3 Riddle, M. C. (2017) "Basal glucose can be controlled, but the prandial problem persists—it's the next target!" *Diabetes Care 40*, 3, 291–300.

4 Riddle, M. C. (2017) "Basal glucose can be controlled, but the prandial problem persists—it's the next target!" *Diabetes Care 40*, 3, 291–300.

postprandial spikes increase the chances of long-term health complications like cardiovascular disease. A recent study showed that postprandial BG numbers are a better predictor of A1c than fasting numbers alone.[5] Other studies show that targeting postprandial glucose reduced cardiovascular disease in T2D, unlike HbA1c and fasting glucose alone.[6] This very study prompted the European Diabetes Policy Group to recommend postprandial glucose levels of 160 mg/dL (8.9 mmol/L) in diabetes to reduce cardiovascular risk, the number one cause of mortality in T1D and T2D.[7]

The moment that I began to pay attention to my postprandial numbers, my A1c dramatically improved. If it were not for a CGM, I may never have become aware of the fluctuations in my levels after eating. The benefit of seeing the trends in my numbers in real time helped me make more appropriate decisions with regard to insulin administration timing to avoid a spike and the implementation of specialized intervention strategies if my BG is spiking, to reduce and nullify the rate of increase. Achieving postprandial numbers under 160 mg/dL (7.8 mmol/L) is challenging but not impossible. It requires quite a bit of self-control and preparation, but if people follow the recommended behavioral steps, they can reduce them.

The biggest barrier to tight postprandial numbers in T1D is the timing of insulin relative to food consumption. When food is digested faster than insulin's activation time, glucose levels will elevate before they stabilize. A longer duration of diabetes slows down the stomach's release of food, adding another level of complication to the timing of food to insulin. It takes about ten minutes for a dietary carbohydrate to have an effect on BG levels and about 15–20 minutes for fast-acting insulin to start working.[8] But this varies from individual to individual, depending on duration of disease, BMI, and insulin sensitivity. In T1D, postprandial hyperglycemia is managed by adjusting the time of insulin to food, which is called "pre-bolusing." For instance, if most short-acting insulin starts working in 15–20 minutes, it would be advantageous

5 Ketema, E. B. and Kibret, K. T. (2015) "Correlation of fasting and postprandial plasma glucose with HbA1c in assessing glycemic control: systematic review and meta-analysis." *Archives of Public Health 73*, 43.

6 Bonora, E. (2002) "Postprandial peaks as a risk factor for cardiovascular disease: epidemiological perspectives." *International Journal of Clinical Practice, Supplement 129*, 5–11.

7 Cosentino, F., Grant, P. J., Aboyans, V., Bailey, C. J., *et al.* (2020) "2019 ESC Guidelines on diabetes, pre-diabetes, and cardiovascular diseases developed in collaboration with the EASD." *European Heart Journal 41*, 2, 255–323.

8 American Diabetes Association (2001) "Postprandial blood glucose." *Diabetes Care 24*, 4, 775–778.

to take insulin before you start eating, so that the insulin kicks in just as the body begins to digest the food. Sometimes this works well, and other times not so well. There are so many variables that can disrupt the efficacy of the equation. A great intermediary strategy if a person notices that their BG is spiking after a meal is to go for a short walk, do some squats, or complete a brief yoga therapy intervention practice.

Diabetic Ketoacidosis (DKA)

Ketoacidosis is a dangerous and deadly condition defined by the absence of insulin and the presence of a highly acidic protein called a ketone. *This is not to be confused with ketosis.*

The body predominantly runs on glucose and without insulin it cannot metabolize glucose, so it instead relies on fatty acids for energy. Ketones are the by-product of fatty acids. DKA happens with severe and persistent hyperglycemia, where too many ketones build up and poison the body. An effect is uncontrollable vomiting, causing severe dehydration and death.

If a person is experiencing severe hypoglycemia, it is recommended that they are tested for ketones (you can easily purchase the strips at the pharmacy). If ketones are present, people need to mindful of being rested, hydrate with electrolytes, and make sure that they are getting adequate insulin.

Severity and Duration

When you live with diabetes, you know that not all hyperglycemia is the same. The longer the duration and severity of hyperglycemia, the higher the risk for conditions like insulin resistance and DKA.

You can experience acute and severe hyperglycemia for short or long durations. For instance, a postprandial reading of 200 mg/dL (11 mmol/L) two hours after a meal is different than a reading of 200 mg/dL (11 mmol/L) all night long or over the duration of several days. Each will affect a person's energetic condition distinctly. A short period of a mild hyperglycemia episode probably won't have that much of an effect on a person, but a long time spent at 200 mg/dL (11 mmol/L) will.

Whenever I am correcting for highs and determining a supportive practice, I consider the severity and duration. I cannot give exact numbers for what constitutes severe, mild, acute, and chronic as they differ from person to person, and are affected by the type of diabetes and other circumstances.

I can tell you what it means for me:

- 190–275 mg/dL (10.6–15.3 mmol/L): mild
- >275 mg/dL (>15.3 mmol/L): severe
- 2–4 hours: acute
- 4+ hours: chronic.

Variables of Hyperglycemia

Hyperglycemia is caused by myriads of reasons—some caused by human error and others that are no fault of our own. I want to mention them because the ability to identify the cause of hyperglycemia is just as important as the ability to avoid it altogether. Some are due to human calculation error and others from outside contributing factors. The ability to identify, preempt, and mitigate the time spent in hyperglycemia is essential for the reduction of diabetes complications and improvement in quality of life.

- Insufficient insulin
- Incorrect timing of insulin to food
- Too much food
- Caffeine (I take 1 unit of fast-acting insulin with black coffee)
- Postprandial high (timing)
- Less exercise than planned
- Hormones
- Somogyi effect (also known as the "dawn phenomenon," this is a release of stored glucose by the liver during the early hours of the morning. This occurs in all people when they are preparing for the day; however, it can cause hyperglycemia with diabetes)
- Insulin resistance

- Stress/anxiety
- Exercise
- Gastroparesis
- Illness
- Medications (like cortisone)
- Malabsorption
- Faulty equipment
- Stale or compromised insulin
- Dehydration
- Divine intervention (when we have no idea)

Symptoms of Hyperglycemia

For the most part, mild hyperglycemia is undetectable and has few to no symptoms. This is why so many people who have *prediabetes* are unaware of it. The symptoms and noticeable effects of hyperglycemia occur at around 180–200 mg/dL (10–11 mmol/L) and vary from person to person. The most common symptoms of hyperglycemia are excessive urination and extreme thirst, although these also vary, just as the acute symptoms do. It is important to identify symptoms, as they can be potential markers of undiagnosed diabetes and can help people who are living with diabetes to be more aware of their own BG fluctuations and treat them accordingly. I really pride myself on my ability to sense my blood sugar going high before my CGM registers it, or awakening in the middle of the night before an alarm goes off. This gives me a leg up on the technology and I can treat highs when they occur. And they will occur; they always do: I have diabetes.

You'll notice that many of the symptoms of hyperglycemia are similar to hypoglycemia, but I can tell you from lived experience that the fatigue from hyperglycemia is distinct from the fatigue from hypoglycemia.

Symptoms

- Dry mouth and throat
- Thirst
- Need to urinate
- Stomach pain
- Nausea
- Vomiting
- Weakness
- Blurred vision
- Headache
- Tingling/pain in extremities
- Fatigue and lethargy
- Mental confusion
- Alert and energized
- Sadness

Long-Term Complications

- Cardiovascular disease
- Alzheimer's disease
- Obesity
- Stroke
- Neuropathy
- Retinopathy
- Death

The Multidimensionality of Hyperglycemia

Hyperglycemia impacts the whole person.

Physical

The effects of hyperglycemia impact life function in both the short and long term. If my BG is high today, I might not feel that great or I may lack the energy I need to show up for my life in the way that I would if my BG was normal. Over the longer duration of the disease, hyperglycemia damages blood vessels, organ systems, and the function of our ANS. Hyperglycemia also damages the endogenous (self-produced) production of insulin. When I was diagnosed in 1998, my BG was severely raised and had been for a long time. My *endogenous* insulin production was exhausted. But some people with T1D, and most with type 2, can maintain some level of insulin production by preventing hyperglycemia. This really helps because then you need less insulin and blood sugars don't swing so violently.

Mental/Emotional

It is incredibly stressful to maintain the recommended BG range of 80–180 mg/dL (4.4–10.0 mmol/L). As people living with diabetes, we are taught to keep our numbers within this tight threshold or suffer the consequences of uncontrolled diabetes, but everyone's BG numbers fluctuate—even without diabetes. It can seem like an impossible goal and can be a source of tension. For the hypervigilant personality, it can create control and anxiety issues. For the avoidant personality, failure to maintain the BG range can perpetuate negative emotions like defeatism and guilt.

The added burden of testing and monitoring BG levels can feel like a full-time job, something that people eschew by ignoring the issue altogether. Eating out, being on the move, and living in the moment are not always conducive to diabetes self-care. However, by applying some simple awareness protocols, and reducing the anxiety and aversion prevalent in diabetes care issues, people can really take charge of their post-meal spikes. By improving their time spent in range, people can assuage the short-term effects of hyperglycemia and positively improve their A1c.

Beyond Diabetes (Spirit)

Hyperglycemia, like any challenge of diabetes, is duḥkha, the experience of avidyā. On the one hand, hyperglycemia is real. Its occurrence damages the nervous system and organs and can eventually cost a person their life if left unmanaged. On the other hand, hyperglycemia is not real. Controversial as it may sound, the effects of hyperglycemia like emotionalism, lethargy, and sensory and mental dullness are the lived experience of avidyā as dukha. Although hyperglycemia is real, it is easy to identify with the experience of hyperglycemia and allow it to sway thoughts, emotions, and actions, perpetuating the incorrect belief that "I am" diabetes.

The goal of yoga therapy is to feel better; practicing for hypers is about not only treating the high, but also reducing its short- and long-term effect on a person's wellbeing. It is also about looking at hyperglycemia objectively as something that is occurring but is not who you are. By creating the subject–object meditative awareness, one can look at a number but not be the number. They can take care of the high BG by correcting it without getting caught up in the cycle of avidyā and dukha.

Reducing actual and perceived suffering means people will be more resilient to hyperglycemia risks. Hyperglycemia happens to everyone with diabetes, and its incidence does not signify uncontrolled diabetes. Small intervention strategies address the effects of hyperglycemia and support the direction of physiological change. This could be avoiding a high by implementing a technique or changing a behavior, curtailing the time above 180 mg/dL (10 mmol/L) and reducing the cognitive and sensory effects that deter life function.

Yoga and Hyperglycemia Research

Most of the yoga for diabetes research has been conducted on people with T2D. I still cannot find a reason why but can only surmise that the population size of people with T2D is substantial compared with that of those with T1D. The argument that researchers posit is that T1D is caused by genetic and environmental factors, while T2D is more varied and is related to modifiable behavioral adaptations. It seems like the effects of yoga on hyperglycemia is a more challenging metric to evaluate because of the relative absence of insulin production. Either way, the statistics are of interest in terms of the implications of yoga as a viable and cost-effective treatment for all types of diabetes.

Twenty-five studies evaluated the effects of yoga with T2D glucose markers, with yogic intervention ranging from 8 days to 12 months.[9] The effects include decreased BG,[10] A1c levels,[11] and postprandial glucose[12] and results showed an improvement in fasting BG levels.[13] A decrease in fasting insulin levels, rise in insulin receptors (where insulin attaches to the cell), and increase in percentage of receptor binding (even before glycemic control) suggests decreased insulin

---

9 Innes, K. E. and Vincent, H. K. (2007) "The influence of yoga-based programs on risk profiles in adults with type 2 diabetes mellitus: a systematic review." *Evidence-Based Complementary and Alternative Medicine 4*, 469–486.

10 Gordon, L. A., Morrison, E. Y., McGrowder, D. A., Young, R., *et al.* (2008) "Effect of exercise therapy on lipid profile and oxidative stress indicators in patients with type 2 diabetes." *BMC Complementary and Alternative Medicine 8*, 21.

11 Khatri, D., Mathur, K. C., Gahlot, S., Jain, S. and Agrawal, R. P. (2007) "Effects of yoga and meditation on clinical and biochemical parameters of metabolic syndrome." *Diabetes Research and Clinical Practice 78*, e9–10.

12 Innes, K. E. (2016) "Yoga Therapy for Diabetes." In S. B. S. Khalsa, L. Cohen, T. McCall and S. Telles (eds) *The Principles and Practice of Yoga in Healthcare*. Pencaitland: Handspring Publishing. p.213.

13 Jain, S. C., Uppal, A., Bhatnagar, S. O. and Talukdar, B. (1993) "A study of response pattern of non-insulin dependent diabetes to yoga therapy." *Diabetes Research and Clinical Practice 19*, 69–74.

resistance and improved sensitivity.[14, 15, 16] Stability in insulin requirements and a reduction in dosage of oral hypoglycemic drugs over time have been observed in type 2 diabetics,[17, 18] displaying yoga as a viable intervention and maintenance strategy for reducing insulin-resistant hyperglycemia. There have been reports of weight loss, decrease in body mass index and waist-hip ratio, stress reduction, and improvement in mood, self-efficacy, and quality-of-life,[19, 20] all contributing factors in hyperglycemia. While these studies are limited to T2D, they are of interest for T1D, because even though the cause and treatment of these two types differ, the physiological effects and long-term cost of unmanaged hyperglycemia are similar.

Yoga nidrā, guided relaxation techniques, meditation, and prāṇāyāma are all yogic tools that contribute to the reduction of long-term hyperglycemia. The implication is that yoga, as a cost-effective method to reduce stress by regulating the HPA axis and restoring ANS function, is a viable approach to improving metabolic control (therefore reducing hyperglycemia) for all types of diabetes. As well as enabling the reduction of oral hypoglycemia medications and insulin, yoga can be considered a cost-effective and complementary therapy that delays the progression of the disease process.[21]

---

14 Sahay, B. K. (2007) "Role of yoga in diabetes." *Journal of the Association of Physicians of India 55*, 121–126.

15 Sahay, B. K. and Sahay, R. (2010) "Lifestyle modification and yoga in prevention of diabetes in India. How far have we come?" *Med Update 20*, 142–146.

16 Gordon, L., Morrison, E. Y., McGrowder, D., Penas, Y. F., *et al.* (2008) "Effect of yoga and traditional physical exercise on hormones and percentage insulin receptor binding in patients with type 2 diabetes." *American Journal of Biochemistry and Biotechnology 4*, 35–42.

17 Jain, S. C., Uppal, A., Bhatnagar, S. O. and Talukdar, B. (1993) "A study of response pattern of non-insulin dependent diabetes to yoga therapy." *Diabetes Research and Clinical Practice 19*, 69–74.

18 Kerr, D., Gillam, E., Ryder, J., Trowbridge, S., Cavan, D. and Thomas, P. (2002) "An Eastern art form for a Western disease: randomized controlled trials of yoga in patients with poorly controlled insulin treated diabetes." *Practical Diabetes International 19*, 164–166.

19 Yang, K. (2007) "A review of yoga programs for four leading risk factors of chronic diseases." *Evidence-Based Complementary and Alternative Medicine 4*, 487–491.

20 Balaji, P. A., Varne, S. R. and Ali, S. S. (2011) "Effect of yoga prāṇāyāma practices on metabolic parameters and anthropometry in type 2 diabetes." *International Multidisciplinary Research Journal 1*, 1–4.

21 Singh, S., Singh, K. P., Tandon, O. P. and Madhu, S. V. (2008) "Influence of prāṇāyāmas and yoga asanas on serum insulin, blood glucose and lipid profile in type 2 diabetes." *Indian Journal of Clinical Biochemistry 23*, 365–368.

General Strategies for Reducing Hyperglycemia

Exercise

If we are looking at hyperglycemia as just a number, exercise is the main intervention and prevention strategy. It is the quickest and most effective way to bring blood sugars down by increasing insulin sensitivity and glucose metabolism. Any kind of movement will help the body metabolize glucose and absorb insulin: walking, shopping, and cleaning the house are all effective methods although not necessarily classified as "working out." Movement is one of the most important self-care strategies to maintain healthy metabolic control. Exercise reduces insulin resistance and can help to potentiate the effect of insulin when BG is high by burning up excess sugar and helping insulin move into the cells.

Exercise counteracts hyperglycemia by potentiating the effect of insulin and reducing insulin resistance as both a short-term intervention strategy and long-term maintenance strategy. People with both types of diabetes are encouraged to exercise regularly to manage BG levels. There's a reason why so many people with diabetes rely on exercise as an important and essential intervention strategy for lowering spiking numbers and improving metabolic control: it really works. But exercise addresses just one layer of hyperglycemia.

Hyperglycemia influences everything from a person's muscles and organ function to the sharpness of their mind and perception of stress. It is true that if we are just looking at diabetes as a number, exercise is an excellent strategy. But it fails to address some of the energetic effects of hyperglycemia and behavioral ramifications of why people have high blood sugars with diabetes. We will now delve a little deeper into hypoglycemia to consider how to empower the whole person.

Red flag: Too much insulin with exercise can be a dangerous variable. As exercise potentiates insulin, people have to be careful not to exercise too much when treating a high BG level because the level will get low. People with T1D have to administer a correction dose to lower BG, but if they exercise intensely on top of that correction, their numbers will crash. Severe lows are dangerous and can cause a rebound effect where a person ends up high again. It is a vicious cycle that should be avoided at all costs, because once it starts, it takes a lot of work and patience to get out of it.

Yoga āsana is a good way to recover from hyperglycemia because its duration and intensity can be adjusted. Breathing offers another layer of benefit in regulating sympathetic overactivation and supporting cognitive and sensory awareness. If I am running at 250 mg/dL (13.9 mmol/L) and take my usual correction shot and then go to practice hot power vinyāsa flow for 75 minutes, the result will be different from that of a 75-minute hatha practice in a non-heated room.

The truth of the matter is that it does not take a lot to get a big result. Just 15 minutes of dynamic movement and increasing heart rate is typically all that I need to wake things up and start to see an arrow moving down. This is why I like using short yoga therapy interventions. They are more manageable, and if the goal is to directly impact BG levels within a short period of time, they can be extremely effective at reducing a spike.

Stress Reduction

The stress response mediated by the ANS and HPA axis elevates blood sugar levels as part of our evolutionary biology. The persistent activation, i.e. chronic stress, continually elevates BG levels and can be a contributing factor in the development of T2D; interestingly, these very pathways contribute to the challenge of managing diabetes, because of insulin resistance.

Diabetes complications as a result of hyperglycemia are associated with an overactive and defective sympathetic response creating both sympathetic overdrive and HPA axis dysfunction, as well as damage to the vagus nerve, the mediator of parasympathetic activation.

The parasympathetic ANS mediates the secretion of endogenous insulin, and any damage to its function can also lead to a decrease in the hypoglycemia effect of insulin (i.e. insulin resistance). In addition, the ANS is recognized as being a major modulator of postprandial glucose metabolism,[22, 23] and any disruptions to its function impact insulin action, the contributing causes of prediabetes and T2D, and the very mechanisms that challenge people with insulin-dependent T1D, insulin resistance. In particular, vagal tone impairment has been shown to be the leading cause of autonomic dysfunction.[24]

---

22 Kalsbeek, A., Bruinstroop, E., Yi, C. X., Klieverik, L. P., La Fleur, S. E. and Fliers, E. (2010) "Hypothalamic control of energy metabolism via the autonomic nervous system." *Annals of the New York Academy of Sciences 1212*, 114–129.

23 Greenfield, J. R. and Campbell, L. V. (2008) "Role of the autonomic nervous system and neuropeptides in the development of obesity in humans: targets for therapy?" *Current Pharmaceutical Design 14*, 18, 1815–1820.

24 Macedo, M. P., Lima, I. S., Gaspar, J. M., Afonso, R. A., *et al.* (2014) "Risk of postprandial insulin resistance: the liver/vagus rapport." *Reviews in Endocrine and Metabolic Disorders 15*, 1, 67–77.

Given the fact that hyperglycemia damages the very mechanisms that help to regulate and reduce hyperglycemia, it is in the interest of the practitioner to recognize the physiological symptoms of hyperglycemia as sympathetic overdrive. This is important to note, and a little confusing when you see the role of the sympathetic response in hypoglycemia. However, both are products of the same mechanism: bring BG levels up. Yoga is one of the few ways that we can voluntarily activate the parasympathetic branch of the ANS, and regularly doing so could potentially be a viable modulator of hyperglycemia's impact on the continued destruction of autonomic function. Yoga may reduce the stress, improve metabolic profile, regulate the ANS, and alter the HPA axis, which acts as the neural mediator of hyperglycemia.[25]

Imbalances in the ANS and HPA axis cause insulin resistance, and insulin resistance as hyperglycemia in diagnosed diabetes continues to damage and accelerate the damage to the CNS. By working with our stress response through yoga-based interventions, we are addressing not only hyperglycemia as a condition, but also the very causes behind hyperglycemia itself.

Diet

The quality and quantity of the food that we put into our bodies is undoubtedly a contributing factor to hyperglycemia. I have many opinions about this and have tried many things—experimenting with what is best for me as an active woman in her 30s who has lived with an autoimmune condition for the majority of her life. Perhaps this will be a topic for another book one day. For the moment, all I have to say is based on what Āyurveda recommends. Eat a healthy, nutritious diet. Keep one third of your stomach for food, one third for water, and one third empty. Pay attention to your digestion and how much you are eating at night.

Behavioral Modifications

A lot of preparation and foresight is needed to avoid the onset of and correct existing hypoglycemia. The more a person is in tune with their body, the better they can fine-tune this process. It is not exact or replicable. So much goes into

25 Mahajan, A. S. (2014) "Role of yoga in hormonal homeostasis." *International Journal of Clinical and Experimental Physiology* 1, 3, 173–178. Accessed on 01/07/20 at: www.ijcep.org/index.php/ijcep/article/view/109.

avoiding hyperglycemia, and when people fail, it is common to hold on to negative emotions about diabetes and/or themselves.

Process of Deduction

There is active behind-the-scenes work a person can do to bring their BG down. Sift through the potential causes of hyperglycemia from dehydration (a common and often over-looked one) to hormones. Once a cause has been inferred, apply behavioral changes to support a change in BG levels. In the case of dehydration I will add an electrolyte to my water. If it is hormonal or an infection, I may increase my rate of insulin, take insulin sooner, and eat simple, easy-to-digest food. This process of deduction is fun (it can be!) and promotes a stronger relationship with diabetes empowerment: self-awareness, self-regulation, self-efficiency, and self-mastery.

Checklist

1. See the number, register it, and scan back in your memory. Is there an obvious reason why you are high? For example, food, insulin, exercise, infection, dehydration, faulty diabetes equipment, a dirty test finger, hormonal cycle, stress, etc.
2. Confirm the number by testing your BG another time or with a different machine.
3. Do you have any insulin on-board (IOB). If so, is it enough to bring your BG down if you wait?
4. How long have you been high? A high BG reading after a meal is different than an all-night high, which will increase insulin resistance.
5. Is there a correlation? Have you experienced a similar pattern before? For instance, I love Brazilian cheese bread, but every time I eat it, I am high several hours later. I have tried taking more insulin, or even changing the way that I take insulin (less upfront, more on the backend), but still cannot avoid the spike. So I limit it or even avoid it.
6. What can you do right now? For example, inject, change your pump set, drink a glass of water with electrolytes, take a ten-minute walk.

7. Regulate your emotions. Recognize that negative thinking about a high BG level will not change anything. If the high is due to your choices in food, commit to not eating the thing that spikes your BG. If the cause is unknown, remember that even "good" diabetics experience high BG. Apply what you can to help bring your sugars back down, practice a short yoga therapy routine, and move on.

Yoga Therapy for Hyperglycemia Practices

My intention for this section is for it to be a menu of comprehensive intervention strategies that address the main challenges that diabetics face with correcting hyperglycemia and recovering from its effects. The long-term benefit of these practices could support improved glycemic control and potentially reduce the cumulative damage of hyperglycemia, which is the cause of so many diabetes complications and, ultimately, detrimental to the quality of a person's life.

Although the goal is to address hyperglycemia, which is an easy metric to observe before and after practice, I encourage people to look beyond the number. How does a person feel afterwards? Do they have more energy? Can they go about their day with more clarity and focus? Do they feel more capable and empowered? Lastly, does the practice provide some level of self-awareness about the causes of and contributing factors in hyperglycemia?

These yoga therapy practices take into consideration the short- and long-term effects of hyperglycemia and that both have physiological and psychological ramifications within each person.

I have outlined three main practice strategies for hyperglycemia. They are beneficial for all types of diabetics and modifiable depending on individual needs and circumstances. For people living with T1D, all three practices are valuable intervention strategies. For people living with T2D, the first practice, which focuses on insulin resistance, is the most applicable as a general maintenance strategy. The practices have the following aims.

1. A general practice for hyperglycemia: reduce insulin resistance and increase insulin sensitivity.
2. Postprandial spike: nip it in the bud.
3. Severe hyperglycemia (over 300 mg/dL, 16.7 mmol/L): recover and move on.

Hyperglycemia (Insulin Resistance)

Hyperglycemia is a hyper condition of glucose in the bloodstream. The primary goal is to metabolize excess glucose and decrease the sensory and cognitive effects of high blood sugar. The long-term goal is to reduce further damage to the ANS and HPA axis, which act to modulate hyperglycemia, and improve life function through the principles of *empowered diabetes resilience.*

Sequencing from the energetic principles of yoga therapy, I recommend a laṅghana (reducing) and shodhana (purifying) orientation for practice, and I will explain why.

Insulin-resistant hyperglycemia is partly a kapha vitiation with a predominance of tamo-guṇa. Like kapha doṣa, the quality of hyperglycemia is heavy and sticky. The effect on the brain is similarly tamasic, represented by sensory and cognitive dullness. Sluggish insulin absorption is blocking (like kapha), and inhibits insulin from attaching itself to the receptor sites and entering the cells from the bloodstream. For this, we want to stimulate, activate, and encourage the elimination of excess sugar by utilizing it through exercise.

We can achieve this through standing āsanas, which emphasize larger-class muscles that require more energy and therefore burn more glucose. Dynamic movements like Sūrya Namaskār A and B can also be applied (if appropriate) to help the muscles metabolize the sugar.[26]

Paradoxically, insulin-resistant hyperglycemia can be caused by sympathetic overdrive. To balance this rajasic orientation, a calming, laṅghana practice is recommended. We can achieve this by lengthening exhale in āsana, including gentle rotation, and using a laṅghana prāṇāyāma practice.

This is where the art and science of yoga therapy converge. The practice begins with movement (a more stimulating orientation) to encourage the muscles to utilize glucose from the bloodstream, decrease sensory and mental dullness, and move progressively towards a laṅghana orientation to calm sympathetic overdrive by moving towards parasympathetic predominance.

A Practice for Hyperglycemia (Insulin Resistance)

Primary goals: Eliminate excess glucose by utilizing it through exercise. Stimulate cognitive function and activate sensory awareness. Create a calming

26 A reason why a person with T1D may practice this is to bring the BG down after a correction bolus (insulin). They can fine-tune the intensity and duration of the practice to avoid hyperglycemia. If there is insulin resistance, many people with T1D take too much correction because their BG won't budge. Please caution people on how much of the "exercise" portion of this practice is needed.

after-effect that will promote sympathetic/parasympathetic balance to help a person recover and reduce the impact of hyperglycemia on the ANS.

Method: A *purifying/stimulating* orientation with standing postures that activate large-class muscles, and vinyāsa flow if applicable to the practitioner. Next, move into laṅghana (calming/reducing) orientation with gentle forward bends and twists to progressively lengthen the exhale.

Prāṇāyāma: This practice has two short prāṇāyāma sequences to stimulate and calm. Begin the practice with 12 rounds of viloma ujjāyī to stimulate and activate the body. End with alternate nostril exhale to calm and soothe through the parasympathetic response.

1	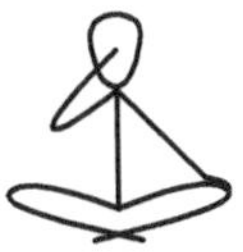	**Viloma ujjāyī:** Alternate nostril inhale, ujjāyī exhale. To stimulate and activate the nervous system.	Sit in a comfortable position and exhale completely. Lift the right hand, close the right nostril with the thumb, and valve the left nostril with the ring finger. Inhale: Left nostril, then lower the right hand. Exhale: Ujjāyī glottal contraction. Lift the right hand, close the left nostril with the ring finger, valve the right nostril with the thumb. Inhale: Right nostril, then lower the right hand. Exhale: Ujjāyī glottal contraction. Repeat six times (total of 12 breaths). *On inhale, expand the chest.*
2	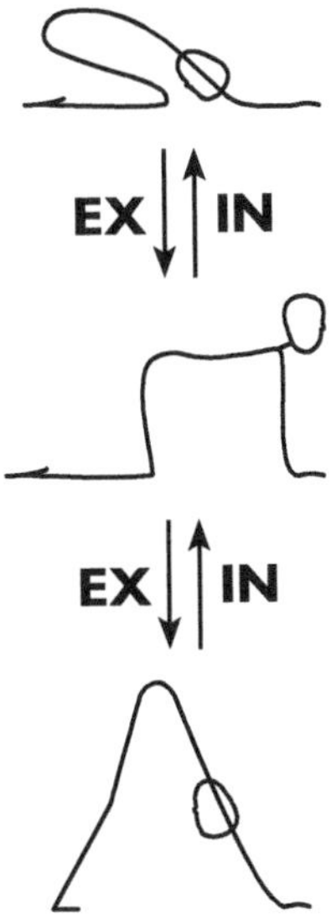	**Cakravākāsana and Adho Mukha Śvānāsana combo:** To warm up the major muscles of the body.	Start in kneeling position with the abdomen on the thighs, and arms extended in front. Inhale: Traction the hands against the ground and lift the body up to all fours, stacking the shoulders over the wrists and the knees over the hips, lengthen the front of the body. Exhale: Press into the hands, lift the knees off the ground, push the hips up and back, lengthen the spine. Inhale: Return to hands and knees. Exhale: Draw the hips back to the heels, bend the elbows lowering the torso to the thighs, returning to the starting position. Repeat four times, lengthening both inhale and exhale.

3	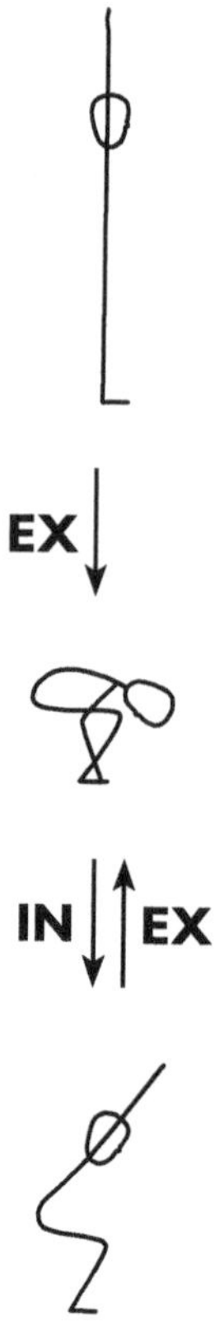	**Ardha Utkaṭāsana and Utkaṭāsana combo:** To strengthen and activate major muscles.	Stand with the feet hip-width apart and arms overhead. Exhale: Sit the hips back, bring the torso to the thighs and the hands on the ground by the sides of the feet. The hips should be just slightly higher than the knees. Inhale: Lift into Utkaṭāsana, keeping the hips low, lift the torso away from the thighs, extend the arms overhead. Encourage the torso to lift as far from the thighs as possible. Exhale: Lower the hands back to the ground, keeping the knees bent (repeat each hold before straightening the legs completely). Repeat six times, moving in and out of Utkaṭāsana/Ardha Utkaṭāsana, before straightening the legs and returning to the starting position. Lengthen the inhale: Four seconds, twice; six seconds, twice; eight seconds, twice.
4	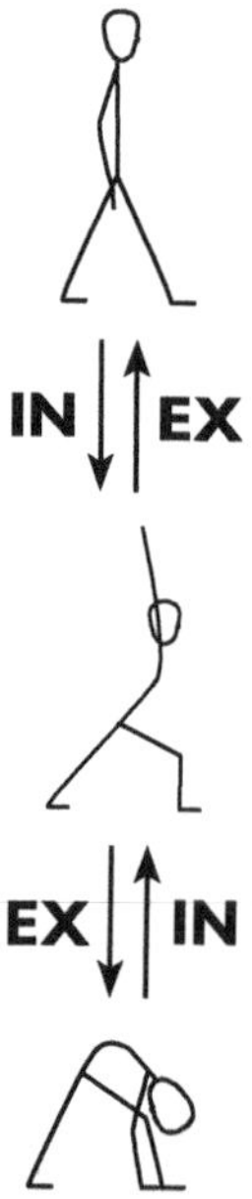	**Vīrabhadrāsana 1 and Parśvottānāsana combo:** To utilize and strengthen the major muscles of the back body, increase circulation, and stretch hamstrings.	Start by standing with the left foot forward, and right foot back. Inhale: Bend the left knee, extend both arms overhead, lengthen the low back, and lift the chest. Exhale: Bend forward, lower the torso to the left thigh, have hands on ground, progressively straighten the left knee. Inhale: Lift the torso, bend the left knee, extend both arms overhead, lengthen the low back, and lift the chest. Exhale: Return to the starting position, lower the arms by the sides while straightening the front knee. Repeat on both sides.

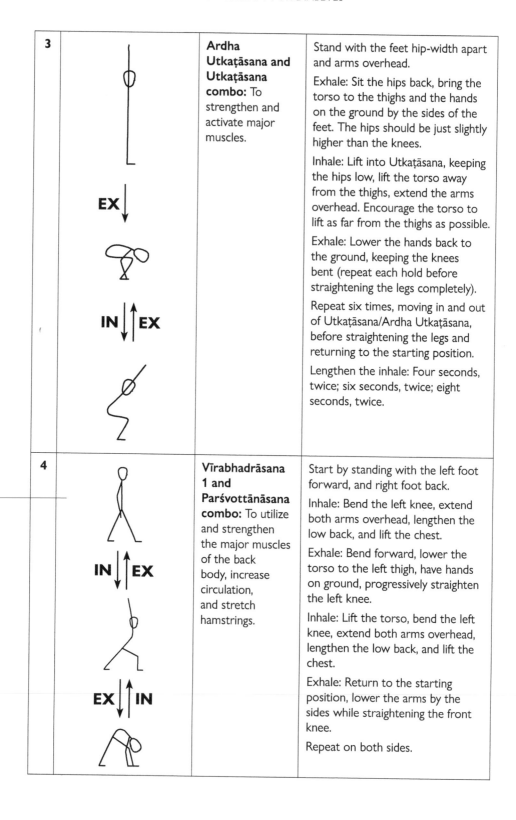

5		**Utthita Trikoṇāsana:** To activate, stretch, and strengthen the body, one side at a time.	Stand with the feet wider than the shoulders. Have the left foot forward and right foot back and turned slightly in. Open the arms and turn the palms to face up. Exhale: Keeping the torso in the same plane, laterally bend to the left, lowering the left hand to the left shin. The right arm is close to the right hip with the palm facing up. Turn the right side of the navel and right shoulder to the ceiling while looking down at the left foot. Inhale: Extend the right arm overhead, looking up at the right hand, and stretch the right side of body. Exhale: Reach the right arm back and slightly behind the body, palm facing up. Look down at the left foot while turning the right side of the abdomen to the ceiling. Repeat six times, and then stay in Utthita Trikoṇāsana for six breaths.
6	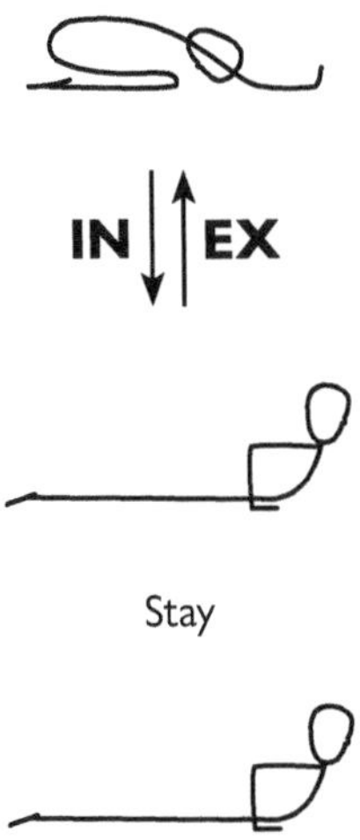	**Bālāsana and Bhujaṅgāsana combo:** To counter pose and transition from standing to the floor.	Start in kneeling forward-bend position, with the abdomen resting on the thighs, knees hip-width apart and arms extended in front with the hands on the ground. Inhale: Move the torso forward and arch the upper back. Keep a slight bend in the elbows, avoid compressing the low back. Exhale: Return to the starting position. Repeat four times, and then stay for six breaths. Inhale: Stay and expand the chest, traction the hands, lengthen the upper back. Exhale: Stay and contract the abdomen.

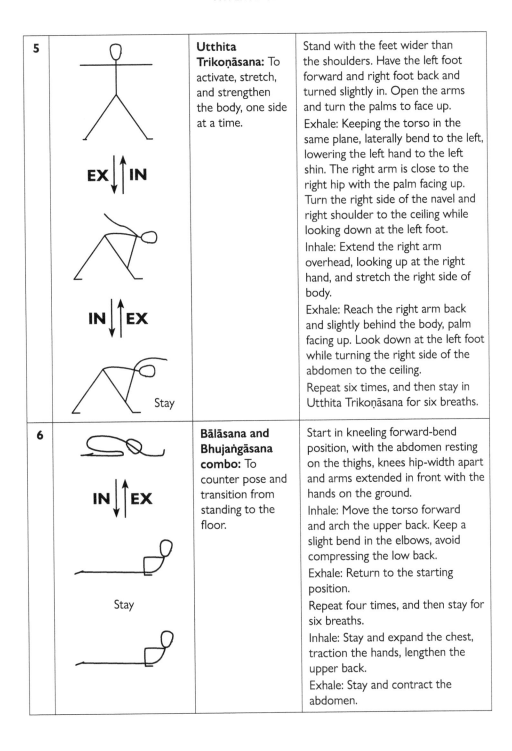

7	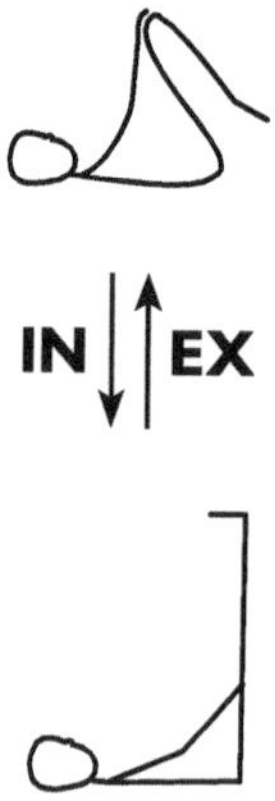	**Ūrdhva Prasārita Pādāsana:** To counter pose from the backbend, compress the abdomen, and stretch the low back and hamstrings.	Lie on the back with both knees lifted towards the chest, feet off the floor, and hands behind the knees. Exhale: Bend the elbows, squeeze the abdomen, draw the thighs into the navel, keep the sacrum on the ground. Inhale: Extend the legs towards the ceiling, flex the ankles. Exhale: Bend the elbows and knees, squeeze the abdomen, draw the thighs into the navel, keep the sacrum on the ground. Repeat six times.
8	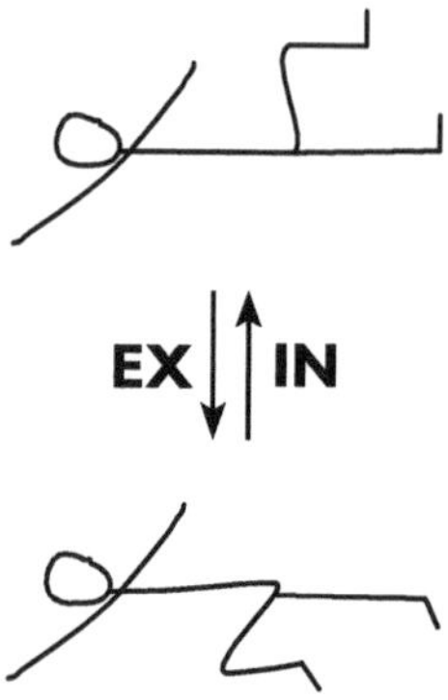	**Jaṭara Parivṛtti:** To prepare for the seated twist and encourage a laṇghana orientation by lengthening the exhale.	Lie on the back, with the arms wide, left knee towards the chest, and right leg straight. Exhale: Twist, bringing the left knee to the right, while turning the head to the left. Inhale: Return to the starting position. Lengthen the exhale: four seconds, twice; six seconds, twice; eight seconds, twice. Repeat on both sides.
9	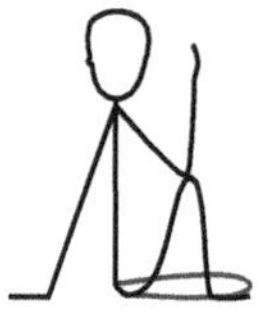 suspend the exhale	**Ardha Matsyendrāsana with exhale suspension:** To reinforce a laṅghana orientation with rotation and breath suspension.	Start in a seated position, with the right leg crossed over the left leg, right sole of foot on the ground, and left knee on the floor with the foot folded towards the right hip. Place the right arm behind the body, and the hand on the ground. Cross the left arm over the right leg, twist, and turn the head to the right. Exhale for eight seconds, suspend for two seconds. Stay for six breaths, and then switch sides.

10	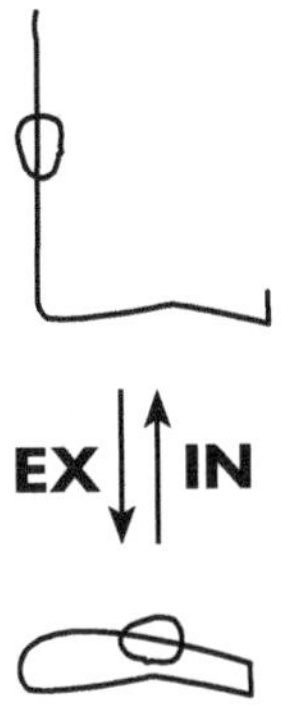	**Paścimatānāsana:** To counter pose for the twists, and stretch the back and hamstrings.	Sit upright with the legs forward, a slight bend in the knees, and the arms overhead. Exhale: Bend forward, lengthening the front of the torso until it reaches the thighs, place the hands on the feet. Inhale: Lift the arms and torso, with a flat back, and return to the starting position. Repeat six times.
11	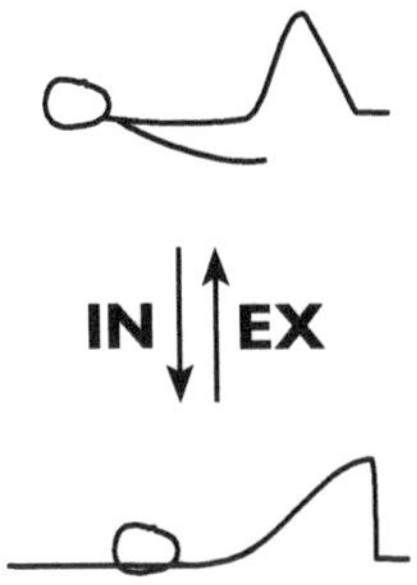	**Dvipāda Pītham:** To counter pose for the spine and prepare for Śavāsana.	Lie on the back with the feet hip-width apart and arms by the sides. Inhale: Press into the feet, lift the hips off the ground while reaching the arms up and behind the head to the floor behind. Exhale: Lower the hips and arms and return to the starting position. Repeat six times.
12	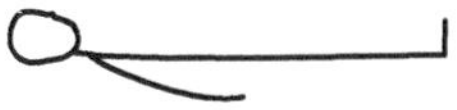	**Śavāsana:** To rest.	Lie comfortably on the back. Relax the breath. Rest in the awareness of the natural breath and sense of aliveness. Rest for three to five minutes.
13	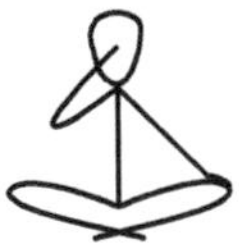	**Anuloma ujjāyī:** Alternate nostril exhale, ujjāyī inhale. To calm and pacify the nervous system.	Sit in a comfortable position and inhale. Lift the right hand, close the right nostril with the thumb, valve the left nostril with the ring finger. Exhale: Left nostril, then lower the right hand. Inhale: Ujjāyī glottal contraction. Lift the right hand, close the left nostril with the ring finger, valve the right nostril with the thumb. Exhale: Right nostril, then lower the right hand. Inhale: Ujjāyī glottal contraction. Repeat six times. *Inhale into the abdomen, relaxing the belly.*

Postprandial Hyperglycemia

I created this practice for myself as an intervention strategy for T1D when BG is spiking rapidly after a meal. It is not uncommon to be high after a meal and stay elevated for several hours. We want to reduce this because it increases the chances of insulin resistance, cardiovascular disease, and delays in cognitive function.

I recommend that individuals work in support with their diabetes care providers to learn how to pre-bolus for their meals. This practice is for the minor slip ups or the times when we need an extra boost. I sometimes do this practice before I eat pancakes, just as an added support strategy. Who does not love pancakes? We should be able to eat them now and again and yoga can help!

Generally, practicing after a meal is not encouraged. It is uncomfortable, and digestion requires energy—energy that otherwise would be going to practice.

This short yoga therapy is an intervention and not a complete practice. It is an exercise-inspired preventative strategy to stop or attenuate a postprandial BG spike once insulin has already been administered for a meal. Anything longer in duration will lose its therapeutic application—increasing the risk of hypoglycemia with post-meal insulin on-board.

We know that there is already active insulin on-board, so the focus is to get that insulin working faster by helping the muscles with the uptake of the available insulin. Anytime a muscle contracts during an activity, it helps your cells with the uptake of glucose from the bloodstream, whether or not insulin is available.[27] Using more muscular activity, and increasing heart rate and breath capacity, can make insulin work better.

Āsana practiced in a strong and dynamic way does not have to be complicated to be effective. Studies reveal that yoga āsana enhances insulin receptor expression in the muscles, causing increased glucose uptake by muscles in T2D.[28] There is little research on T1D, but I can tell you from direct experience that it is no different. This practice is inspired by high intensity intervals, which has been proven to improve BG levels for one to three days post exercise. What is really cool about a short and quick intervention is that

27 American Diabetes Association (n.d.) *Blood Sugar and Exercise*. Accessed on 08/07/20 at: www.diabetes.org/fitness/get-and-stay-fit/getting-started-safely/blood-glucose-and-exercise.

28 Raveendran, A. V., Deshpandae, A. and Joshi, S. R. (2018) "Therapeutic role of yoga in type 2 diabetes." *Endocrinol Metab (Seoul)* 33, 3, 307–317.

it gets insulin working but helps avoid hypoglycemia, which can often occur after hyperglycemia corrections during longer-duration exercise.[29]

A Practice for Postprandial Hyperglycemia

Primary goals: Reduce or attenuate a postprandial BG spike using the least amount of time and effort as possible.

Method: Stimulate and activate circulation, heart rate, and major muscle groups. Encourage the metabolization of glucose and uptake of insulin. Focus on postures that will activate the core, legs, and back muscles. Incorporate dynamic movement with some body weight holds if applicable.

1	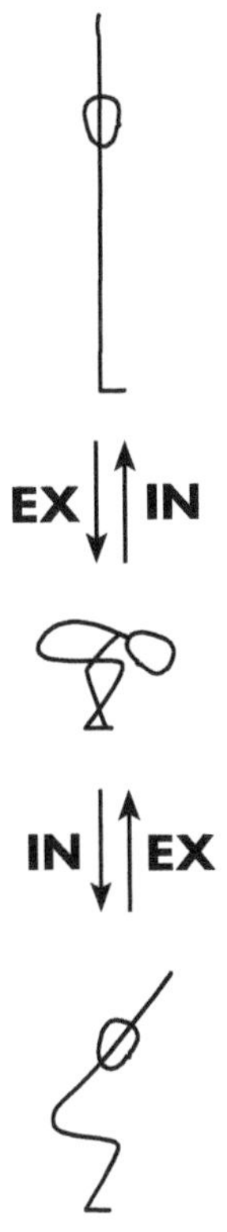	**Ardha Utkaṭāsana and Utkaṭāsana variation:** To strengthen and activate major muscles.	Stand with the feet hip-width apart and arms overhead. Exhale: Sit the hips back, bring the torso to the thighs and the hands on the ground by the sides of the feet. The hips should be just slightly higher than the knees. Inhale: Lift the torso into Utkaṭāsana, keeping the hips low, lift the torso away from the thighs, extend the arms overhead. Encourage the torso to lift as far from the thighs as possible. Exhale: Lower the hands back to the ground, keeping the knees bent (repeat each hold before straightening the legs completely). Inhale: Lift the torso into Utkaṭāsana but continue straightening the legs, returning to the starting position. Repeat six times.

29 Adams, O. P. (2013) "The impact of brief high-intensity exercise on blood glucose levels." *Diabetes, Metabolic Syndrome and Obesity* 6, 113–122.

2	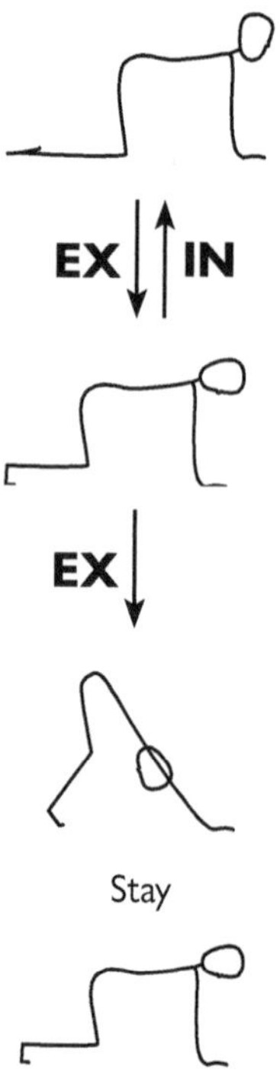	**Bhārmanāsana and Adho Mukha Śvānāsana combo:** To activate the arms, and major muscles of the back and abdomen.	Start on all fours—with the hands under the shoulders and the knees under the hips. Exhale: Press into the hands, broaden and abduct the shoulder blades, and lift the knees off the ground a few inches (Bhārmanāsana). On the same exhale, press back into a modified version of downward facing dog with the knees bent and spine long. Inhale: Return to all fours with the knees on the ground. Repeat four times, and then stay in Bhārmanāsana (knees hovering) for several breaths. Feel the activity in the body, and maintain a smooth and even breath.
3	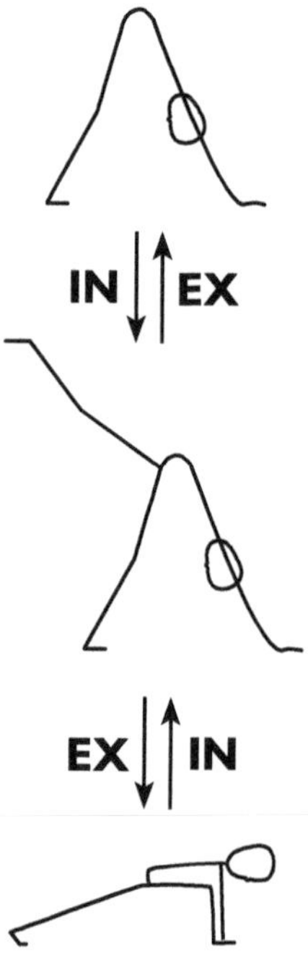	**Adho Mukha Śvānāsana and high lunge vinyāsa:** To increase stimulation, circulation, and activation of the major muscles of the body.	Start in Adho Mukha Śvānāsana, press the hands forward and lengthen the spine. Inhale: Lift the right leg up off the ground, maintain the level of the hips. Exhale: Step the right leg forward towards the right thumb. Inhale: Return to Adho Mukha Śvānāsana with the right leg lifted. Exhale: Lower the right leg, return to the starting position. Repeat eight times, alternating the legs with the breath.

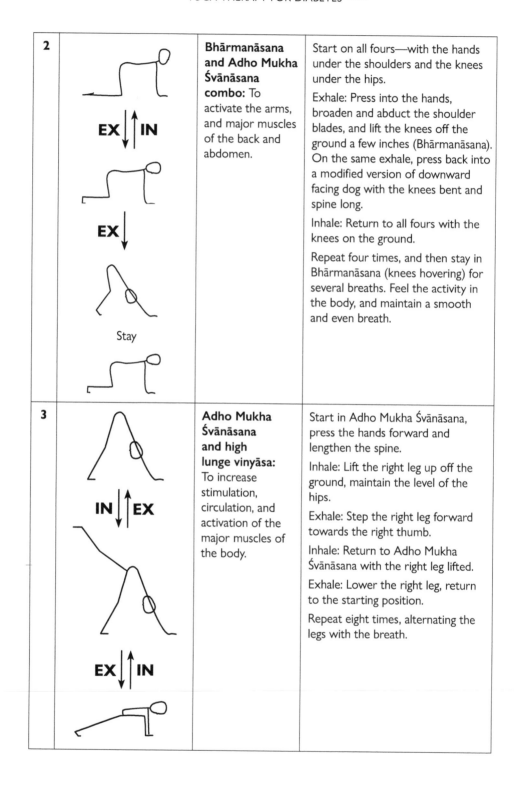

4	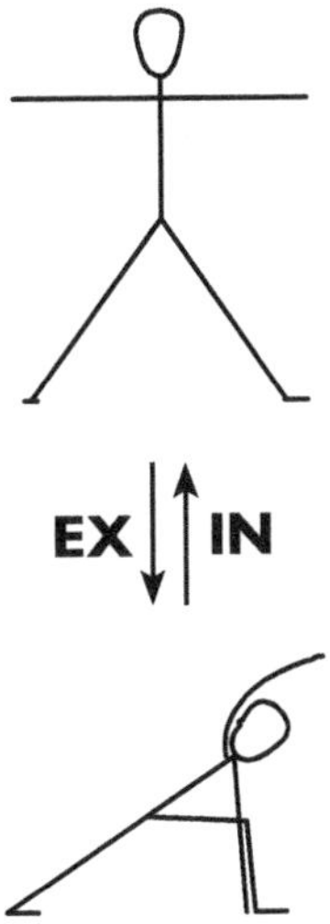	**Utthita Pārśvakoṇāsana:** To stretch and isolate each side of the torso while strengthening the legs.	Stand with the legs wider than the shoulders, left foot turned out, right foot parallel. Inhale: Open the arms parallel to the ground, palms face up. Exhale: Bend the left knee to 90 degrees, laterally bend, bring the left arm and torso towards the inner left leg, extending the right arm overhead. Inhale: Return to the starting position. Equal inhale to equal exhale: Four, five, six, seven, and eight seconds, progressively. Do this eight times and then switch sides.
5	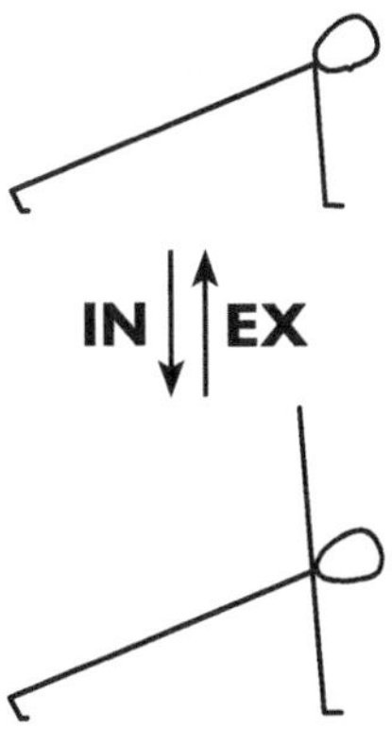	**Daṇḍāsana and Vasiṣṭhāsana combo:** To use the body weight to increase energetic demand.	Start in plank position, with the arms and legs straight, abdomen engaged, and back flat. Inhale: Keeping feet slightly apart, turn the heel to the right, rolling to the outside edge of the right foot, rotate the torso, and reach the left arm overhead. Turn by squeezing the abdomen. Exhale: Return to plank, repeat on the opposite side. Repeat four times, alternating the right and left sides.
6	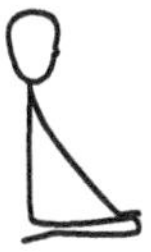	**Vajrāsana:** To rest and allow the heart rate to slow down.	

7	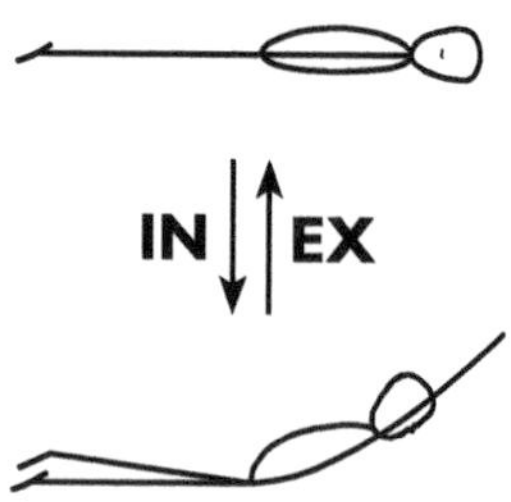	**Ardha Śalabhāsana variation:** To transition to the floor, counter pose for weight bearing postures, strengthen the back, and mobilize the shoulders asymmetrically.	Lie down on the belly, with the head to one side, the hands at the sacrum, a slight bend in the elbows, and the palms facing up. Inhale: Lift the chest, sweep the right arm wide and forward, bending the arm into a salute, lift the right leg off the ground. Exhale: Return to the starting position, turning the head to the right—away from the sweeping arm. Repeat eight times, alternating the arm and leg.
8	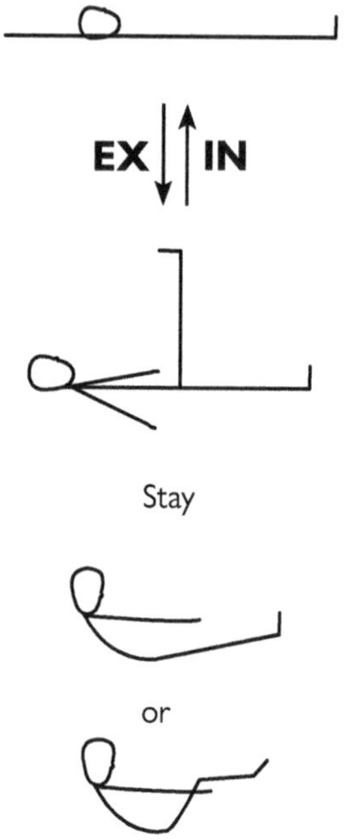	**Conscious core activation and Ardha Nāvāsana:** To strengthen the abdominal muscles.	Lie flat on the back, with the legs straight, arms overhead on the ground, and feet flexed. Exhale: Lower the arms and lift the right leg towards the ceiling by engaging the abdominal muscles. Inhale: Return to the starting position. Repeat six times, alternating the leg lift. Stay in Ardha Nāvāsana. Lift both legs a few inches off the ground, and use abdominal strength to lift the head and shoulders off the mat, reaching the arms forward. Stay for 1 breath, 2 breaths, 3 breaths, 4 breaths.
9	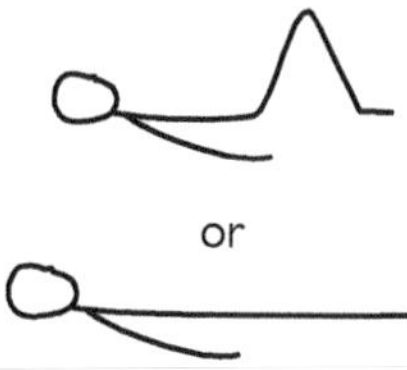	**Rest:** Up to one minute.	

10	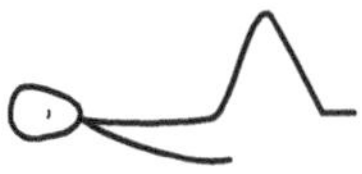 or 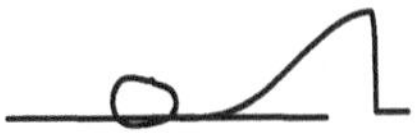	**Dvipāda Pītham variation:** To counter pose for the spine, neck, and shoulders, and prepare for final relaxation.	Lie on the back, feet hip-width apart and arms by the sides. Inhale: Press into the feet, lift the hips off the ground while reaching the right arm behind the head to the floor, gaze at the ceiling. Exhale: Simultaneously lower the hips and the right arm and turning the head to the left to return to the starting position. Repeat four times, alternating arm and head rotation.
11	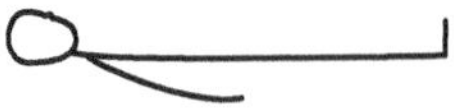	**Śavāsana (optional):** Three minutes.	

Severe Hyperglycemia (over 300 mg/dL (16.7 mmol/L))

Severe hyperglycemia has an entirely different orientation once BG is higher than around 300 mg/dL (16.7 mmol/L), and I will explain why. The brain relies on glucose, and any massive changes affect cerebral function. Severe hyperglycemia occurs rapidly in T1D, while in T2D it is more progressive and less severe if a person is on medication. People with T1D are at increased risk for ketoacidosis and should check their ketones and hydrate with electrolytes before practice.

The swift change in BG levels increases irritability and feelings of diminished wellbeing. When I am high, I feel like a truck hit me. I am weepy and depressed.

We want to nourish the whole system, but a nourishing practice is a bṛṁhaṇa orientation, which is too strong in this compromised energetic state. I recommend a laṅghana orientation to calm as well as soothe the nervous system and the mind. Under the right circumstances, laṅghana creates a bṛṁhaṇa (nourishing) effect, and that is our goal with this practice. The practice could lead up to balancing prāṇāyāma like nāḍī śodhana or alternate nostril inhale (slightly stimulating) with bhramari (humming breath) on exhale to continue the calming orientation. Should there be time, you could end with an extended yoga nidrā practice.

A Practice for Severe Hyperglycemia

Primary goals: Nourish and soothe the nervous system without overstimulating the SNS.

Method: Laṅghana to bṛṁhaṇa. Start slow, preferably on the back, and work your way up to kneeling. Emphasize a longer stay in gentle restorative postures. Progressively lengthen the exhale. Chant in low pitches on exhale if applicable. Follow up with a balancing prāṇāyāma practice like nāḍī śodhana and yoga nidrā relaxation supported on the back if time allows.

The practice is similar to the practice for hypoglycemia recovery (Chapter 9).

CHAPTER 9

Hypoglycemia

Hypoglycemia is a condition represented by the *deficiency* of BG—below the standard threshold of around 70 mg/dL (3.9 mmol/L). Glucose is the primary fuel of the brain, which is so glucose reliant that even in a resting state it requires up to 60% of the available glucose.[1] Unlike the liver, the brain cannot store glucose and is dependent upon a steady trickle of glucose at all times to maintain its function. When glucose levels drop below the standard threshold, the brain goes into emergency mode, creating a variety of neuroendocrine responses to bring levels back up. During a "low," as we call them, a person can experience uncomfortable and debilitating effects, resulting in cognitive and neurological impairment. These effects vary from person to person and according to the severity of the low. If left untreated, severe hypoglycemia can even result in *death*.

Frederick Banting, the co-discoverer of insulin, in a 1925 Nobel laureate speech, described the first indicators of hypoglycemia as "unaccountable anxiety and the feeling of impending trouble associated with restlessness."[2] Some other examples of hypoglycemia symptoms are shakiness, extreme hunger, profuse sweating, dizziness, confusion, and irritability. The symptoms can come on rapidly, inhibiting our ability to make rational and swift decisions, and sometimes requiring assistance from others.

Luckily, most people do not get low enough to even feel these symptoms. *Why?* Our evolutionary biology devised specific counterregulatory steps to keep BG levels from dropping.

1 Berg, J. M., Tymoczko, J. L. and Stryer, L. (2002) "Section 30.2, Each Organ Has a Unique Metabolic Profile." In *Biochemistry*. Fifth edition. New York: W H Freeman. Accessed on 08/07/20 at: www.ncbi.nlm.nih.gov/books/NBK22436.

2 Freir, B. M. (2014) "Impaired Awareness of Hypoglycaemia." In B. M. Freir, S. R. Heller and R. J. McCrimmon (eds) *Hypoglycaemia in Clinical Diabetes*. Third edition. Chichester: John Wiley & Sons Ltd. p.117.

The steps are:

1. Stop the production of insulin and pull it out of circulation.

2. Signal the pancreas to produce glucagon (the antagonist of insulin). Glucagon, just like insulin, is a hormone produced by the pancreas. Its principal function is to raise BG levels. It does this by traveling to the liver, where it harvests stored glucose reserves in the form of glycogen and turns it back into glucose. It then releases the glucose into the bloodstream and avoids hyperglycemia.

3. Produce additional counterregulatory hormones. If numbers continue to fall, the sympathetic nervous system steps in and produces norepinephrine and epinephrine to expedite glucagon's effect. The HPA axis, our longer-acting friend, helps out too, releasing cortisol to buffer the impact of the sympathetic response, increasing the potency of glucagon for hours to come.

Sounds kind of familiar, right? This is an *acute* stress response. Its activation increases BG levels and is our primary counterregulatory protection mechanism against hypoglycemia. It raises the BG levels as a protection mechanism.

In this conversation on hypoglycemia, our orientation is a little different from that described in the last chapter. *Whereas elevated BG levels can be a result of the stress response, hypoglycemia causes the stress response.*

The Stages of Hypoglycemia

There are three stages of hypoglycemic symptoms. The first stage involves neurogenic or adrenic symptoms, and it is our first indicator of hypoglycemia, turning on some time after 70 mg/dL (4 mmol/L) and before 55 mg/dL (3 mmol/L). It's considered to be a mild level of hypoglycemia. I struggle to call the symptoms "mild," because sometimes they are wildly uncomfortable, and they should be. This is when we really want a fight-or-flight response, when we are in immediate danger.

It is like when you narrowly miss being in an accident. Your heart rate increases, face turns beet red, body temp goes up, and mind is in a daze. This is *not* unintentional. It is a *sympathoadrenal* response. As we learned, the SAM system is in charge of our *acute* stress response. The hypothalamus commands the pituitary gland to signal the adrenals to produce the hormones epinephrine and norepinephrine for immediate counterregulatory action. So what you feel during the first phase of hypoglycemia is a result of epinephrine (adrenaline). These hormones potentiate glucagon's arrival to the liver and also sound the alarm that you are getting low, so *act fast*!

During the first stage, the brain still has sufficient glucose, so you can function. It is the periphery of the body that is deficient in glucose. People can usually make logical decisions at this point. When BG drops to around 55 mg/dL (3.1 mmol/L), the brain is in glucose deficit. The secondary moderate stage, called *neuroglycopenia*, is the deficiency of glucose to the brain. Although the symptoms vary, it involves the loss of cognitive and motor function. You get confused, can't make appropriate decisions, act belligerent, and end up eating the whole kitchen (not guilty!).

The tertiary stage is not really a stage; it is the eminent result of untreated hypoglycemia, seizure or even death.

Could you imagine living with the condition that causes BG levels to rise and also plummet, with debilitating disorientation and a threat of death if left untreated? Imagine experiencing hyperglycemia and hypoglycemia several times a day and night for the rest of your life.

The real-time experience of highs and lows is one thing; the after-effect is another. It is a complete energy suck, rendering you physically, mentally, and spiritually void.

Who Gets Low?

Now, let's back up a step and talk about who *actually* experiences hypoglycemia, because this is a chapter about helping *those* people.

People with T1D!

Not only are people with T1D chasing the highs, but they *also* have to avoid the lows. Not to mention, they need to be prepared to treat a low at any moment. The state is so intense at times and comes on so quickly that you have to stop whatever you are doing, address the low, and wait to recover. Depending on the severity, it could be anywhere from 15 minutes to a whole day!

This is just one reason why T1D is a recipe for exhaustion. The nature of it is very anxiety provoking.

Unless you are taking insulin, you probably will not experience hypoglycemia *ever*. This is why most people with T2D do not get low: they do not take insulin, as their pancreas still makes it. The drugs that they do take help them use their self-produced (endogenous) insulin better. Some people with long-duration T2D end up taking insulin to help with metabolic control, and hypoglycemia happens to these individuals too.

Let's Talk About Why

When you have diabetes, there is intense pressure to keep BG levels under 7.0% to avoid the long-term complications of hyperglycemia. With this pressure to keep levels under a specific level, people are more vigilant about keeping glucose levels within range, which increases their risk of hypoglycemia. The A1c test is an indicator of improved diabetes management, but that number can be skewed by frequent hyperglycemia. So a person may have an excellent A1c reading, but when you look at their daily totals, they are low all of the time. On a subtle level, frequent reoccurrence of hypoglycemia impacts quality of life.

Now, let's talk about physiology, again... Remember how the first step in the counterregulatory process is to stop the production of insulin? This has to happen first, because whenever there is active insulin, the counterregulatory power of glucagon will not work; insulin will always override it.

Here lies the first reason why people with insulin-dependent diabetes get low: *they have to take insulin from an outside source* because they do not produce insulin on their own (or at least very little of it). The insulin they inject has an active duration time, which means that if their BG drops, they can't stop the production of insulin. It is already in the body. Therefore, the presence of artificial (exogenous) insulin inhibits the counterregulatory effect of glucagon, and a person has to eat some type of carbohydrate to counteract the low. The truth of the matter is that all insulin will inhibit glucagon.

In a non-insulin-dependent individual, the pancreas stops the production of insulin before it can secrete the counterregulatory hormones glucagon and epinephrine, giving insulin time to leave the bloodstream and blood sugars to rise naturally. But for a person with diabetes who is undergoing insulin therapy, this is not the case. Self-administered insulin (exogenous) is not subject to a standard feedback loop. Too much insulin causes hypoglycemia, even if their CRR is intact.[3]

This is a particular issue during exercise. Let's say you ate lunch a couple of

3 Freir, B. M. (2014) "Impaired Awareness of Hypoglycaemia." In B. M. Freir, S. R. Heller and R. J. McCrimmon (eds) *Hypoglycaemia in Clinical Diabetes*. Third edition. Chichester: John Wiley & Sons Ltd. p.117.

hours ago and administered fast-acting insulin to cover the nutrient content of that meal. Your friend calls you up and asks if you want to go on a bike ride or go to a yoga class. Unless you take a specific preemptive action, you will get low during this activity. Depending on the amount of active insulin, duration, and intensity of the exercise, and starting BG, you will probably need to "carb load" to prevent hypoglycemia.

Only two things can reduce insulin in the bloodstream: time and carbohydrates. All insulin has an active duration time. Most fast-acting insulin, the type a person takes for a meal, has a duration time of three to four hours with a potency peak about halfway. If a person miscalculates the insulin needed for a meal, they have too much active insulin on-board. BG levels drop, and they need to supplement with additional carbohydrates.

Exercise adds an extra layer of complication to BG balance. During physical activity, you are burning glucose for immediate energy, so you need less insulin. If you already have active insulin in your system and move your body, not only will that insulin work faster, but it will also burn any remaining available glucose. As a type 1 athlete who loves to mountain bike, ski, backpack, and do a lot of fun, crazy things, it has been a long journey of making a lot of mistakes and getting low. We should never let these things stop us from living our lives fully.

Insulin pump therapy is the best way a person can mimic pancreatic suspension of insulin. These systems, called closed-loop insulin pumps, work in synch with a CGM and constantly adjust insulin dosage per BG levels. These systems can suspend exogenous insulin and then allow the counterregulatory hormones to work. But they are not fail-safe. During exercise, a person should adjust their pump to keep the slow rate of insulin at a lower dose. More often than not, when a person inadvertently takes too much insulin, they need to find glucose from outside sources.

The second reason why people with insulin-dependent diabetes get low is a *damaged CRR*. The main hormones involved in the CRR are glucagon, epinephrine, and cortisol. Glucagon brings BG up, and the other hormones expedite it. Epinephrine is also responsible for the first warning signs of impending hypoglycemia, like sweating, hunger, dizziness, etc.

Like anything with diabetes, the duration of the disease inflicts damage on our regulatory systems. Within the first five years, many (not all) people with T1D lose their ability to secrete *sufficient* glucagon in response to hypoglycemia.[4]

4 McCrimmon, R. J. (2014) "Counterregulatory Deficiencies in Diabetes." In B. M. Freier, S. Heller and R. McCrimmon (eds) *Hypoglycaemia in Clinical Diabetes*. Third edition. Chichester: John Wiley & Sons Ltd. p.48.

Once glucagon's response is damaged, a person becomes reliant upon the support of epinephrine to stimulate a CRR.

It is essential to maintain these responses, because they signal a self-directed behavioral intervention, often the last resort for people with T1D to treat their low. Unfortunately, persistent lows damage sympathetically activated alarms, and people become "desensitized" to their lows. This is a condition of hypoglycemia—impaired awareness of hypoglycemia (IAH). It could fit into the second category of impaired CRRs, but as it is a condition I will give it a classification of its own.

IAH affects about 30% of adults with T1D. If people who do not have this awareness, the preliminary warning signs of hypoglycemia are weakened or do not occur at all. IAH increases the risk of severe hypoglycemia by as much as six times.[5] Symptoms may not be identifiable until a person is severely impaired and cannot make decisions. If a person cannot feel their lows, the margin for error is small. It is like walking along a cliff on a moonless night;[6] one small misstep can be life threatening. These individuals function at low levels of BG concentrations that would trigger symptoms in other people.

Thanks to the first stage of hypoglycemia symptoms (neurogenic), and its internal alarm clocks, a person can "feel" their low and respond before it becomes a problem. People with IAH lack the sensitivity to perceive the signs, and they drop dangerously low before they notice any symptoms. They virtually bypass the first stage and move into the second stage, where the brain is affected and response is attenuated. The problem is two-fold: first, the lack of sensitivity to symptoms increases their risk of severe hypoglycemia and the ability to treat it without auxiliary assistance. Second, every time a critical low occurs, it damages the autonomic stress response and makes a person even more susceptible to recurrent severe lows.

---

5 Gonder-Frederick, L., Cox, D., Clarke, W. and Julian, D. (2005) "Blood Glucose Awareness Training (BGAT-2): Long-Term Benefits." In F. J. Snoek and C. T. J. Skinner (eds) *Psychology in Diabetes Care*. Chichester: John Wiley & Sons Ltd. p.175.

6 Freir, B. M. (2014) "Impaired Awareness of Hypoglycaemia." In B. M. Freir, S. R. Heller and R. J. McCrimmon (eds) *Hypoglycaemia in Clinical Diabetes*. Third edition. Chichester: John Wiley & Sons Ltd. p.125.

Why Does This Happen?

Throughout human evolution, the nervous system has adapted to environmental changes. Energetic efficiency is implicit in the survival of the species; the less energy expended to achieve a metabolic goal, the higher the survival rate. This conditioning enhances evolutionary fitness, but it can also dull sensory awareness.

Whenever I travel to a big city, I cannot sleep for the first few nights because all I hear are sirens, honking cars, and people. But after a few days, my senses adjust. The hustle and bustle no longer bother me. I might not even notice the noise at all. The city doesn't stop being chaotic, but I change. Why? I adapt to a new normal. My sympathetic alarms become conditioned and what used to prompt a stress response no longer does.

Conditioning also applies to hypoglycemia. If someone is continually experiencing low BG levels, even mild ones, the nervous system adapts to this new normal. Even if that new normal is not healthy, the nervous system does not discriminate. The person is, more often than not, arriving at a low level, so the nervous system incorrectly mistakes those lower levels for the new baseline. It does not send out preemptive stress alarms in the form of hunger, sweat, and dizziness. The same thing can happen with high BG levels.

For instance, if a person has been at a high BG level for an extended amount of time when their BG finally returns to normal, they may experience the same symptoms as they would with a low BG. This is because the nervous system has been conditioned to the state of being high and misidentifies normal as low.

How Do We Fix It?

The easiest way to correct hypoglycemia unawareness is to reduce the frequency of hypoglycemia. This is a testament to our nervous system's resilience. When we allow it to heal, it does.

CGMs are the most widely prescribed tool for this but they are expensive and out of reach for the vast majority of the world's diabetics.

Another exciting pathway is to stimulate glucose sensors. "Gluco-sensing" is a term used to refer to the parts of the nervous system and brain that sense hypoglycemia. Stationed throughout the body are specific neurotransmitters in charge of detecting when glycemic levels are low. The hypothalamus is the most important area. It is the connection between the nervous system and the endocrine system. Within it lies the primary hypoglycemia sensors.

These neurotransmitters experience a type of neuropathy, diminishing their ability to sense glycemic danger and generate an adequate stress response.

The central and most important of these sensors are located in a part of the hypothalamus known as the ventral medial hypothalamus (VMH). Studies show that if this part of the brain is stimulated, the CRRs return to normal function.[7] These studies are limited to animal models with T1D. Still, they are interesting enough to mention as we look towards the future of diabetes health as well as a potential pathway in which yoga-based interventions can be of service.

It is no secret that yoga-based exercises, especially prāṇāyāma, have a profound effect in regulating neuroendocrine responses. We do *not* have sufficient evidence to link yoga-therapy-based practices to the reactivation of *glucose-sensing* neurons and potentially improving the CRR in insulin-dependent diabetes. But I am leaving this as an open-ended question, and I hope the area will one day be studied in greater depth.

Hypoglycemia is just as much a part of diabetes management as hyperglycemia. When it comes to hypoglycemia, acquiring and maintaining sensitivity to the onset of a low is an essential and life-saving tool. Without it, there is an increased risk of severe hypoglycemia, and every acute episode escalates the chance of another by damaging the neural sensors.

To maintain existing counterregulatory responses, we also have to reduce the time spent in hypoglycemia and sympathetic overdrive. The very mechanisms behind creating hypoglycemia resilience are protecting the role of an *appropriate* stress response. Hypoglycemia produces sympathetic overdrive, damaging the remaining CRRs that ward off hypoglycemia, as well as increasing the risk for subsequent hyperglycemia. It's a catch-22 and incredibly frustrating for a person living with diabetes who just wants to be healthy.

The Lived Experience of Hypoglycemia

For a person living with insulin-dependent diabetes, hypoglycemia is an ever-present reality, whose symptoms and effects can impact every aspect of daily life. The fear of hypoglycemia is always on the mind, and with due cause: hypoglycemia can be deadly. Whenever I am asked to explain the experience

7 McCrimmon, R. J., Fan, X., Cheng, H., McNay, E., *et al.* (2006) "Activation of AMP-activated protein kinase within the ventromedial hypothalamus amplifies counterregulatory hormone responses in rats with defective counterregulation." *Diabetes* 55, 6, 1755–1760.

of hypoglycemia, I say that it feels like you are dying. First, you lose control of your body, your impulses; then, you lose your mind. It is not a pretty picture, but I cannot come up with a better description that connotes the same weight.

The worst low I ever experienced happened early on in my teaching career. Let me just preface the story by saying that this was before CGMs. Back then, you relied on internal sensing and finger prick testing to know if you were low. I was teaching a private yoga session to a new client and felt myself going low near the end of our time. That day I was unprepared, without glucose tabs in case of emergency. For some reason, I decided not to burden the client and request juice. Perhaps I was embarrassed or shy because we had just met. Maybe I was worried that they would judge me. Regardless, our session was almost over, and I lived only five minutes away. I stuck it out, like a disciplined (and stupid) yogini.

By the time I made it home, I was a wreck and could barely make it up the stairs to my apartment. I remember thinking I needed to do something, but could not connect my mind with my body. Somehow, out of habituation, I ended up stuffing my face with protein bars and crawling to bed. Lying there waiting for the remedy to take effect was an other-worldly experience and not in a positive way. Colors, patterns, and psychedelic shapes floated by as I closed my eyes.

When I recall this story, it scares me how ignorant I was. So many things could have gone wrong. Being unprepared happens with diabetes, but not communicating it for fear of judgment is stupid. I am lucky that I was able to treat the low and have learned from that situation what *not* to do. The even scarier thing about it was that I thought I was in control, when, in fact, I was not at all. It just shows you how the symptomatology of severe lows poses a particular challenge when a person needs to make swift and grounded decisions. You may think you are fine, until you aren't. When a person is this low, all rationale goes out the door, even if you know better.

Next, we'll look at the emotional impact of hypoglycemia and why changing our attitudes may be the answer to transforming behavior.

The risk and reality of hypoglycemia leave an indelible mark on how a person lives with diabetes, and the attitudes they form about it. Ask anyone with insulin-dependent diabetes if they would rather be high or low, and most people would probably say that they would rather be high. Highs don't express nearly the intensity of symptoms that hypos do.

Hypoglycemia is one of the most challenging obstacles to diabetes management for several reasons that extend beyond short-term discomfort.

First, it's unpredictable. Hypoglycemia can creep up slowly or hit all at once. A person may feel the low coming on or be completely asymptomatic. The second is its debilitating nature. It knocks you for a punch. You have to stop whatever you are doing and take care of yourself. Communicating hypoglycemia to others when you are low is challenging but also an essential skill of hypoglycemia management. People need to know what is going on, especially if they need to be of assistance. Many diabetics do not want to attract unnecessary attention, which ends up being more of a burden than a boon. If you can educate those around you in a calm and precise manner, it is freeing. I am now at a point where I do not care what anyone thinks or says. I'll be teaching to a large audience, my BG drops, and I'll demonstrate a pose while explaining that I am low and eating glucose tabs. I like to say stuff like "Don't mind me. I'm just trying not to pass out." No one can argue with that!

During hypoglycemia, the body and the brain no longer connect; it impairs all internal reasoning skills and pushes a person into a fight-or-flight survival mode. If left untreated, severe hypoglycemia can cause heart arrhythmia, coma, seizure, and even death. With this in mind, it makes sense that the fear of going low is always in the background of a diabetic's mind and can influence their decisions, performance, and quality of life. Exposure to recurrent hypoglycemia negatively impacts self-confidence, which fuels anxiety and pessimistic beliefs about diabetes management and, ultimately, a sense of hopelessness.[8] The physiological effects disrupt cognitive, emotional, and behavioral performance.[9] Even mild events can impact normal daily activities and function. The effects of hypoglycemia, including nausea and intense fatigue, stick around long after the restoration of BG levels.[10] This is why hypoglycemia is one of the leading risk factors for diabetes burnout,[11] something you will learn more about soon.

An acute fight-or-flight response is a biological imperative. In yoga

8 Snoek, F. J., Hajos, T. and Rondagas, S. (2014) "Psychological Effects of Hypoglycaemia." In B. M. Freir, S. R. Heller and R. J. McCrimmon (eds) *Hypoglycaemia in Clinical Diabetes*. Third edition. Chichester: John Wiley & Sons Ltd. p.323.

9 Snoek, F. J., Hajos, T. and Rondagas, S. (2014) "Psychological Effects of Hypoglycaemia." In B. M. Freir, S. R. Heller and R. J. McCrimmon (eds) *Hypoglycaemia in Clinical Diabetes*. Third edition. Chichester: John Wiley & Sons Ltd. p.324.

10 Snoek, F. J., Hajos, T. and Rondagas, S. (2014) "Psychological Effects of Hypoglycaemia." In B. M. Freir, S. R. Heller and R. J. McCrimmon (eds) *Hypoglycaemia in Clinical Diabetes*. Third edition. Chichester: John Wiley & Sons Ltd. p.324.

11 Snoek, F. J., Hajos, T. and Rondagas, S. (2014) "Psychological Effects of Hypoglycaemia." In B. M. Freir, S. R. Heller and R. J. McCrimmon (eds) *Hypoglycaemia in Clinical Diabetes*. Third edition. Chichester: John Wiley & Sons Ltd. p.324.

psychology, one of the aims of practice is to rewire our ingrained reactions to stressors and to assert conscious control over them. The physiological condition of hypoglycemia triggers our most deep-seated survival mechanisms, and the urge to treat the low can at times outweigh all rational decision-making skills.

Hypoglycemia can also induce rapid changes in mood, which come out of nowhere and can seem irrational to those who live with the person. Mood swings are an indicator of low blood sugar, especially if a person is desensitized to the first stage of hypoglycemia. This poses a challenge to loved ones who recognize the symptoms and want to help. The mood changes that occur can influence the cooperation and willingness of the affected individual to accept help, making it challenging to get them to take a snack or juice. People with diabetes need a reliable support system, but these instances can severely burden the spouses and damage relationships.[12]

Effective and efficient treatment of hypoglycemia amid an intense primitive urge to eat requires an enormous amount of willpower. Over-treating hypoglycemia is common and results in hyperglycemia. Once the high-low-high-low cycle starts, it takes a lot of willpower to stop it. The general rule of 15g of carbs, 15 minutes of rest before eating more carbohydrates, is a proper self-treatment measurement. But unless we address the biological urge and develop the willpower to treat hypoglycemia by learning to wait in the discomfort until it passes, people will continue to overeat and end up high, further perpetuating the vicious cycle of crazy ups and downs.

Kelly McGonigal, Ph.D, a professor at Stanford University, author, and yoga therapist, recommends a practice called "Surfing the Urge"[13] *for developing willpower in the midst of a stressful occurrence.* It is a real-time meditation practice that I find useful for myself and clients who have a tendency to overeat or overreact during hypoglycemia.

---

12 Snoek, F. J., Hajos, T. and Rondagas, S. (2014) "Psychological Effects of Hypoglycaemia." In B. M. Freir, S. R. Heller and R. J. McCrimmon (eds) *Hypoglycaemia in Clinical Diabetes.* Third edition. Chichester: John Wiley & Sons Ltd. p.325.

13 McGonigal, K. (2012) *The Willpower Instinct: Talks at Google.* Accessed on 08/07/20 at: https://youtu.be/V5BXuZL1HAg. (Jump to 50:33 on the video to hear about the practice.)

Hypoglycemia Willpower

1. Notice the thought, craving, or feeling.
2. Accept and attend to the inner experience.
3. Breathe and give your brain and body a chance to pause and plan.
4. Broaden your attention and look for an action that will help you achieve your goal.

I've added these steps for hypoglycemia.

1. After you complete the action (which is to treat the low with 15g of carbs), sit or lie down and repeat steps one to three.
2. Broaden your attention, witness the feeling of hypoglycemia, and recognize that you have completed everything that you need to do. The feeling is temporary. You are safe.
3. Observe your breath for 15 minutes. If your number is still low, eat another 15g of carbohydrates and repeat the steps.

The Lingering Stain of Fear

For every severe low a person has, there is physical and emotional consequence. Consistent severe lows damage the vital alarm systems necessary to induce a behavioral response and increases future susceptibility to frequent and dangerous lows. But beyond human biology, there is a more insidious and troublesome effect of hypoglycemia. Severe lows are traumatic, and like any negative experience, there is a psychological impact carving deep grooves in the subconscious.

Like so many things in life, the way we see something determines our response to it.

Hypoglycemia can be anxiety provoking, both in the experience of it and the anticipation of it. If hypoglycemia is not anticipated, the symptoms of falling BG are less likely to be perceived and interpreted accurately. A study conducted on non-diabetic individuals experimented with injecting subjects with either saline or insulin. Half were told they were getting insulin when in fact they were getting saline. Those who expected to experience hypoglycemia reported more symptoms like weakness, drowsiness, and headache,[14] even with a saline injection. It just shows the power of suggestion.

A belief is created by past experiences, and even those past experiences are influenced by something prior. Fearful, avoidant thoughts may precipitate anxious emotions and behaviors, to a point where the thought about getting low may be as detrimental to blood sugars as hypoglycemia itself. Whether these thoughts are real or perceived, the body does not discriminate: both physical and mental stressors stimulate the same hormonal response. Constant anxiety and negative thought patterns about hypoglycemia cause more stress and weaken diabetes resilience. People will do everything they can to avoid hypoglycemia; from running their BG higher and suffering the long-term consequences or avoiding exercise and activities that they might otherwise enjoy. Without the opportunity to rest, reflect, and soothe the ANS, an individual is more susceptible to other illnesses, ailments, and mental disturbances, blocking their ability to recover from even mild hypoglycemic episodes. It seems like the people who are most resilient to hypoglycemia are the ones who can disassociate with the experience and treat their symptoms without emotion. They are less likely to view hypoglycemia as a threat and more likely to see it as a consequence of living a full life with diabetes. With preparation, awareness, and adaptability, hypoglycemia is more easily navigated.

Symptom perception and awareness

When I was diagnosed, diabetes care was different. I think it was both easier and harder. We did not have all these gadgets that warn of approaching highs and lows. You had to sense your body and really feel what was going on. You had to test your BG levels several times a day and log the numbers on a chart. The purpose of this was to watch BG trends and adjust dosage accordingly, with your doctor. Sensitization to BG was an asset.

Now, people just have to look at a screen to tell them where they are at. I am not saying that's a bad thing; I am grateful for technology and would not choose to live without it. These advances have saved many lives and reduced the rate of severe hypoglycemia. But on the other hand, like all technology intended

14 Snoek, F. J., Hajos, T. and Rondagas, S. (2014) "Psychological Effects of Hypoglycaemia." In B. M. Freir, S. R. Heller and R. J. McCrimmon (eds) *Hypoglycaemia in Clinical Diabetes*. Third edition. Chichester: John Wiley & Sons Ltd. p.324.

to help us, it can also dull awareness. I still pride myself on my ability to sense where I am at and accurately confirm that number with a test. Symptom perception reflects a person's awareness and interpretation of their bodily and mental sensations, which is described as interoception.[15]

While once this was a highly coveted diabetes skillset, with the advent of CGMs and closed-loop insulin pump systems, it has become a non-essential, antiquated thought. Call me old-fashioned, but I think it remains an essential skillset to be developed and refined with practice. We cannot become so reliant on a screen to dictate what is going on or what we really feel or need. The ability to sense a low is no different than the power to accurately interpret emotion from an unconscious fear, or right from wrong. Diabetes awareness teaches us life skills.

Sensitization helps people with all types of diabetes to be more in tune with themselves and with diabetes. Whether a person is high or low, when they can recognize the sensations associated with the number, they can also create a cognitive separation from the feeling and the emotional experience. Then, a person rises above diabetes and rests in the observer where they can respond to diabetes masterfully.

Yoga Therapy for Hypoglycemia

Before anyone begins a yoga therapy practice for hypoglycemia, their BG levels should not be low. Treat the low first, and then practice. The only exception to this rule is an awareness-based practice like the hypoglycemia willpower practice (below) to reduce the impulse to over-treat the low, and remain steadfast and emotionally even-tempered as the observer.

The goal is to support the whole person and their personal experience of hypoglycemia. Just like *hyperglycemia*, practice depends on the individual. For some, hypoglycemia can trigger anxiety and fear; for others, it is more of an energetic drain, sucking out their vitality and productivity; it could be both. Sometimes, the fear of hypoglycemia is subtle and shows up with avoidant tendencies like keeping BG levels higher or refraining from exercise. While this may help to reduce hypoglycemia in the short term, in the long term it will create its own set of problems, mainly from hyperglycemia.

---

15 Snoek, F. J., Hajos, T. and Rondagas, S. (2014) "Psychological Effects of Hypoglycaemia." In B. M. Freir, S. R. Heller and R. J. McCrimmon (eds) *Hypoglycaemia in Clinical Diabetes*. Third edition. Chichester: John Wiley & Sons Ltd. p.324.

That being said, it is a reminder that the practices are potential pathways for improving a person's quality of life by reducing the mental and physiological effects of hypoglycemia.

I have designed three central themes for working with hypoglycemia. The first practice, a recovery practice for a post-hypoglycemia episode, is a general strategy to attenuate the physiological energy drain of hypoglycemia.

Like all yoga therapy practices, it is essential to first address what is out of balance. A helpful starting point if you are unsure is to ask your client whether or not they feel their lows. If they say no, they could benefit from the second practice, an awareness and sensitivity-based practice to awaken perception of hypoglycemia symptoms. This practice is not an intervention strategy but rather a preventative strategy. Improving interoceptive sensitivity is a way of reducing the risk of hypoglycemia onset, which can come on quickly even with the use of CGM technology. By improving sensitivity, and rebalancing sympathetic and parasympathetic activation, we are not only retraining the nervous system to be more "sensitized," but also allowing a person to be more "awake" in their life.

The final practice is to witness hypoglycemia, abide in steadfast, determined awareness, and treat the low appropriately rather than give in to the impulse to overeat, freak out, or whatever the physiological sensations of hypoglycemia trigger as a threat response. To be proficient at hypoglycemia recovery is the ability to abide the intense symptoms of low BG while remaining steadfast and apply appropriate action. You can say that this is a skillset to be developed for all humans; something that can be used in many circumstances. The goal is to help individuals witness biological urges and recognize them as a passing phenomenon. You can revisit this practice in Chapter 9. The practices are as follows.

1. Hypoglycemia recovery
2. Hypoglycemia awareness
3. Hypoglycemia willpower

Hypoglycemia Recovery

This practice is designed to reduce the effects of hypoglycemia after BG levels have returned to normal. After a hypoglycemia episode, it is common to feel energetically drained, deranged, and "hungover" from an intense hypoglycemia episode. We want to use the practice to alleviate some of these physiological symptoms and recover faster. On a psycho-emotional level, hypoglycemia is a trigger for fear and hypervigilance, making it challenging for a person to release the gas pedal to their stress response and simply let go of effort. So, on one level, we are addressing the immediate physiological impact of hypoglycemia and, on another, we are training the nervous system to turn off or down-regulate the stress response.

Hypoglycemia is a condition represented by the deficiency of BG, and the *result* is sympathetic overdrive, a true and *necessary* fight-or-flight response as the symptoms of hypoglycemia are intended to warn of danger. Without this sensitivity, people run the risk of future and chronic hypoglycemia, but it does not make it any easier. The experience zaps vitality and engenders a psychological trigger for many.

The first stage of hypoglycemia is an acute stress response with *heightened sympathoadrenal* symptoms like increased heart rate, intense hunger, and dizziness. The second stage, represented by the absence of glucose to the brain, results in cognitive impairment like confusion and disorientation.

The after-effects of hypoglycemia are kind of like what I would consider adrenal fatigue to be: physical exhaustion and weakness with sensory and cognitive overstimulation. The severity of the low and mental derangement will determine certain aspects of the practice, like duration and intensity, but the general pathway for recovery is similar. It is also important to note that after a severe episode of hypoglycemia, there is an increased chance of recurrent lows, so do not over activate the body.

Sequencing from the energetic principles of yoga therapy, I recommend a laṅghana orientation for recuperation. This is one of those instances where a laṅghana orientation, which is generally calming, can have a post-digestive effect that can be bṛṁhaṇa—nourishing and energizing. The key to a successful sequence is to start where a person is at, slowly, cautiously, and lovingly. Create physical and mental calm and stability (laṅghana), and soothe and balance sympathetic overdrive while allowing the individual to progressively build their energy back up (bṛṁhaṇa).

Typically, hypoglycemia is a vāta vitiation with rajo-guṇa predominance. Psychologically, hypoglycemia can increase mental rajas (fear and anxiety) and a sense of not being safe (also rajas). This psychological state can lead to hypervigilance, and an inability to trust and truly let go of perpetuating physical and mental exhaustion. To recuperate, a person has to feel safe and supported in their body so they can turn off the vigilance and turn towards surrender. Practice should help a person feel safe, so they can relax, let their guard down, and not be so self-reliant. As hypoglycemia may be anxiety provoking for some, we want the practice to create an environment where the individual feels supported from within. Be cautious not to over activate with too many postures or sophisticated breathing practices.

To balance mental rajas, we have to move it towards sattva, but we cannot do this in a hypervigilant state. Bringing in some grounding qualities of sattwic-tamas creates physical stability and, secondarily, promotes mental space (sattva). The pathways to treat and balance mental rajas and vāta doṣa are similar: restoratives, forward bends, and postures closer to the ground. The mantra *Om Mā Om* calls to the divine mother, *mā*, in all of her nurturance, to hold the individual in full support. Chanting at lower pitches in the lower regions of the body from the navel down encourages this orientation.

A Practice for Hypoglycemia Recovery

Primary goals: To restore physiological and psychological balance after a hypoglycemia episode.

Theme: A laṅghana orientation to calm, reduce, and relax. Cultivate a safe space, where a person can let go of effort and trust, and receive nurturance.

Method: Sound in āsana, grounding postures, and lengthening exhale all have an inherent parasympathetic orientation. To build and increase vitality, apply slight inhale retention should a person be up to it.

Breath-centric āsana: Gentle forward bends in supine and kneeling positions. Backbends are applied in a restorative fashion with longer holds and never pushing.

Śavāsana: A version of pratyāhāra, withdrawing of sensory awareness from an external orientation to an internal restfulness.

1	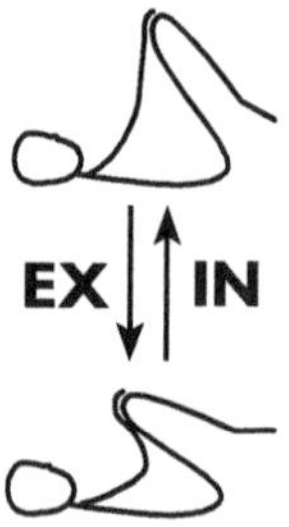 chant on exhale	**Apānāsana:** To stretch the low back and encourage the calming effect of exhalation with sound.	Lie on the back, bend the knees into the body. Place the hands on or behind the knees. Exhale: Gently pull the legs into the body while chanting. Inhale: Return to the starting position. Chant: *Om Mā Om.* Repeat eight times.
2	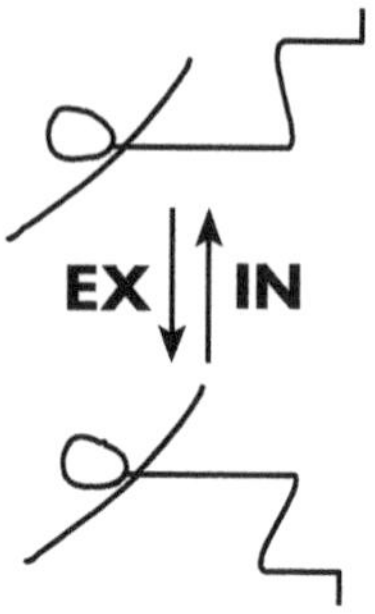	**Jaṭara Parivṛtti:** To stretch and strengthen while compressing the abdominal organs and supporting exhalation.	Lie on the back, with both arms wide and the knees bent into the chest. Exhale: Twist, gradually contract the abdomen, bring the legs over to the left side, and turn the head to the right. Inhale: Return to the starting position. Alternate sides eight times.
3	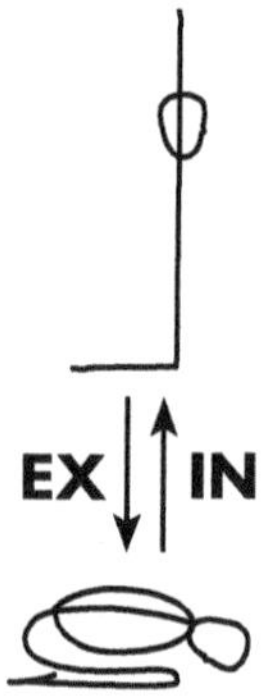 chant on exhale	**Vajrāsana:** To counter pose for the twist, transition from the back, progressively build energy.	Start in a kneeling position with both arms overhead. Exhale: Bend forward, sweep both arms wide and behind the body, lower the torso to the thighs, rest the hands on the sacrum with the palms of the hands facing up, and have the forehead on the ground. Inhale: Return to the starting position. Chant: *Om Mā Om.* Repeat eight times.
4	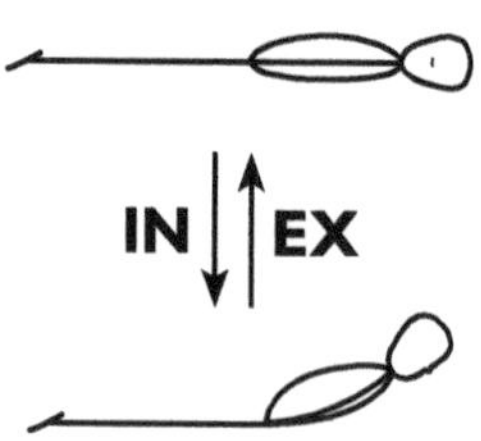 retain 2s, 4s	**Bhujaṅgāsana variation:** To slightly build uplifting energy with a gentle backbend and inhale retention.	Lie facing down, with the head to one side, hands at the sacrum, a slight bend in the elbows, and palms facing up. Inhale: Lift the torso, rotate the head to center. Exhale: Return to the starting position, turning the head to the opposite side. Repeat twice with no retention, twice with a two-second retention, twice with a four-second retention.

5	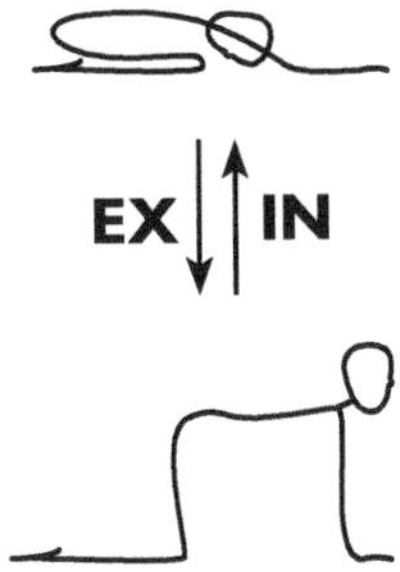 chant on exhale	**Cakravasana:** To compensate for the backbend, gently stretch, and strengthen the back body, while chanting to encourage calming orientation.	Start in a kneeling position with the abdomen on the thighs, and arms extended in front. Inhale: Pull back on the hands and rise to hands and knees. Stack the shoulders over the wrists and the knees over the hips. Lift the chest slightly, broadening the collarbone. Exhale: Draw the hips towards heels, bend the elbows, lower the torso to the thighs, returning to the starting position. Chant: *Om Mā Om* eight times.
6	stay 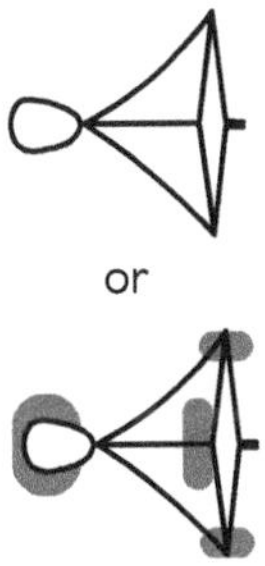 1:2 breath	**Supta Baddha Koṇāsana—restorative:** To gently open the chest, with a laṅghana prāṇāyāma ratio of 1:2 to encourage parasympathetic activation.	Lie flat on the back, place the soles of the feet together, splay the knees wide. Optionally, place a block under each knee, a bolster under the back, and a blanket under the head for support. Place the hands on the abdomen. Inhale: Four seconds, and expand the belly. Exhale: Eight seconds, from the belly, gently pulling in and up. Stay for five minutes.
7	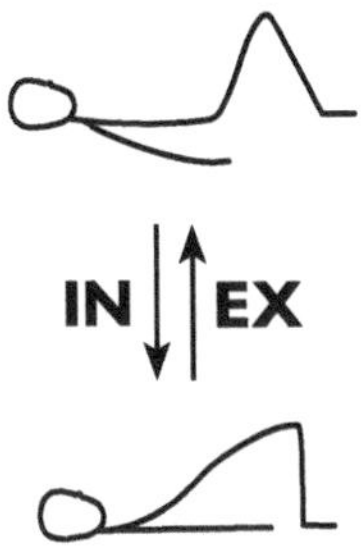	**Dvipāda Pītham:** To counter pose the back from the previous posture.	Lie on the back, feet hip-width apart and arms by the sides. Inhale: Press into the feet, lift the hips off the ground, rising into the upper back. Exhale: Lower the hips and return to the starting position. Repeat eight times.
8	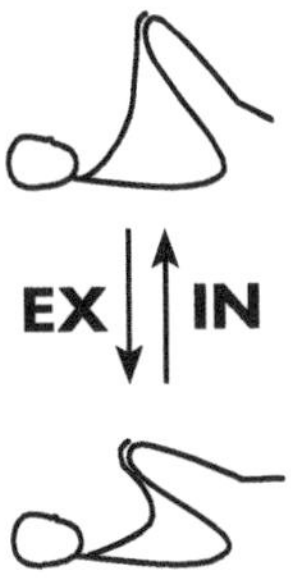 chant on exhale	**Apānāsana:** To stretch the low back, counter pose for the backbends, and encourage the calming effect of exhalation with sound.	Lie on the back, bend the knees into the body. Place the hands on or behind the knees. Exhale: Gently pull the legs into the body while chanting. Inhale: Return to the starting position. Chant: *Om Mā Om.* Repeat eight times.

9	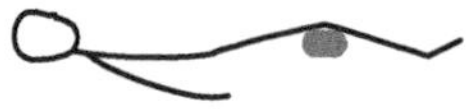	**Śavāsana:** To rest and internalize awareness. To abide in effortlessness.	Lie flat on the back using prop support as necessary. Pay attention to sound—trace awareness in attention to how you are holding the body—relax all contraction. Pay attention to the breath at the navel—watch the effortless rise and fall of the belly and the breath. Inhale vitality and health, exhale out contraction, effort, and tension, relaxing deeply. Rest for five to ten minutes.
10	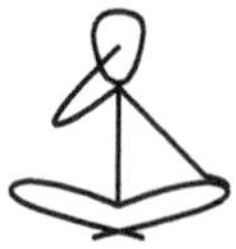	**Nāḍī śodhana:** To promote balance between the sympathetic and parasympathetic nervous systems.	Sit up in a comfortable position, with the spine long. Open the mouth and exhale. Lift the right hand into mṛgī mudrā (Chapter 5). Close the right nostril with the thumb and valve the left with the index finger. *Inhale* through a valved left nostril. Close the left nostril, valve the right, and *exhale* out through a valved right nostril. *Inhale* through a valved right nostril. Close the right nostril, valve the left, and *exhale* out through a valved left nostril. Repeat for nine rounds. *Rest in awareness for as long as you would like.*

Hypoglycemia Awareness

Reducing hypoglycemia risk has a lot to do with *prevention*. We can only avoid something if we can identify it. For many with long-duration diabetes, recurrent hypoglycemia has desensitized their detection of internal bodily cues designed to stave off hypoglycemia. In normal daily activity, detecting hypoglycemia is more challenging because your focus is elsewhere. With a robust CRR, these cues eventually become so intense that a person can no longer ignore them. But for many—those who lack sensory awareness—they do not.

It may seem contradictory that, on one level, hypoglycemia creates sensory overstimulation and, on another, its reoccurrence dulls the senses. I know it is confusing, but if you look at what type of hypoglycemia challenge you are addressing, it makes sense.

Building hypoglycemia sensitivity is a preventative strategy for those who are at risk of developing IAH or those who already have it. When a person is unaware of the physical cues associated with hypoglycemia, it is hard for them to accurately interpret the symptoms and take appropriate action.

Appropriate hypoglycemia detection is developed through interoceptive awareness. Correct perception in yoga (viveka) is the ability to see things correctly as they are. Individuals need to be sensitive enough to detect the symptoms of low BG and interpret them correctly to stave off hypoglycemia. When this doesn't happen, they are at increased risk for severe hypoglycemia and subsequent development of IAH.

It is somewhat ironic. Hypoglycemia leads to hypoglycemia, and awareness begets awareness. We may not know the starting point, but the cause is also the effect. If IAH is a defect in the afferent feedback loop from the body into the brain, improving interoceptive awareness through āsana and prāṇāyāma may serve to strengthen internal sensors, increase self-awareness, and improve action. Afferent neurons are the neurons that run from the body back into the brain. They are mediated by the vagus nerve, part of the parasympathetic branch of the ANS.

Sensory dullness is a result of damaged sympathetic responses over the long duration of diabetes. By allowing the ANS to alternate between sympathetic and parasympathetic activation, we can potentially modulate and improve sympathetic function. Also, by inviting a pause between sides and between different postures, you develop sensitivity to internal cues as sensations.

Identifying the Symptoms

Re-sensitization is developed through various mind-body practices with a focus on perceiving sensation as information. Internal cues associated with neurogenic and neuroglycopenic symptoms vary from person to person. These cues can also be swayed by external influences. Actual hunger, caffeine, and exercise are all potential conflicting markers of hypoglycemia. It is cognitive as well as sensory. Even mild episodes can delay cognitive motor function. As a writer and teacher, I notice that when my BG is dropping, my words lack fluidity. That is my first awareness of BG fluctuations—before my sensor even reads them. A helpful tool is to have your client verbalize the feeling of being low in their body. Verbal cues can be powerful tools to help them link with the symptoms on a more regular basis.

For this practice, we will focus on the energetics of activating the SNS and pacifying it by allowing for pauses to slow the heart rate down and check-in. This will create an equalizing effect between sympathetic and parasympathetic nervous systems. Hypoglycemia unawareness is a product of chronic sympathetic overdrive and damaged sympathetic responses with cognitive and sensory dullness. We want to be cautious not to overstimulate the sympathetic responses; we will only stimulate it so much and then back off. We will achieve this with activation and relaxation. After each activation, pause and do an internal scan. Notice the sensations flowing and pulsating throughout the body. This will attune the individual to the presence of prāṇa. The primary goal is not to lower BG levels but to heighten and stimulate sensory awareness.

L.H., a 43-year-old type 1 diabetic for over 30 years, came to see me several years ago. During our sessions, his BG would regularly fall low, pretty much every time. When his alarm on the CGM would sound, naturally I would look to my own out of habit. But L.H. barely glanced at his. I mentioned something at one point, asking him if he was okay to continue. He said yes, he felt okay with his BG in the low 60s, mentioning that he was used to running low and functioned just fine. An active individual, L.H. ran about six miles daily and spent his weekends mountain biking. When I read his pulse, his heart rate was through the roof. During our initial consultation, I asked him to close his eyes and feel the breath in the body. He immediately opened his eyes and asked me, "What does that mean?" I knew I had my work cut out.

A couple of months into our time working together, L.H. had a motor vehicle accident. His BG was low, and his levels dropped without warning because he was used to running low. Disoriented, he crashed his van into a phone pole. Luckily, he came out of the accident unscathed but he was definitely shaken up emotionally by the experience.

After this, L.H. finally admitted that he needed help with improving his glucose sensitivity. Together we designed a practice for improved responsiveness to not only hypoglycemia but also awareness in general. I witnessed a dramatic change in L.H. throughout our time together. He came prepared for lows during our session, and the mid-practice alarms were less frequent. Whenever I see him around town, he tells me that he continues to do this practice regularly. His wife thanks me more.

Hypoglycemia Awareness

Primary goals: Eliminate or reduce sensory dullness through modulation of sympathetic and parasympathetic activation. Improve interoceptive awareness, the internal awareness to physical bodily cues. Long-term goal: reduce hypoglycemia risk by improving detection, interpretation, and appropriate action.

Theme: A *samāna* (balancing) orientation for physiological equilibrium. Stimulate and then relax, sensitizing perception of prāṇa, circulation, and interoceptive awareness.

Method: Balance sympathetic and parasympathetic activation with quick stimulation and pauses between postures to reintegrate and notice sensations. Focus on contra-lateral (alternate arm and leg) variations, lateral bends, and axial extension. Pause briefly between sides and after repetition of poses to cue into internal sensation. Learn to relax into the presence of the body, linking with the subtlety and nuance of sensations.

Breath-centric āsana: Focus on an equal inhale to exhale ratio (*samavritti*) 1:1 in all poses. Add slight inhale retention and suspension. Lateral bends and axial extension poses to link with sides of the body and the spine.

Prāṇāyāma: In *Mahāmudrā*, a *samāna* ratio of 2:1:2:1 for physiological balance.

Śavāsana: Relax into the presence of the body, feeling of sensation as the awareness of being.

1	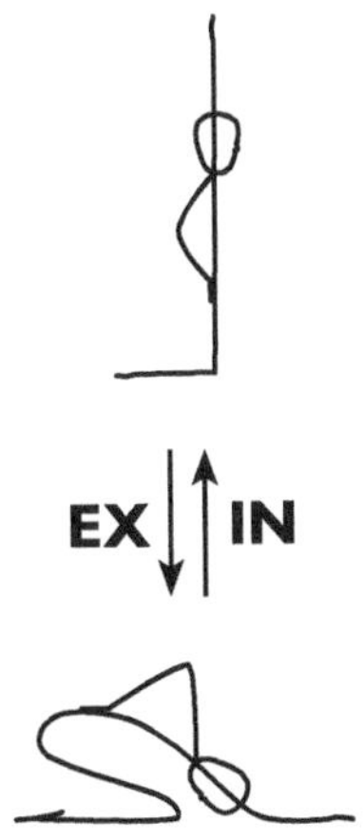	**Varjasana variation:** To stretch and strengthen the back, one side at a time.	Start standing in a kneeling position, with the right arm overhead, the left arm folded behind the body, palm facing out. Exhale: Bend forward, contracting the abdominal muscles, squeezing the right arm, simultaneously lowering the torso to the thighs, the hand and forehead to the ground. Inhale: Challenge the back body to lift the torso and arm at the same time returning to the starting position. Repeat four times each side.

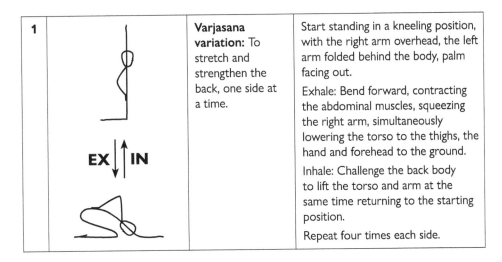

2	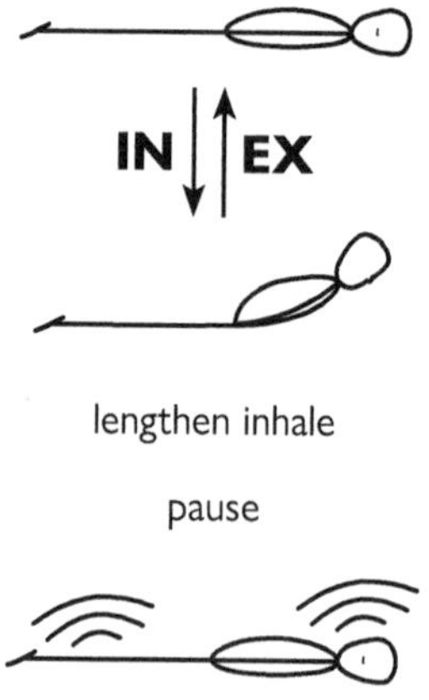	**Bhujaṅgāsana variation:** To strengthen the low back, open the upper back and chest, while developing inhalation.	Lie down on the belly, head to one side, hands at the sacrum, slight bend in the elbows and palms facing up. Inhale: Lift the torso, rotate head to center. Exhale: Return to the starting position, turning the head to the opposite side. Lengthen the inhale: 5 seconds, 6 seconds, 7 seconds, 8 seconds progressively. Repeat four times, then rest in awareness.
3		**Cakravākāsana and Adho Mukha Śvānāsana:** To strengthen the arms, stretch the hamstrings, promote axial extension (length) in the spine, counter pose for the backbend, and transition to standing.	Start in kneeling position with abdomen on thighs, arms extended in front of you. Inhale: Lift up to hands and knees, stack shoulders over wrists and knees over hips, lengthen the sternum from the navel, and broaden the collarbone. Exhale: Tuck the toes, press into the hands, and lift knees off the ground moving into downward facing dog (Adho Mukha Śvānāsana) while lengthening the spine. Inhale: Return to hands and knees. Exhale: Lower hips to heels, torso to thighs, softening the elbows, returning to the starting position. Repeat four times.

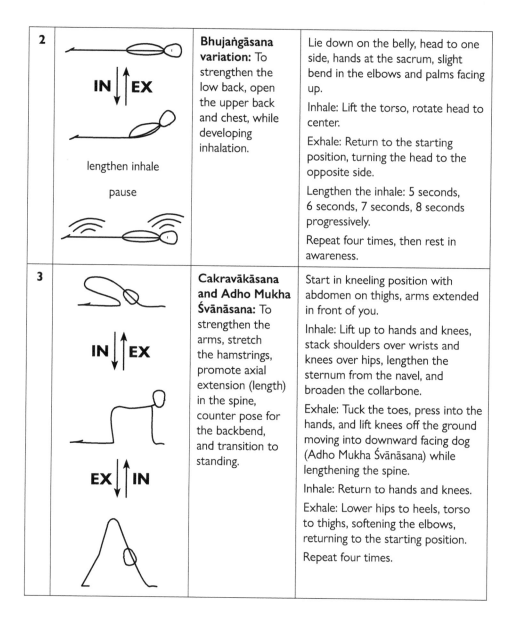

4	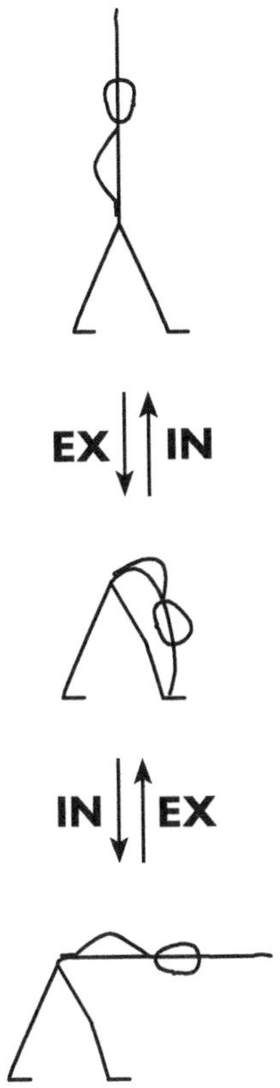 retain 2s, 4s pause 	**Parśvottānāsana and Ardha Parśvottānāsana combo:** To stretch and strengthen the low back, lengthen the spine, and promote stability of body and mind.	Stand a few feet apart with the left leg forward and right leg back, maintain right heel on the ground. Fold the left arm behind the body, palm facing out, right arm overhead. Exhale: Bend forward, squeezing the right elbow, lengthening the right side. Torso to thigh, right hand on the ground by the foot. Try to lengthen the spine rather than dive forward. Inhale: Simultaneously lift the torso and arm until parallel with ground, lengthening the spine and squeezing the right arm muscles to activate the right side of the body. Retain the inhale. Retain 0 seconds two times. Retain 2 seconds two times. Retain 4 seconds two times. Exhale: Bend forward, torso to thigh, right hand on the ground by the foot. Inhale: Return to the starting position, lifting the arm and torso simultaneously. Repeat six times on both sides. Rest between sides, feel the sensations in the side body.

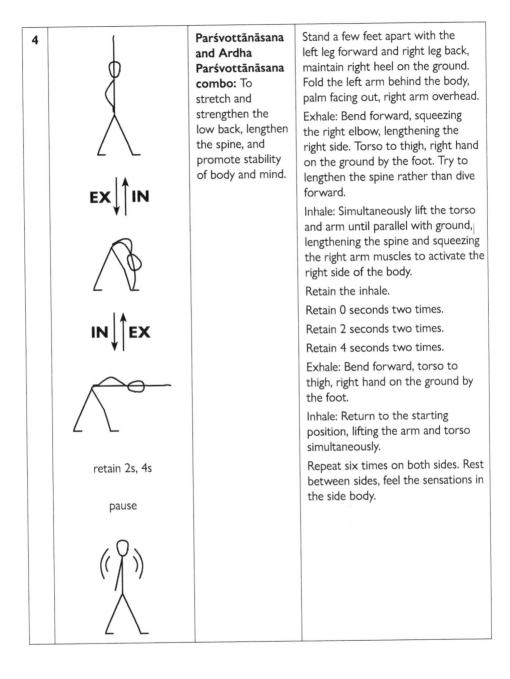

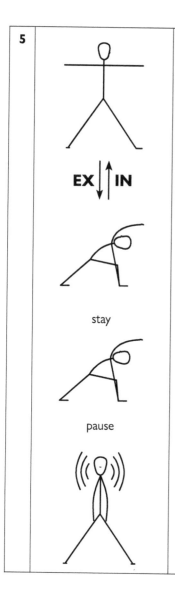

5	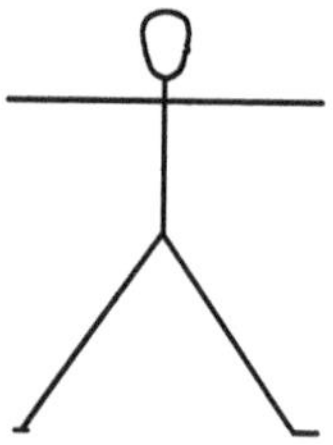 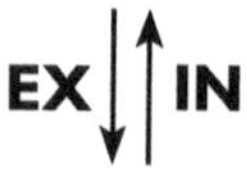 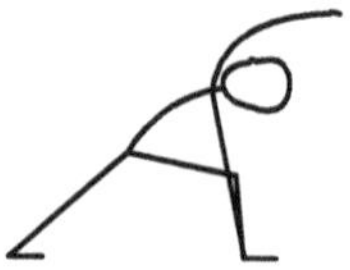 stay 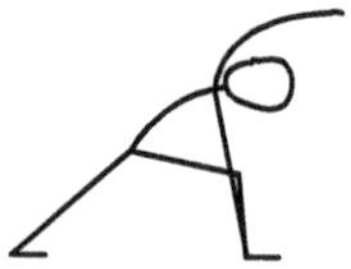 pause 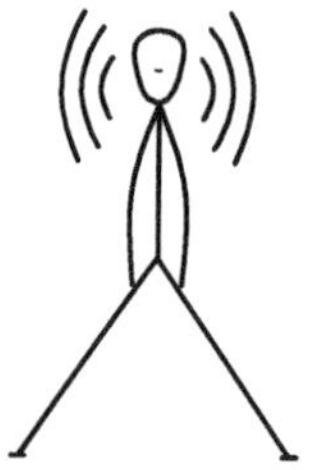	**Utthita Pārśvakoṇāsana:** To stretch the torso and strengthen the legs, especially the hips, one side at a time. An emphasis on exhale will prepare for the next posture.	Stand with legs wider than the shoulders, left foot forward, right foot back. Open the arms parallel with ground, palms face up. Exhale: Bend the left knee to 90 degrees, laterally bend, bring the left arm and torso toward the inner left leg, reaching the right arm overhead. Inhale: Return to the starting position. Lengthen the exhale—5 seconds, 6 seconds, 7 seconds, 8 seconds progressively, then stay in the pose for six breaths. Press the left inner leg into the left arm, activating the hip muscles. Repeat both sides, rest between sides for several breaths. Close eyes, notice and observe sensations.

6	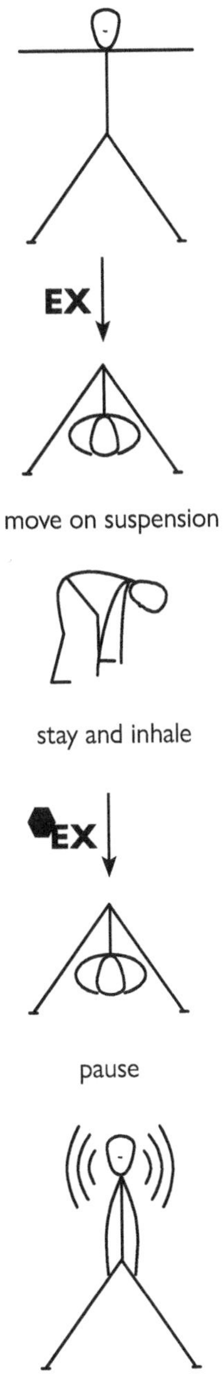	**Prasārita Pādottānāsana and Ardha Prasārita Pādottānāsana combo with uḍḍiyāna-bandha 'like' movement:** To create a specific energetic effect (slightly stimulating and intensifying) and physiological response by suspending the exhalation.	Stand with feet wider than the shoulders and parallel. Exhale: Bend forward with a little bend in the knees, glide the hands down the legs, place hands under shoulders. Suspension: Holding the breath out, lift the torso until back is flat and arms are straight. Keep the chin in. Try to draw the abdomen in and up creating a vacuum-like suction in the upper and lower abdomen. Hold empty for a few sections without creating tension. Stay in the pose, relax the abdomen, and inhale. Exhale: Bend forward. Repeat eight times before returning to the starting position. Rest for several breaths, allowing the nervous system and breath to recalibrate before moving on.

7	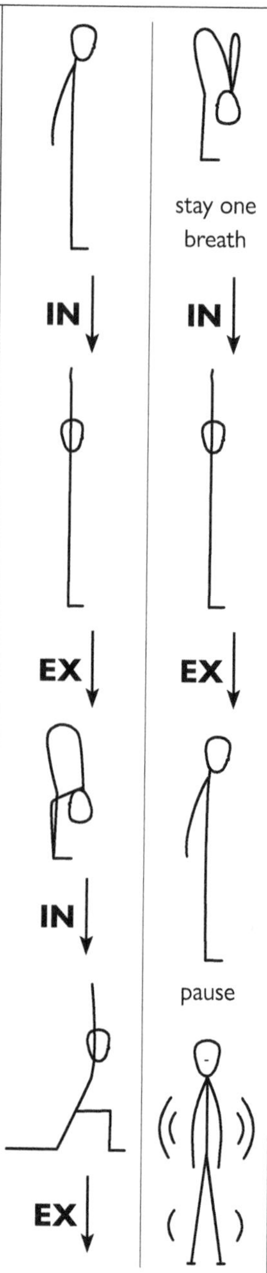	**Candra Namaskār variation:** To counter pose from the previous pose, redistributing energy throughout the body. To prepare the hip flexors, upper back, and arms for subsequent postures.	Start in Tāḍāsana, feet together, arms by the sides. Inhale: Reach arm overhead, lengthen the low back and sides of the body. Exhale: Bend forward, lower the torso to the thighs, hands on the ground. Inhale: Step the right leg back, right knee on ground, lift the torso, arms overhead. Exhale: Bend forward, lower the hands to the ground, step the right leg to meet the left. Slight bend in the knees, interlace the hands behind the back, lifting away from the low back. Stay for one breath. Inhale: Open arms, lift torso, and return to standing with the arms overhead. Exhale: Lower arms by sides, return to the starting position. Repeat eight times, alternating legs. Pause between each round, take a few breaths. Last round, stay in the lunge and forward bend with hands interlaced for five breaths.

8	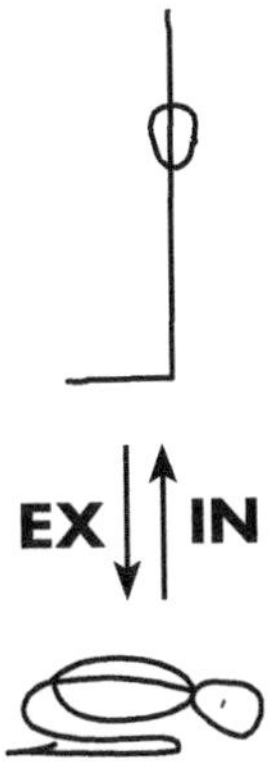EX IN	**Vajrāsana:** To transition to the floor.	Start standing in a kneeling position with both arms overhead. Inhale: Sweep both arms wide, lift torso, and stand up on the knees, reaching arms overhead. Exhale: Return to the starting position. Repeat four times.
9	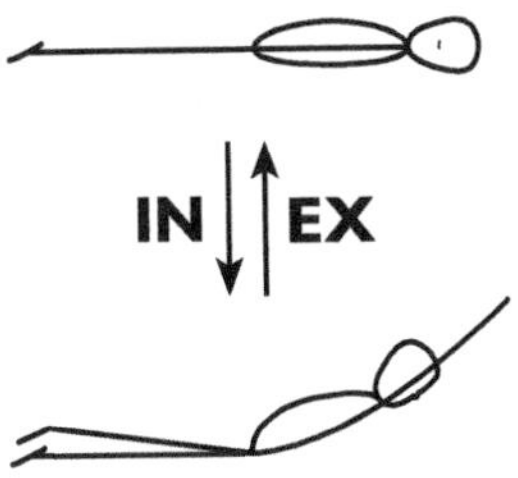IN EX	**Ardha Śalabhāsana variation:** To combine asymmetrical movements of upper back, neck, shoulders, and low back.	Lie down on the belly, head to one side, hands at the sacrum, slight bend in the elbows, and palms facing up. Inhale: Lift the chest, sweep right arm wide and forward, bending the arm into a salute, lift the right leg off the ground. Exhale: Return to the starting position turning the head to the right away from the sweeping arm. Repeat eight times alternating arms and legs.
10	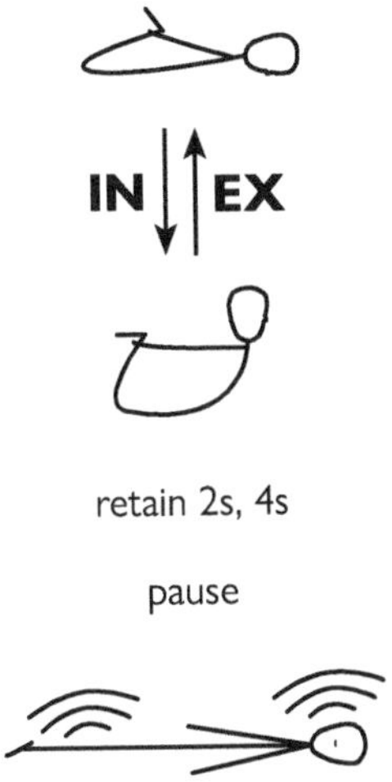IN EX retain 2s, 4s pause	**Dhanurāsana:** To create an opening and expansive quality without over-stimulating the nervous system.	Lie down on the belly, bend knees, reach back and grab ankles. Take a breath in and out, anchor the pelvis to the mat, lengthen the low back. Inhale: Lift the chest and kick the feet into the hands. Retain: 0 seconds two times, 2 seconds two times, 4 seconds two times. Exhale: Lower back down. Repeat six times, then release the pose and rest for several breaths, feel presence at heart.

11	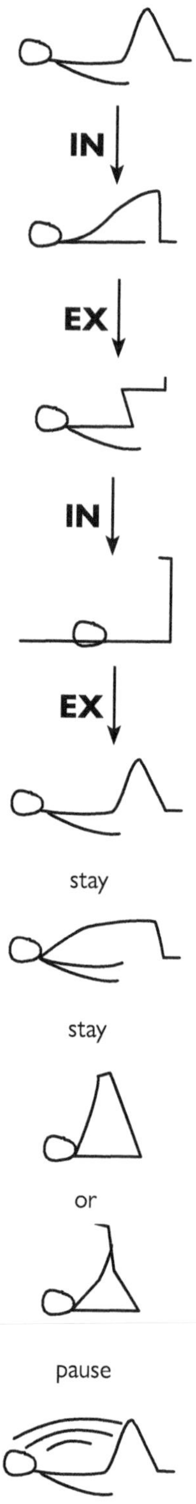	**Dvipāda Pītham and Ūrdhva Prasārita Pādāsana combo:** To counter pose, lengthen the spine, strengthen the low back, internalize the mind, and prepare for maha mudrā.	Lie on back, feet on the mat hip-width distance apart, arms by the sides of the torso. Inhale: Press into the feet, lift the hips off the ground, rise to upper back. Exhale: Lower hips and lift the feet off of the ground drawing the knees into the chest. Inhale: Straighten arms behind the head and straighten legs to the ceiling keeping the sacrum on the ground. Exhale: Lower arms and legs, bend the knees, and place the feet on the mat. Repeat six times. On the last round, stay in each pose for four breaths. Then rest for one minute before transitioning to being seated.

12

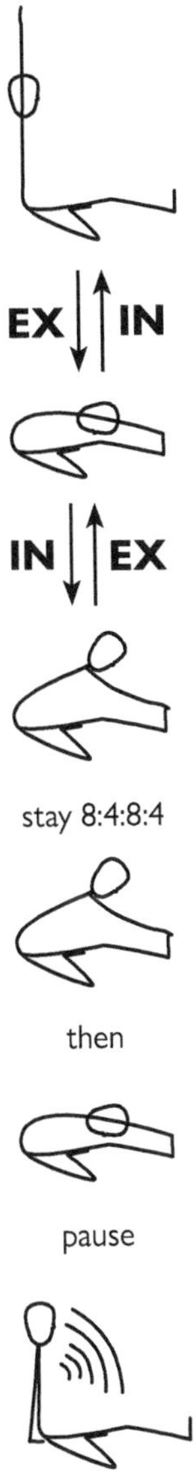
EX
IN
IN
EX
stay 8:4:8:4
then
pause

Jānu Śīrṣāsana and Mahāmudrā with prāṇāyāma ratio: The apex of the practice. To bring attention to the spine, the central channel, and the presence which rides along the wave of the breath. This pose is strengthening, stabilizing, internalizing, and expansive. To encourage interoceptive awareness and sensitivity.

Sit with right knee bent, heel to inner left thigh, left leg extended forward and arms overhead.

A: Jānu Śīrṣāsana and Mahāmudrā

Exhale: Bend forward, bring belly and chest to left leg and hands to foot.

Inhale: Holding the foot with both hands, lean back, lift the torso as far away from the thigh as possible, chin in, spine long.

Exhale: Bend forward, bring belly and chest to left leg and hands to foot.

Inhale: Return to the starting position.

Do four times.

B. Mahāmudrā with prāṇāyāma

Exhale: Bend forward, bring belly and chest to left leg and hands to foot.

Inhale: Holding the foot with both hands, lean back, lift the torso as far away from the thigh as possible, chin in, spine long. Stay and breathe 8:4:8:4 for 6–8 breaths (see table and instructions below).

Inhale	Hold (R)	Exhale	Hold (S)	Number
8	4	8	4	6–8 times

Then:

Exhale: Bend forward, bring belly and chest to left leg and hands to foot. Stay for a few breaths.

Inhale: Return to the starting position.

Repeat A and B on one side before switching sides. Pause between sides for a few breaths and notice sensation, presence, awareness of the body.

13	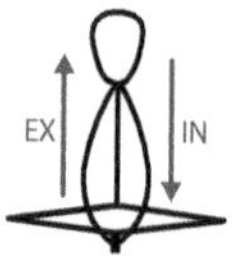	**Baddha Koṇāsana:** To counter pose for Mahāmudrā, stretch the hips, lengthen the spine, and bring attention to the presence which rides along the wave of the breath.	Grab feet, sit up tall. Maintain the abdomen slightly firm. Inhale and expand the chest and grow tall. On exhale, reengage the abdomen, sit even taller. Notice how the effect of exhale (drawing the abdomen in) prepares for the inhale, and how the inhale effect (expanding the chest) is felt on the exhale. Stay for 6–8 breaths.
14	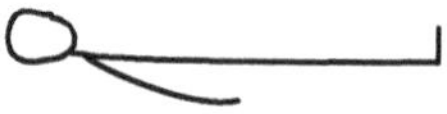	**Śavāsana:** To rest in sensitivity to presence (interoceptive awareness).	Attention to presence in the: right foot—pause left foot—pause right hand—pause left hand—pause right foot and left hand—pause left foot and right hand—pause right foot, left hand, right eye—pause left foot, right hand, left eye—pause the whole body—pause. Rest in the infinite presence of the whole body—pause.

CHAPTER 10

Neuropathy

Hyperglycemia damages blood vessels and nerves. A common effect of longer-duration diabetes is neuropathy. There are two main forms of neuropathy: peripheral and autonomic. The former is painful nerve damage felt in the body's bodily extremities, and the latter is neurological damage to the afferent nerve ANS. For instance, a person can experience autonomic neuropathy in their stomach. This causes a very uncomfortable condition called gastroparesis, where the stomach takes forever to release food, making it very difficult to manage diabetes with insulin. Neuropathy can damage the vagus nerve, which is responsible for regulating the ANS and other parts of the brain. The ventral medial hypothalamus is a part of the hypothalamus, which helps people sense their low blood sugars. Without this function, people are at increased risk of dangerously low BG episodes.

Digestion

Digestion problems, gastroparesis, and GI discomfort are some of the most common effects of diabetes. As many as 50% of diabetic patients with long-duration diabetes have severe gastrointestinal issues.[1] Symptoms can include postprandial fullness and discomfort, nausea, vomiting, bloating, early satiety, and abdominal pain.[2] Hyperglycemia in diabetes causes microvascular damage, which results in severe peripheral, autonomic, and central neuropathy. Diabetic autonomic neuropathy can affect various systems of the body, including cardiovascular, gastrointestinal, and urogenital systems. We talked a little

1 Brock, C. (2013) "Diabetic autonomic neuropathy affects symptom generation and brain-gut axis." *Diabetes Care* 36, 3698–3705.

2 Brock, C. (2013) "Diabetic autonomic neuropathy affects symptom generation and brain-gut axis." *Diabetes Care* 36, 3698–3705.

about a symptom of diabetic autonomic neuropathy when we discussed IAH (impaired awareness of hypoglycemia) (see Chapter 9). One of the effects of this type of nerve damage is an attenuated response to hypoglycemia symptoms resulting from damage to the ANS.

Our digestion is also regulated by the ANS, in particular the vagus nerve, which provides parasympathetic innervation of the various organs responsible for stimulating muscular activity, enzyme secretion, and acid production for digestion.[3] When the vagus nerve is damaged from autonomic neuropathy, the stomach has a hard time digesting food. It stops moving in the way it needs to, and the base of the stomach, where food is released into the small intestine, closes in spasm. The result is an incredibly slow release of food, resulting in acid back up. Not everyone experiences this abdominal discomfort, but people can notice complete unpredictability in their BG numbers after a meal. With normal digestion, we begin to digest our food immediately and can finish about three hours after a meal. It can become quite challenging to anticipate how much insulin to take for a meal. You never know when your stomach will decide to release food. You can crash low after a meal only to see that your BG levels are really high eight hours later.

There are some things that we can do to reduce stomach discomfort. One is to shorten the time spent in hyperglycemia; however, that can be challenging, for the reason I just explained. Other modifiable changes could be to reduce stress, and limit caffeine, fat, and alcohol, which can all slow down gastric emptying. It is important to note that not all diabetes stomach issues are attributable to autonomic neuropathy. In fact, irritable bowel syndrome (IBS), leaky gut, candida overgrowth, hypothyroidism, and celiac disease are all common with diabetes. So it is crucial to get tested to figure out what is going on.

No matter what the cause is, the result is attenuated and compromised digestion with abdominal discomfort. We know from Āyurveda that so much of our health starts in the gut. The abdomen is the seat of agni, our digestive fire. We want yoga therapy to support gut motility and digestion in the short term and improve long-term digestion through parasympathetic predominance and vagal activity. We can try to replicate gastrointestinal motility through specific

3 Bernstein, R. K. (2011) *Dr. Bernstein's Diabetes Solution: The Complete Guide to Achieving Normal Blood Sugars*. Fourth edition. Boston, MA: Little Brown Publishers. p.65.

breathing techniques and āsanas, simultaneously compressing and stretching the abdominal region.

Some other intervention tools are uḍḍiyāna-bandha, agni sara, and movement on suspension. These are all techniques that encourage the lifting of the abdominal organs and diaphragm. These techniques can simulate the action of the stomach. Just a side note: When applying uḍḍiyāna-bandha, you hold mūla-bandha after releasing uḍḍiyāna-bandha. If you want to increase apāna (elimination), release mūla-bandha when you release uḍḍiyāna-bandha. Otherwise, you will do the opposite of apāna—udāna, which holds prāṇa in and up.

E.O., a young woman in her late 20s, came to me complaining of cyclical bouts of late-night stomach aches, gas, and bloating. Besides the discomfort, she reported slow digestion and a challenge in knowing how much insulin to dose for her meals. She was continually waking up in the morning with fasting glucose over 200 mg/dL (11 mmol/L) and reported that when this happened, she lacked the energy for her day. She guesstimated that it could sometimes be three or more hours before her stomach would begin to digest the food from her meal, and she knew this because her BG would spike at that time. A1c was right under 7.0%, but she admitted to me that it had not always been so good, especially during her teenage years. E.O. had been practicing yoga for several years and had seen several specialists who could not figure out her problem. Doctors had rebuked claims that she had a condition known as gastroparesis, common in diabetes patients, and she tested negative for celiac disease. I was not entirely convinced that she was not experiencing mild-grade gastroparesis or, at least, a product of slight autonomic neuropathy after 20-plus years with T1D.

Together, we developed this practice to help encourage digestion (stimulate digestive fire), activate vagal tone, and massage her abdominal organs. I wanted to support the action of apāna, the downward and outward flow of prāṇa, to help her elimination, and also samāna vāyu, the movement of prāṇa inward, to promote assimilation of food. The energetic focus of the practice has a laṅghana orientation to activate the parasympathetic branch regulated by the vagus nerve. I added longer exhale suspension to stimulate digestive fire and encourage the stomach's motility.

While sluggish digestion could be viewed as a kapha condition, in this case, an active individual with T1D exhibiting gas and bloating, I see it as a vāta imbalance.

Sometimes poor digestion is also a result of anxiety, so I emphasized a laṅghana orientation to help reduce and calm any excessive rajas of the mind. As our relationship developed, E.O. admitted to having anxiety about falling low from the insulin, and, as a result, she ate her meals way too fast, causing digestive distress. A symptom of hypoglycemia is hunger, and E.O. confused the hunger with hypoglycemia.

We discussed her eating her dinner mindfully and slowly, with the absence of external distractions like the TV or a phone. She would begin her meals by taking a moment to look at her food and asking that it nourish her body. Each bite would be a mindful meditation of being present in the moment.

I also recommended that E.O. tracked her cycles in a journal (as hormones could impact digestion and insulin absorption). I suggested she try a khecharī (adapted for diabetes) recipe (see Chapter 6) during her flare-ups to help neutralize the abdominal discomfort. Over time E.O.'s bouts of going to bed with stomach pain, gas, and discomfort, only to wake up with hyperglycemia, greatly diminished and her energy improved.

A Practice for Slow Diabetes Digestion

Primary goals: Encourage elimination (apāna vāyu movement down and out) and proper assimilation (samāna vāyu movement to the center) of food, tonify the vagus nerve through parasympathetic activation.

Method: A laṅghana orientation. Activate the parasympathetic nervous system to encourage digestion via exhalation.

Breath-centric āsana: Focus on forward bends and spinal rotation, as they are executed on the exhalation, and massage and compress the abdominal organs. First, introduce segmented breath and movement. Then, add short exhale suspension and movement on suspension, creating an uḍḍiyāna-bandha "like" suction to massage and compress the abdomen. Make sure to release mūla-bandha, as this will inhibit elimination.

Prāṇāyāma: Lengthening the exhale to be longer than the inhale promotes parasympathetic activation and supports digestion. Exhale does not always originate naturally from the abdomen, so we need to train it. A method is viloma krama: a 2-part exhale. For example: exhale halfway, pause, exhale remainder, pause, then inhale.

Meditation: Niṣṭhā dhāraṇā (navel-gazing meditation) with mantra: *Om Ram*

Agnaye Namaha. It means: *om*, giving reverence; *ram*, the bija mantra of the navel; *agni* (*Agnaye*), the fire of transformation and of health, which abides at the navel; *namaha*, "not by me" but "by You," where You represents the Highest for us.[4]

1	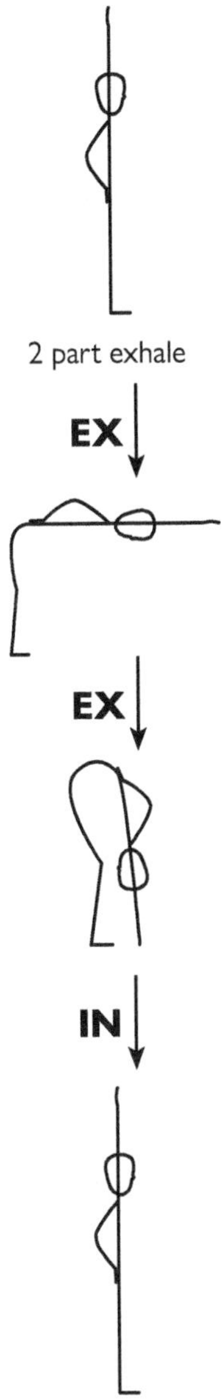	**Uttānāsana variation with two-part krama exhale:** To compress the abdomen and lengthen the exhale, one side at a time.	Stand at attention with the feet slightly separated. Place the left hand at the low back, with the palm facing out, and have the right arm lifted overhead. Exhale: For half a breath, bend forward halfway, with slight flexion in the knees, lengthen the spine, keep the chin in. Pause briefly. Exhale: For the second half of the breath, bend forward all the way, lower the torso to the thighs, place the right hand on the ground by the foot. Inhale: Simultaneously lift the arm and torso, returning to the starting position. Repeat three times on both sides.

4 Kraftsow, G. (2002) *Yoga for Transformation: Ancient Teachings and Holistic Practices for Healing Body, Mind, and Heart*. New York: Penguin Compass. p.226.

2	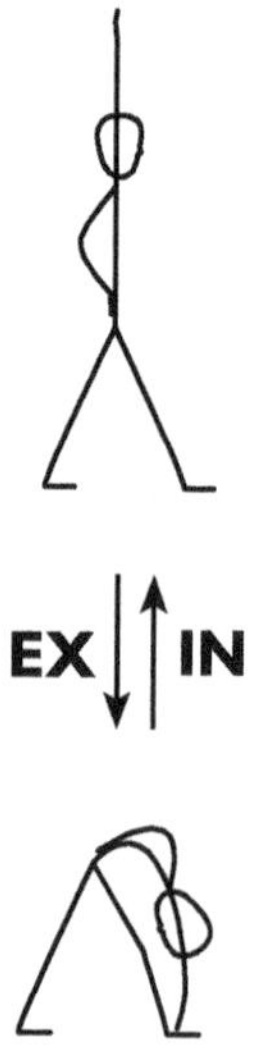	**Parśvottānāsana variation:** To strengthen the back and compress the abdomen one side at a time, introduce exhale suspension and movement on suspension.	Stand with the feet apart with the left leg forward and right leg back, and keep the right heel on the ground. Place the left hand at the sacrum, with the palm facing out, and have the right arm overhead. Exhale: With a slight bend in the front knee, bend forward, squeezing the right elbow and lengthening the right side on the transition, lower the torso to the thigh, have the right hand on the ground by the foot. Inhale: Return to the starting position with length, using the back muscles to lift up. a. Free breath, twice. b. Suspend the breath for two seconds, twice. c. Exhale in the starting position, move into the pose while suspending the exhale, suction the abdomen in and up. Do this twice. Do this on both sides.
3	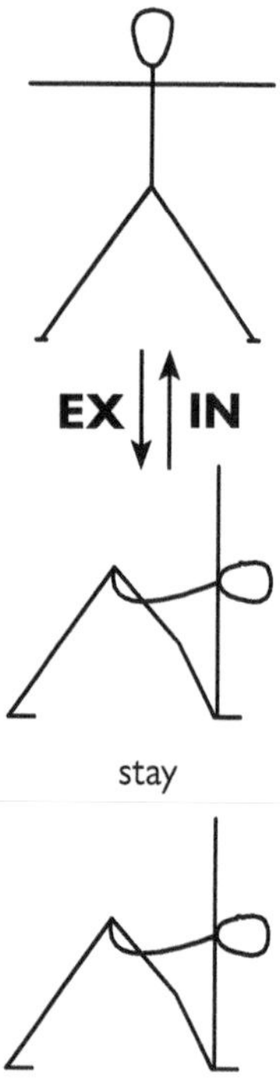	**Parivṛtti Trikoṇāsana:** To compress the abdomen, one side at a time.	Stand with the feet wider than the shoulders and parallel, and the arms out to sides, level with the floor. A: Exhale: Twist to the left, place the right hand on the floor, reach the left arm vertically, and twist the navel to the left. Inhale: Return to the starting position. Repeat six times, alternating sides. B: Stay in the twist with the right hand down and the left arm up. Inhale: Lengthen the torso. Exhale: Stay and twist from the navel. Stay for six breaths and then return to the starting position and repeat on the other side.

4		**Cakravākāsana and Adho Mukha Śvānāsana combo:** To counter pose after a twist, transition to the floor, compress and relax the abdomen.	Start in a kneeling position with the abdomen on the thighs, and the arms extended in front. Inhale: Lift up to hands and knees, stack the shoulders over the wrists and the knees over the hips, lengthen the sternum from the navel, and broaden the collarbone. Exhale: Tuck the toes, press into the hands, and lift the knees off the ground, moving into downward facing dog (Adho Mukha Śvānāsana) while lengthening the spine. Inhale: Return to hands and knees. Exhale: Lower the hips to the heels, the torso to the thighs, soften the elbows, and return to the starting position. a. Free breath, twice. b. Pause after exhale, suspend the breath for four seconds, twice. c. Exhale in the starting position, move into the pose while suspending the exhale. Try to suction the abdomen in and up, twice.
5	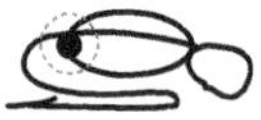	**Vajrāsana with hands in abdomen:** To manually massage the abdominal organs.	Sit on the shins. Wrap four fingers around each thumb, making fists with the hands. Bring the knuckles of both hands together and placing them in the abdomen. Bend forward and bring the torso to the thighs. Spend some time breathing into the hands and pressing the fists up and into the abdomen, massaging around. When you feel discomfort, breathe into it; notice if it subsides. Stay for several minutes, maintaining a smooth and even breath.

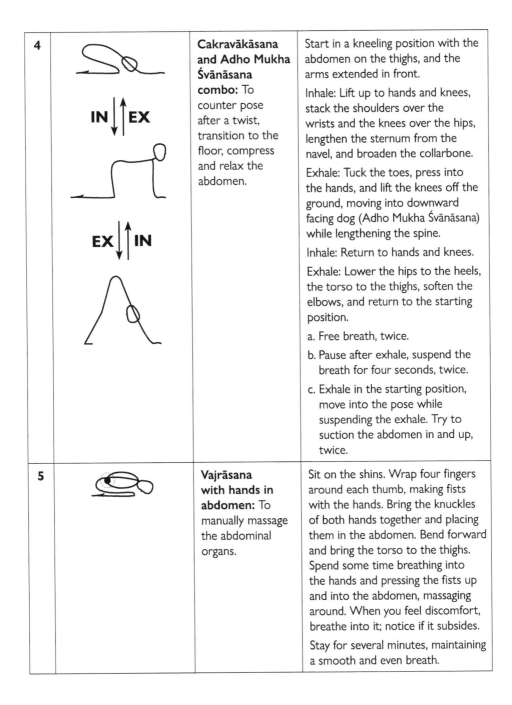

6	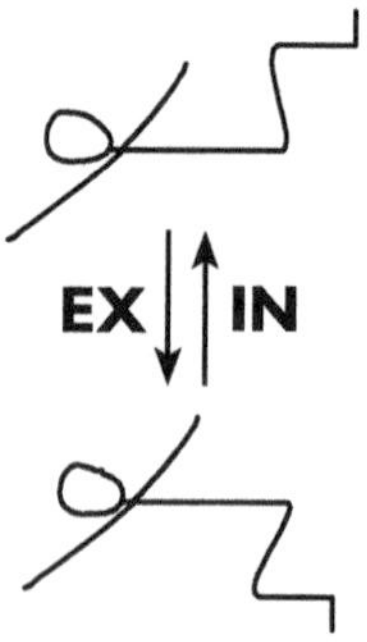 EX IN	**Jaṭara Parivṛtti:** To stretch the sides and compress the abdomen, one side at a time.	Lie on the back, with both arms wide and the knees bent into the chest. Exhale: Twist, bring the legs over to the left side, and turn the head to the right. Inhale: Return to the starting position. Repeat six times, alternating sides.
7	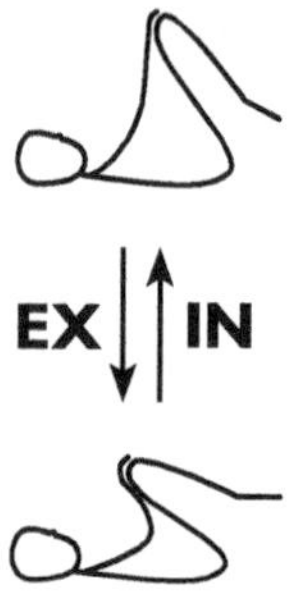 EX IN	**Apānāsana:** To counter pose for the supine twist, compress and relax the abdomen.	Lie on the back, and bend the knees into the body. Place the hands on the knees. Exhale: Gently pull the legs into the body. Inhale: Return to the starting position. a. Free breath, twice. b. Pause after exhale, suspend the breath for four seconds, twice. c. Exhale in the starting position, and move into apānāsana on suspension, twice.
8	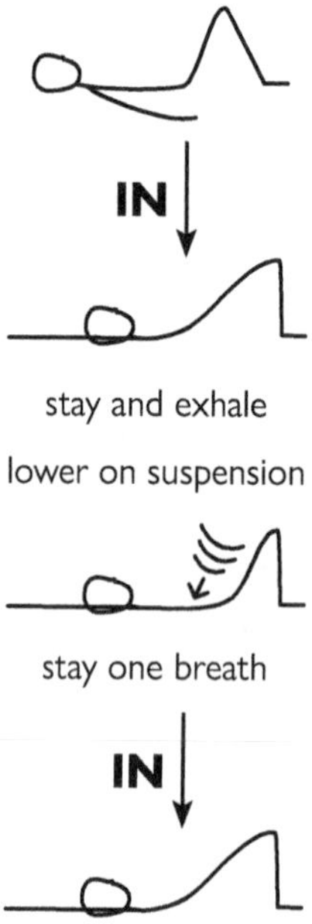 IN stay and exhale lower on suspension stay one breath IN	**Dvipāda Pītham variation with uḍḍiyāna-bandha "like" movement:** To unwind the spine, compress and relax the abdomen through uḍḍiyāna-bandha like activation.	Lie on the back with the feet hip-width apart and arms by the sides. Inhale: Press into the feet, lift the hips off the ground while reaching the arms up and behind the head to the floor. Exhale: Stay in the pose. Suspension: Slowly lower the hips, keeping the arms behind, suction the abdomen in and up. Inhale: Stay and relax the abdomen. Exhale: Stay. Repeat six times.
9	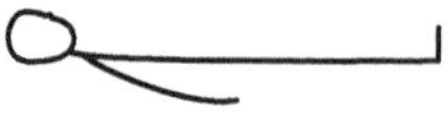	**Śavāsana:** To rest.	Soften the abdomen, relax the breath. Stay for three to five minutes minimum.

10	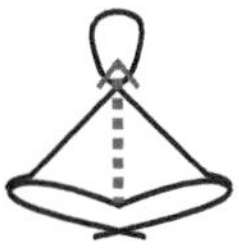	**Prāṇāyāma two-part segmented exhale:** To contract and relax the abdomen through segmented exhale.	Sit in a comfortable position with the spine long. Deepen and lengthen the breath. Exhale: Half of the exhalation in five seconds. Pause: Five seconds. Exhale: The rest of the exhale in five seconds. Pause: Five seconds. Inhale: Slowly and completely. Do 12 rounds.
11	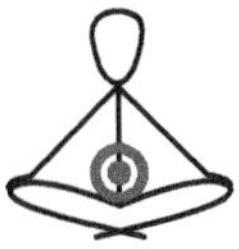	**Niṣṭhā dhāraṇā meditation:** To rest in the abdomen and link with the presence of agni, the assimilative and digestive fire.	Relax the shaping of the breath. First, establish prāṇa dhāraṇā in the abdomen. Sense a warm, glowing presence at the navel, like expanding from the navel on the natural inhale and returning to center of the navel on the natural exhale. Continue for several minutes, and then relax the technique and rest in awareness at the abdomen. Feel the mantra emerge at navel center. Repeat mantra: *Om Ram Agnaye Namaha.* Stay as long as your time allows.

Peripheral Neuropathy

Peripheral neuropathy from long-duration hyperglycemia is damage to the PNS, resulting in discomfort, pain, tingling, and lack of awareness in the limbs. Standing āsana is often difficult and painful. With lack of awareness and sensitivity in the limbs, people are at higher risk for complications that result in infection.

M.B., a client in his late 60s with T2D, came to see me. Diagnosed ten years prior, he was becoming increasingly frustrated about weight gain and pain in his feet. A once vibrant and active man in the community, M.B. spent less time socializing and more time at home. He wanted to be dynamic like he once was, but the neuropathy was limiting his movement.

His view on diabetes was ambivalent. He did not do much to "manage" diabetes other than taking an oral medication. I asked him whether or not he changed his diet much after diagnosis. He said that he was watching his carbohydrate intake—reducing bread and pasta. But when he explained his diet he reported eating cereal for breakfast, a sandwich for lunch, and over 6oz of alcohol at night.

I could tell that M.B. had a great sense of humor but he was easily discouraged and had a hard time following verbal instruction. He had no prior yoga experience and was sedentary, although he once was active. I observed that he got aggravated by too much verbal instruction and more "strenuous postures," exhibited when he hastily pulled out of a pose or exposed his anger beneath his breath. He overworked whenever he felt remotely challenged by a pose, breathing rapidly and sweating.

M.B. was mentally anxious and physically sedentary. The pain in his limbs and weight gain put additional pressure on his cardiovascular system. I devised this modified chair adaptive practice to help M.B. increase sensitivity to his limbs by stretching and strengthening the leg and hip muscles.

The goal for M.B. was to awaken awareness in his legs, hips, feet, and abdominal muscles. We worked with a particular emphasis on the legs and built up his practice over several months to standing balancing poses.

M.B. has gotten his A1c down, reducing pain in his feet, and is able to take daily walks around his neighborhood with his wife and dog. He still visits me, although less frequently. Now, he is more interested in prāṇāyāma and meditation. The foundation of this practice helped him feel more empowered to influence change in his body and set the stage for deeper practices.

A Practice for Diabetes Peripheral Neuropathy

Primary goal: Reduce pain, improve circulation and strength in the hands, legs, and feet as a result of peripheral neuropathy.

Secondary goal: Improve self-awareness and self-efficacy through intentional practice.

Method: Stretch and strengthen the hips, hamstrings, calves, feet, upper back, and wrists.

1	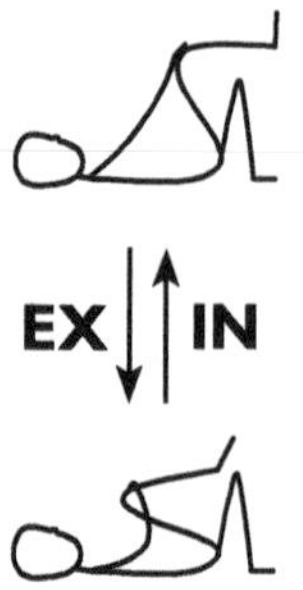	**Ardha apānāsana variation:** To stretch the musculature of the hips and low back.	Lie flat on the back with the left foot on the floor. Have the right foot lifted, the hands holding the right knee, and the elbows straight. Exhale: Bend both elbows and pull the right thigh into the body. Inhale: Return to the starting position. Repeat eight times each side; stay for four breaths on the last repetition.

2	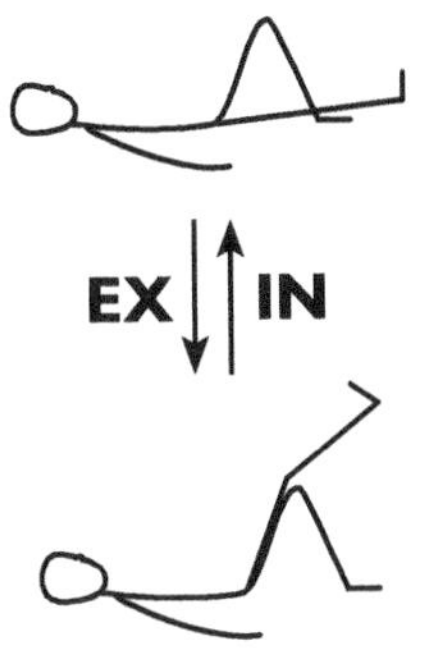	**Supta Eka Pādāṇguṣṭhāsana variation:** To stretch the hamstrings, strengthen deep abdominal musculature, promote circulation in the feet.	Lie flat on the back with the right leg straight, the left knee bent and foot on the floor, and arms by the sides. Lift the right leg off the ground a couple inches, activating the leg muscles. Exhale: Extend the leg up about 45 degrees, flex the foot. Inhale: Lower the leg to hover in the starting position. Repeat eight times on both sides. Try to keep the body still and shoulders relaxed. Use abdominal and leg strength to lift the leg.
3	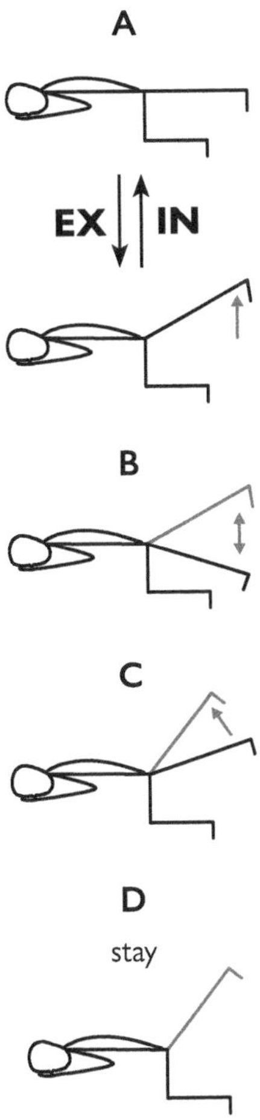	**Side lying pose variations:** To stimulate the abductors and gluteus maximus while stretching the hip flexors.	Lie on the right side of the body, support the head with the right arm, have the right knee bent to 90 degrees, the left hand on the left hip, and the left leg straight. a. Exhale: Lift the left leg off the ground until it is just beyond parallel with the ground. Inhale: Lower to the starting position. Repeat four times. b. Return to the previous position with the leg lifted and level with the ground. Exhale: Bring the leg back behind the body, stretch the front of the leg, and squeeze the gluteus maximus. Inhale: Return to the starting position. c. Return to the previous position with the leg lifted level and behind the body. Turn the toes of the foot down so the thigh is internally rotated. Inhale: Lower the leg just below level. Exhale: Lift the leg just above level. d. Stay with the leg back and toes down for four breaths.

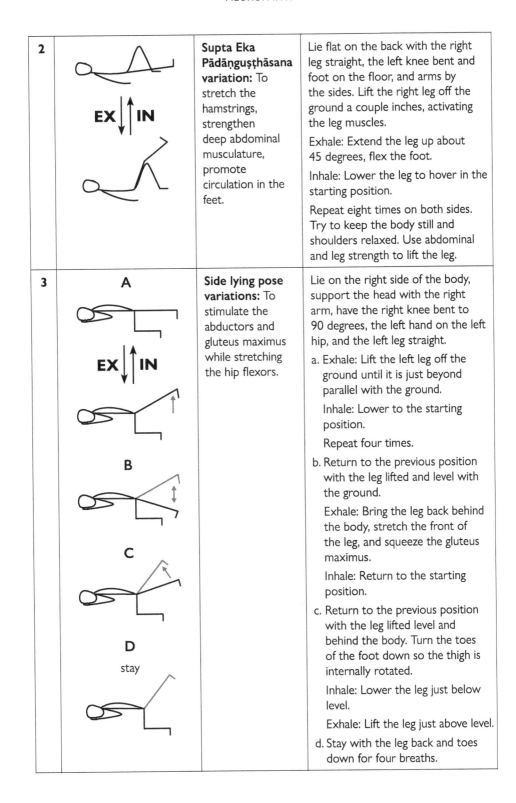

4	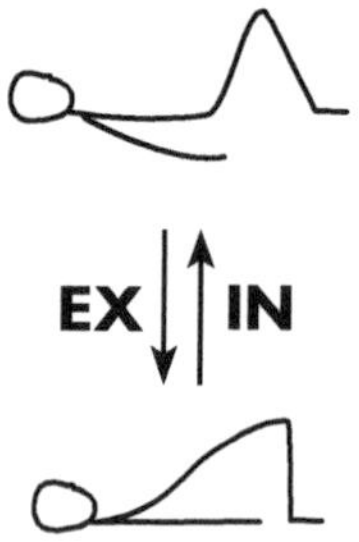	**Dvipāda Pītham variation:** To strengthen the back, hamstrings, adductors, and glutes.	Lie on the back, with the feet hip-width apart and arms by the sides. Flex the ankles so just the heels are on the ground. Exhale: Press into the heels and lift the hips off the ground. Inhale: Return to the starting position. Repeat eight times.
5	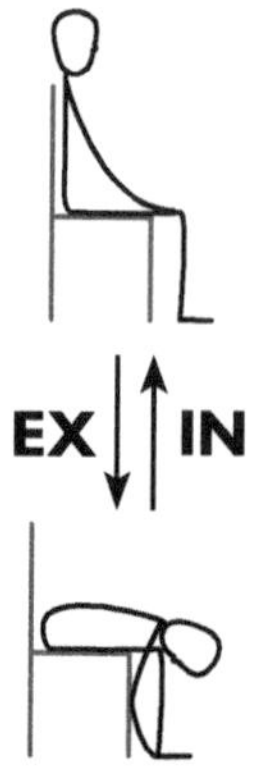	**Cakravākāsana variation:** To stretch and contract the back body, lengthen the exhale for abdominal strength.	Sit on the edge of a chair, with the feet on the ground, hands on the thighs, and arms straight. Inhale: Lift the torso, traction the hands against the thighs, reach the collarbone forward. Feel the back and side bodies contracting. Exhale: Bend forward, gliding the hands down the legs. Inhale for six seconds, exhale for eight seconds. Repeat eight times.
6	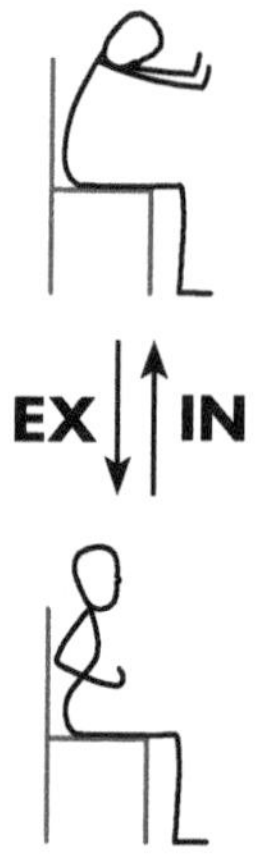 retain 2s, 4s	**Vīrabhadrāsana variation:** To stretch and strengthen the upper back, hands, and wrists.	Sit on the edge of a chair, with the feet on the ground. Inhale: Displace the chest forward, bend the elbows into the sides, squeeze the scapulae, adducting the shoulder blades, and make fists with the hands, palms face up. Retain: Lift the chest and chin slightly. Retain or hold the inhale in for two seconds and then for four seconds. Exhale: Push the hands forward, straighten the arms, flex the wrists, lower the head between the arms, lower the chin, abduct the shoulder blades. Repeat eight times.

7	**A**  **B** 	**Tāḍāsana variation:** To work on balance and stability, and improve awareness of the feet.	Stand with the feet hip-width apart. Place the left hand on the chair and right arm by the side. a. Inhale: Lift both heels and rise up onto the balls of the feet, reach the right arm overhead. Exhale: Lower to the starting position. Repeat four times, alternating arms. b. When (a) is mastered, try doing this with one leg lifted and the knee bent. Do this four times on both sides.

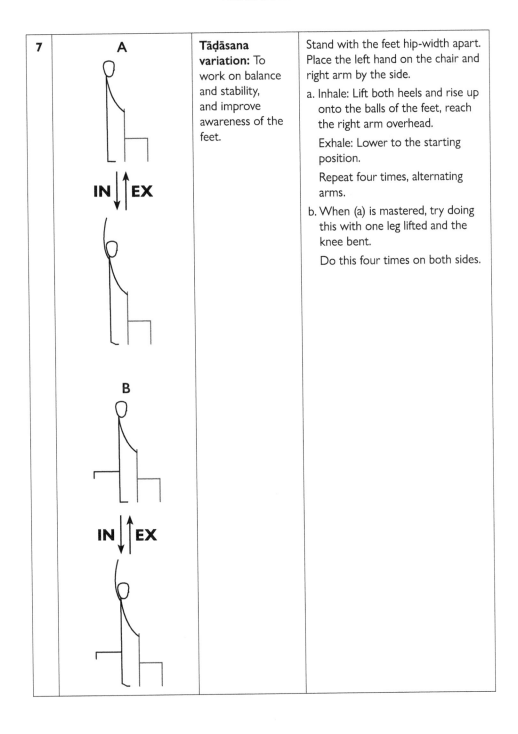

8	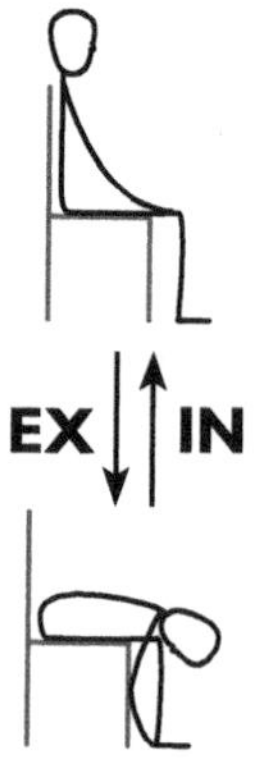 IN 6s EX 8s	**Cakravākāsana variation:** To counter pose from standing balance, stretch and contract the back body, lengthen the exhale for abdominal strength.	Sit on the edge of a chair, with the feet on the ground, hands on the thighs, and arms straight. Inhale: Lift the torso, traction the hands against the thighs, reach the collarbone forward. Feel the back and side bodies contracting. Exhale: Bend forward, gliding the hands down the legs. Inhale for six seconds, exhale for eight seconds. Repeat eight times.
9	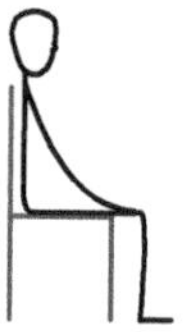 or 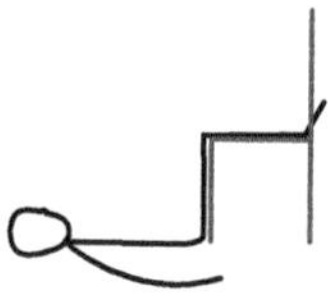	**Śavāsana with support:** To take pressure off of the feet and to relax.	Lie flat on the back, placing a chair under the legs for support or remain seated with the eyes closed. Rest for three to five minutes.

CHAPTER 11

Diabetes and Mental Health

A diabetes diagnosis at any age is, in a way, a sort of death. We mourn when we lose something or someone important to us. There is a time when we experience grief and longing, a persistent sadness known as melancholy. We reminisce about what we have lost and desire to have it back or relive the past. But with time, this passes. In the case of a diagnosis, it is a way of life that once was and that will never be again. While coming to terms with the loss, your whole life as you once knew it is turned around, and you have to think about living in a whole new way. All of a sudden you are expected to be aware of everything you do, eat, feel, and think, to enable you to manage your "condition."

We are not really given a manual about how to make the shift; we just do it. The transition can be awkward and sloppy. After all, you are learning a whole new way of living but there is not much forgiveness in the learning process, and you are expected to automatically get it. Suddenly, you have to think about food in a whole new way: survival. Labels like good, bad, right, and wrong pop up. Your attachments to a lifestyle once lived take time to truly change so that the old patterns and desires are replaced with new and diabetes-supportive ones. This takes time and effort. At first, the work is constricting. It feels so uncomfortable, and you are likely to slip. It can be an extra cookie that turns into five, too many glasses of wine, binge-watching Netflix for hours rather than taking a walk. All of these "things" that you used to do and not think about are now wrong, and you are bad too because you still do them.

You may feel like there will be an end to the madness. Once you acclimatize and figure it out, the discomfort will subside. But as time goes on, you realize that you will always be in a constant state of transition. You try hard to implement new changes, to get it right, but you get in the way of yourself. At times the impulse to continue in the way you lived before diabetes is more durable than your desire to change. Or you try and it does not work, so there's a great rationale for slipping up.

In the back of your mind, you are aware of what you are doing wrong, but you lack ability to find anything positive in this experience. Feelings of hopelessness, overwhelm, anger, and sadness linger—now the new normal. You try to connect with your family and friends but they do not understand your burden. The doctors lack empathy and do not praise your efforts; all they see is a number that has yet to be reached. A person lives in a perpetual state of mourning a life that once was, and so there is no growth. It is like being caught in a battle with no way out. When all a person sees is negative, the focus will be on that rather than on the positive. The positive is always present but it requires more work to access.

There is a high emotional burden on people who live with diabetes. To stay healthy requires tremendous work, sacrifice, and effort. People need to develop a high level of willpower and awareness to achieve the recommended parameters, and many need help in developing these skills. It is not all about achievement. There is a legacy of stressful emotions that stay in the body and influence the way a person sees and responds to diabetes. Developing qualities like forgiveness, adaptiveness, rest, and relaxation—to let go of mistakes and depersonalize diabetes from their sense of self—is as important as willpower. It is imperative for people with diabetes to have outlets to resolve their grief, sadness, and frustration with diabetes. I will argue again that the mind-body component of yoga is a comprehensive tool that mollifies the physiological and psychological sources of stress, empowering individuals to dually observe diabetes and who they are, and inform intelligent action. When this occurs, diabetes transforms into opportunity.

The ramifications of diabetes are physical and psychological, and they tap so profoundly into behavior that it is not uncommon for people with diabetes to be burned out and depressed because of all that goes into self-care. This further perpetuates the risk of long-term diabetes complications, significantly increasing when a person does not or cannot adhere to the strict guidelines.

The ADA's recommendations for glycemic control are A1c <7.0% for adults with T1D and T2D, and <7.5% for youths with T1D. But for many, these goals are not met. About half the people with T2D meet the <7.0% requirements, and the rates are even lower in T1D, with about 16% of youths, 25% of young adults, and 50% of older adults meeting the criteria for glycemic targets.[1]

While the suggestions are correct in that improved glycemic control will reduce diabetes-related complications and improve the quality of a person's life, without adequate tools to process diabetes stress, people are at an increased risk of psychological disturbances and adverse outcomes like reduced quality of life, increased mortality, increased financial burden, and decreased productivity. The latter could be about a person's vocation and also their sense of purpose in life. Who does not want to live a life without meaning or purpose?

Diabetes is a highly personalized disease because requirements are self-administered. Therefore, when personal efforts fail to meet the challenges, people take it as an affront to their self-worth. A number can become a grade, and, depending upon their personality, this can create mechanisms for hypervigilance and/or aversion. When these persist beyond a need for survival, energy and vitality are depleted. Stress hormones stay in the body, distorting thinking and perception, and subsequent behavioral responses increase and perpetuate distress. Studies show that emotions like defeatism and helplessness lead to the activation of the HPA axis, causing endocrine abnormalities and insulin resistance.[2] Without appropriate support systems, coping skills, and self-awareness, people with diabetes are at a higher risk for developing psychosocial disorders like anxiety, depression, and sub-clinical conditions like diabetes distress and burnout.

Half of all people with diabetes will have a diagnosable psychological disorder at some point in their lives.[3] Depression and anxiety are the most common and occur far more frequently in people with diabetes than in the general population of America.[4] It is estimated that one in five people with diabetes will develop depression, and 40% of people with diabetes have depressive symptomatology, although not clinical.[5] We do not know as much about the rates of anxiety, but studies show that they are as high as depression.

1 Hilliard, M. E., Yi-Frazier, J. P., Hessler, D., Butler, A. M., Anderson, B. J. and Jaser, S. (2016) "Stress and A1c among people with diabetes across the lifespan." *Current Diabetes Reports 16*, 8, 67.

2 Lloyd, C., Smith, J. and Weinger, K. (2005) "Stress and diabetes: a review of the links." *Diabetes Spectrum 18*, 2, 123–124.

3 Rubin, R. R. (2009) "Psychotherapy and Counselling in Diabetes Mellitus." In F. J. Snoek and C. T. J. Skinner (eds) *Psychology in Diabetes Care*. Chichester: Wiley & Sons Ltd. p.248.

4 Rubin, R. R. (2009) "Psychotherapy and Counselling in Diabetes Mellitus." In F. J. Snoek and C. T. J. Skinner (eds) *Psychology in Diabetes Care*. Chichester: Wiley & Sons Ltd. p.248.

5 Rubin, R. R. (2009) "Psychotherapy and Counselling in Diabetes Mellitus." In F. J. Snoek and C. T. J. Skinner (eds) *Psychology in Diabetes Care*. Chichester: Wiley & Sons Ltd. p.248.

Sub-clinical disorders, diabetes distress, and diabetes burnout hold similar qualities to anxiety and depression but differ in that they only show up with the burden of diabetes management.

People with diabetes need to take care of their mental health just as they would take care of their BG levels. They are interrelated. Studies show that psychiatric disturbances impact metabolic control and the ability of a person to lead a healthy and prosperous life with diabetes. Psychological problems affect metabolic control on three levels. First, the neuroendocrine and physiological effects of stress, the release of stress hormones, increase insulin resistance and make a person more sensitive to stressors. Increased sympathetic activity reduces muscle blood flow, reducing glucose uptake and increasing insulin resistance. Chronic stress increases the release of glucocorticoids, increasing the HPA axis and sympathetic overdrive. These hormonal conditions increase BG and heighten sensitivity to stressors, fueling the cycle of reactivity and constant stress.

It is well hypothesized that there is an inherent link between diabetes, mental health issues, and dysregulation of the HPA axis. Chronic stress and increased allostatic load exhaust the HPA axis, confusing its release of cortisol. In a way, cortisol is responsible for our daily rhythm, and when the rhythm is disturbed, either due to its increased production or "blunting" of the diurnal cortisol release, individuals are susceptible to insulin resistance and depression.

Dysregulation in the neuroendocrine responses negatively impacts self-care adherence and diabetes management, essential for achieving recommended BG requirements, leading to a dramatic decrease in wellbeing and quality of life.

Understanding the association between BG control and psychological disturbances is critical in applying intervention strategies to break the cycle of suffering.

If we can resolve the blood sugars, perhaps we can reduce the distress, or if we can reduce the causes of distress, we may be able to improve blood sugars. Either way, whichever doorway is the entrypoint, the goal is the same: whole-person wellness.[6]

6 Gilsanz, P., Karter, A. J., Schnaider Beeri, M., Quesenberry, C. P. and Whitmer, R. A. (2018) "The bidirectional association between depression and severe hypoglycemic and hyperglycemic events in type 1 diabetes." *Diabetes Care 41*, 3, 446–452.

A Need for Effective Therapy

Diabetes management requires complicated, demanding, and relentless treatment routines that impact many dimensions of people's lives.[7] Effective self-management is a critical step in achieving both physiological and psychological balance. The intensity of self-care requirements is dependent upon the type of diabetes (T1D or T2D), duration of the disease, and the existence of complications or co-morbidities. It also depends on the kind of lifestyle a person leads.

A lack of coping skills, social support, and other protective processes increases the individual risk for mental health issues. It is recommended that people with diabetes have psychological support systems, but many of these systems are reliant on others helping. People with diabetes need to be self-reliant and find ways to cope with diabetes stress in healthy and productive ways by developing protective mechanisms to identify potential diabetes stressors and resolve existing psychological disturbances.

Stability and clarity of mind are essential for everyone, with or without diabetes. Still, when your daily function relies on appropriate self-care, problem-solving, and action-oriented skills, it is non-negotiable. People with diabetes are at a higher risk for developing sub-clinical and clinical psychological problems for many reasons. The psychological burden of diabetes, combined with new complications, functional impairment, lack of social support systems, and passive coping skills, are all potential contributing factors to the onset of mental health issues. We also know that hyperglycemia has a direct effect on the hippocampus, which regulates mood and cognition.[8]

The fact of the matter is that diabetes will always be stressful until a person can gain control over their emotional responses to diabetes changes. They will remain identified with diabetes as a part of "who they are" and will suffer. This suffering perpetuates negative stress responses via the neuroendocrine system and the psychological misappraisal of threat versus non-threat. Yoga teaches us how negative emotions are all based on misunderstanding. The practice purifies the mind and enables it to not give in to the impulses that are driven mostly by emotion. As we learned in Chapter 3, there are various reasons to

7 Butkiewicz, E., Carbone, A., Green, S., Miano, A. and Wegner, E. (2016) "Diabetes Management." In M. A. Burg and O. Oyama (eds) *Behavioral Health Specialist*. New York: Springer Publishing Company. p.84.

8 Golden, S. (2016) "Why are diabetes and depression linked?" *Johns Hopkins Medicine*. Accessed on 09/07/20 at: www.youtube.com/watch?v=HZ6aYCRcfeE.

be "stressed out" by diabetes, but that is mostly perception. The people who manage diabetes the most successfully can create positive coping strategies to help them offset diabetes-related stress and find more beneficial ways of perceiving their lives in relationship to and with diabetes.

The answer to the quandary of managing diabetes and psychological disturbances is two-fold: biological and behavioral. We need to regulate the mechanisms behind dysfunctional HPA axis/SAM responses by training the ANS to down-shift to the parasympathetic rest-and-repose response, improving heart rate variability and vagal tone. This offers the nervous system an opportunity to recuperate but also affords the mind a spacious pause to reflect and reassess. Next is cognitive awareness. Practice that encourages the rebalancing of the HPA axis/SAM to downshift to a parasympathetic response helps people get out of their impulsive reactions and separate from them. They recognize their saṁskāra-s (patterns) and from a new vantage point can reassess their triggers (svādhyāya) and apply healthier patterns for coping with diabetes stress (saṁkalpa and praktipaṣa bhāvanā).

Diabetes Distress and Burnout: More Than a Worry

There is a hidden emotional burden that people with diabetes carry. It can be hard to identify because it shares some elements of depression and anxiety. These conditions develop in response to the relentless emotional burden of managing chronic illness. Although sub-clinical, distress and burnout can be dangerous because they directly impact how a person views and responds to diabetes.

In some medical circles, *diabetes distress* and *diabetes burnout* are synonymous, but I view them separately. In this book, we will be qualifying diabetes distress as the emotional burden (stress) of coping with unabating diabetes management demands, akin to the feeling of overwhelm and anxiety. Feelings of being overwhelmed are reasonable but also need to be addressed and relinquished by coping positively. Otherwise, these untethered emotions will be harmful to metabolic control, self-care, and quality of life.

The symptoms of diabetes distress are:

- emotions like anger and frustration about diabetes and its management requirements
- persistent fear and worry about one's health with diabetes, but an inability to implement behavioral changes

- avoidant behaviors concerning checking BG or administering insulin
- feeling isolated and alone
- continuously making choices that are not in the best interest of the diabetes.

People with all types of diabetes experience diabetes distress. Diabetes distress is widespread in diabetes: as many as one in four people with T1D and one in five people with type 2 experience it.[9] It is believed that people with T1D experience more diabetes distress because of hypoglycemia.

When *diabetes distress* goes unchecked it can result in *diabetes burnout*, and burnout can result in depression. When burnout occurs, people are so overwhelmed by diabetes demands that they stop taking care of themselves and diabetes. The implications of this are obviously life threatening. People need to have their heads on right to muster up the daily effort to manage diabetes.

People who experience diabetes burnout may exhibit a complete disregard for diabetes management practice. Burnout can occur simultaneously with stress, anxiety, and depression, although many of its symptoms most similarly resemble depression with physical exhaustion and emotional withdrawal.

Its symptoms resemble depression, but it is different than depression. First of all, it is not a major depressive disorder or even on the spectrum of a clinical disease, which touches every avenue of a person's life. Diabetes burnout is a depression about everything that has to do with diabetes from the experience of it to the self-management requirements for it. When a person with diabetes burnout reflects on other areas of their life, they may remain optimistic and positive. When it comes to diabetes, they are "over it." It does not mean that a person has stopped taking care of themselves with diabetes, it just means that they are really struggling emotionally with the cost of diabetes.[10]

People with diabetes burnout tend to cut corners—to put diabetes on the back-burner so to speak. There is an avoidant and resistant tendency in these individuals, which can resemble depression. They might make poor food choices, lie about their blood sugars, skip insulin, intentionally allow their BG to run high, and harbor intense emotions like being really scared or

9 Diabetes UK (n.d.) *What Is Diabetes Distress and Burnout?* Accessed on 09/07/20 at: www.diabetes.org.uk/guide-to-diabetes/emotions/diabetes-burnout.

10 Vieira, G. (2019) "Diabetes burnout vs. depression: what's the difference?" *Insulin Nation*. Accessed on 09/07/20 at: https://insulinnation.com/living/diabetes-burnout-vs-depression-whats-the-difference.

extremely angry about diabetes.[11] It may not seem like a big deal, but it is very common. I have experienced mild forms of it and also witnessed friends lose their health, wellbeing, and even their lives over it. Luckily, it is manageable with support from healthcare providers, psychiatrists, and, yes, yoga therapists. The progressive balancing of the stress responses via the HPA axis/SNS, and emotional, cognitive reappraisal, and self-awareness practices, helps people cope more effectively, because diabetes is not going away anytime soon.

As diabetes distress and burnout are sub-clinical, they are not reliant upon medications and therefore can be managed with positive coping strategies to release tension. It is possible that, left untreated, these sub-clinical mental health conditions could develop into clinical diagnoses. Recognizing these key distinctions will help you and your clients to make the most appropriate plan of action regarding self-care and yoga therapy recommendations. While treatment may overlap, diabetes distress/burnout are sub-clinical and typically not treated with medication. Burnout holds similar qualities to depression, but burnout extends just to the experience of diabetes, whereas depression impacts the whole person.

The PAID (problem areas in diabetes) scale is a useful survey for assessing the emotional burden of diabetes management. I have adapted some questions for a diabetes-sensitive intake form in Chapter 7. If you think that a client has diabetes distress or burnout, it is a helpful tool that can help you to understand how to meet the client's (or your) emotional needs. In my case, I realized that a problem area I have concerns healthcare, which explains why I have such an aversion to calling my provider.

Sub-clinical mental health challenges are common and pervasive, and they can dramatically affect the lives of people with diabetes. I have witnessed myself and so many others suffer from diabetes burnout, and without adequate tools it can be life threatening. Why? People stop caring about and doing the necessary things to make sure that diabetes does not win. The good news is that, while it is common, it is not clinical, and yoga therapy interventions can be an effective coping strategy to ensure the stress does not evolve into anything more.

It is natural to feel frustration and sadness with diabetes, but when it is a persistent feeling of "I can't do this," it negatively impacts how a person copes. Not addressing the symptoms of diabetes burnout is dangerous in the

11 Vieira, G. (2019) "Diabetes burnout vs. depression: what's the difference?" *Insulin Nation*. Accessed on 09/07/20 at: https://insulinnation.com/living/diabetes-burnout-vs-depression-whats-the-difference.

short term because a person is less likely to do what they need to do to take care of diabetes, and in the long term because diabetes burnout can turn into depression. Although yoga therapy can serve people with diabetes burnout and depression, if symptoms carry on even with attempts to stop them, a person should seek out a mental health professional.

Anxiety

Anxiety is a fundamental misappraisal of the perception of danger. It is a type of hypervigilance that induces overreactive responses to stressors. The essential correlating factor between diabetes and anxiety is hypervigilance that attention to diabetes and especially self-care creates.[12] Clinical anxiety disorder is diagnosed when people have been uncontrollably anxious for at least six months. Some of the symptoms include: restlessness and being on edge, being easily fatigued, having difficulty concentrating, irritability, muscle tension, and sleep problems such as falling asleep or staying asleep.[13]

Anxiety is a common psychological disorder in people with diabetes because they live every day of their lives with higher levels of stress than most other people, so they experience more perceived stress and, subsequently, anxiety. Studies reveal that 14% of patients have a general anxiety disorder (GAD), while up to 40% exhibit signs of elevated anxiety symptoms compared to the general population.[14] Anxiety is a condition in which people do not feel safe, and because of this, they remain in a fight-or-flight state, always on guard and prepared to respond to the next attack. The sympathetic fight-or-flight response was biologically adapted to ensure the survival of the individual, placing all long-term projects on hold and increasing the production of catecholamines (epinephrine and norepinephrine). These hormones increase heart rate, blood pressure, and BG levels to produce energy for a response.

The effect of these hormones makes people jittery and nervous. Cortisol acts as a buffer for catecholamines, but during chronic stress, like anxiety, cortisol

12 Butkiewicz, E., Carbone, A., Green, S., Miano, A. and Wegner, E. (2016) "Diabetes Management." In M. A. Burg and O. Oyama (eds) *Behavioral Health Specialist.* New York: Springer Publishing Company. p.93.

13 Rubin, R. R. (2009) "Psychotherapy and Counselling in Diabetes Mellitus." In F. J. Snoek and C. T. J. Skinner (eds) *Psychology in Diabetes Care.* Chichester: Wiley & Sons Ltd. pp.252–253.

14 Kalra, S., Jena, B. N. and Yeravdekar, R. (2018) "Emotional and psychological needs of people with diabetes." *Indian Journal of Endocrinology and Metabolism 22*, 5, 696–704.

is depleted. This gives people a feeling of always being on edge, nervous, and, yes, anxious.

Excessive, inadequate, or faulty stress responses, as we see in high anxiety,[15] influence the mind and its perceptions. People are more likely to have an exaggerated emotional response to everyday diabetes stressors[16]—the stuff that is not going to go away.

The limbic brain is the epicenter of all fear processing. The physical and psychological effects of anxiety are generated when the higher processing centers (cerebellum) fail to properly regulate over-reactivity in the amygdala-hippocampal complex, triggering an immediate stress response via the hypothalamus. Modulating how the brain receives information (bottom-up) and how it sends it out (top-down) through yoga practices may reduce the pathophysiological processes of anxiety that contribute to diminished diabetes self-care, reduced quality of life, and challenging metabolic control.

Yoga helps individuals suffering from diabetes-related stress to promote self-regulatory behaviors and down-regulate allostatic load, resulting in increased self-control during an acute stress response. As we learned in Chapter 3, chronic stress and allostatic load can be mediated by strengthening the vagus nerve's function through yogic-based practices, especially prāṇāyāma. Prāṇāyāma has a more substantial effect on down-regulating the stress response towards the parasympathetic predominance than sustained postures or meditation. A regular breathing practice focused on down-regulation trains the ANS to be more adaptable, turning on the brakes to stress just as readily as it can rev up the gas pedal (sympathetic activation) when needed.

The more regularly an individual can train their nervous system to establish balance, the easier it will be to control their responses during acute stress. Maintaining a steady breath during challenging moments, like hypoglycemia, is an opportunity for individuals to apply "non-reactive" awareness in the face of diabetes challenges. That being said, yoga practices teach people how to implement an anxiety antidote in the moment of a real stress response and how to create an inner state of equanimity on and off the mat.

This is but one step in the process. As stress is psychologically and hormonally driven, the "pause" created by breath regulation improves diabetes

15 Rubin, R.R. "Psychotherapy and Counselling in Diabetes Mellitus." In F.J. Snoek and C.T. Skinner (eds) *Psychology in Diabetes Care*. John Wiley & Sons Ltd. pp.252–253.

16 Rubin, R.R. "Psychotherapy and Counselling in Diabetes Mellitus." In F.J. Snoek and C.T. Skinner (eds) *Psychology in Diabetes Care*. John Wiley & Sons Ltd., pp.252–253.

self-care by renegotiating the ingrained stress responses. People have an opportunity to change impulses with cognitive reappraisal. Out of the impulse-trigger-oriented sympathetic state, people can reevaluate their thoughts, emotions, and behaviors, changing their interpretation of a stressor into a non-stressor. Relaxation training has been shown to have a significant benefit for people with T2D—reducing anxiety, and improving glucose tolerance and long-term hyperglycemia. Results of relaxation-based interventions in T1D are less straightforward but report similar findings.[17]

Depression

When someone is depressed, their responses are blunted and they cannot derive joy or pleasure from life experiences. The causes of depression are varied and can be related to various factors like genetic vulnerability, stressful life events, medications, hormones, and medical problems like diabetes. Depression is a biopsychosocial disorder, with both biological and psychological factors, is characterized by faulty mood regulation, and can co-occur with anxiety.[18] When a combination of genetics, biology, and stressful life events come together, and there is a lack of coping strategies, depression can result.[19] There are many proposed causes of depression, and just as many types. Even the same type of depression will represent itself differently from person to person. Depression is commonly linked to faulty release neurotransmitters (serotonin, norepinephrine, and dopamine) but that does not even begin to cover the complexity of depression. Even though we know that depression is much more than faulty neurotransmitters, we cannot completely discredit them either.

Depression is associated with decreased production of gamma aminobutyric acid (GABA), a primary inhibitory neurotransmitter in the brain. GABA acts like the brakes on excessive brain activity, turning off the neurotransmitters that "overthink" and ruminate, which may play a role in anxiety and the development of depressive disorders. Psychology also plays a role. Depression is a faulty neuroendocrine response to stress, represented by impaired emotional

17 Rubin, R. R. (2009) "Psychotherapy and Counselling in Diabetes Mellitus." In F. J. Snoek and C. T. J. Skinner (eds) *Psychology in Diabetes Care*. Chichester: Wiley & Sons Ltd. pp.252–253.

18 Uebelacker, L., Lavretsky, H. and Tremont, G. (2016) "Yoga Therapy for Depression." In S. B. S. Khalsa, L. Cohen, T. McCall and S. Telles (eds) *The Principles and Practice of Yoga in Healthcare*. Pencaitland: Handspring Publishing. p.73.

19 Harvard Health Publishing (2019) *What Causes Depression?* Accessed on 10/07/20 at: www.health.harvard.edu/mind-and-mood/what-causes-depression.

regulation. Something goes off that tells the brain that the individual is under siege and, with time, allostasis is compromised. In a normal stress response there is a feedback loop that turns off when the perception of a threat has subsided. Like chronic stress and anxiety, in depression there is a dysregulation of this loop, and the stress response does not turn off. This compromises the system, increasing allostatic load.

The HPA axis is designed to awaken the body during physical or emotional threats. When a threat is continuous, or at least perceived to be continuous, the hypothalamus secretes corticotropin-releasing hormone (CRH), which tells the pituitary gland to secrete adrenocorticotropic hormone (ACTH) to the adrenals and stimulates the production of cortisol.[20] CRH also impacts other parts of the brain that help process emotion and behavior in the cerebral cortex, amygdala, and brainstem. Functioning throughout various neural pathways, CRH influences the gathering of neurotransmitters that are related to depression. This suggests that the HPA axis hormones may also affect neurotransmitters, and neurotransmitters may affect the hormonal responses.[21]

T2D, obesity, and depression are all HPA-axis dysfunctions and are linked with an excessive production of cortisol. Cortisol is a very important hormone that in many ways regulates our daily cycle but also provides that extra energy we need to go the long distances. When it functions properly, cortisol is an anti-inflammatory and helps the diurnal cycle taper off in order to receive the benefits of a good night's sleep. A normal cortisol release is higher in the morning and winds down in the evening. It is shown that in depression, however, the release of cortisol is the inverse: it is very low in the morning and steadily increases throughout the day.[22] This could relate to depression's effect of tiredness in the day and restlessness at night. The dysregulation of the diurnal cortisol curve increases individual risk factors for depression, diabetes, cardiovascular problems, and increased A1c levels.[23]

People with diabetes are about twice as likely to develop depression as

20 Harvard Health Publishing (2019) *What Causes Depression?* Accessed on 10/07/20 at: www.health.harvard.edu/mind-and-mood/what-causes-depression.

21 Harvard Health Publishing (2019) *What Causes Depression?* Accessed on 10/07/20 at: www.health.harvard.edu/mind-and-mood/what-causes-depression.

22 Golden, S. (2016) "Why are diabetes and depression linked?" *Johns Hopkins Medicine*. Accessed on 09/07/20 at: www.youtube.com/watch?v=HZ6aYCRcfeE.

23 Joseph, J. J. and Golden, S. H. (2017) "Cortisol dysregulation: the bidirectional link between stress, depression, and type 2 diabetes mellitus." *Annals of the New York Academy of Sciences 1391*, 20–34.

non-diabetic populations.[24] This statistic extends to both T1D and T2D. The stats are similar for anxiety. And the question of why remains.

The causes of diabetes depression are varied, just like the causes of depression itself, but the development of depression in diabetes is generally related to high BG levels and behavioral factors, which include negative coping strategies and self-care practices. Meta-analyses link depression in diabetes to hyperglycemia and suboptimal medical management,[25] corroborating the connection between biology and behavior. High blood sugars atrophy and damage the neuronal receptors in the hippocampus that are responsible for learning and memory.

Depression is associated with poor diabetes self-management and treatment adherence, like checking BG and taking insulin for food. Such lapses in self-care are linked to the effects of depression, like poor concentration and memory, difficulty collaborating with others, and general fatigue. It can also lead to negative coping mechanisms like cigarette smoking and emotional eating.

Diabetes distress and depression can occur together and have serious implications for the treatment of diabetes, making people feel unable or unmotivated to follow through on important self-care behaviors. A group of researchers identified both diabetes-related stressors and other life stressors as contributing factors in evaluating self-care. Those who reported feeling out of control because of diabetes, or that their lives were too chaotic to deal with diabetes, were less likely to follow through on self-care behaviors.[26] There are a lot of similarities between the symptoms of diabetes and the symptoms of depression, making it confusing to identify which is which. Such examples would be that depression can mimic and intensify diabetes symptoms, like increased thirst, blurred vision, and hunger. People with depression are more likely to complain of diabetes symptoms, even when their A1c is in control.

Although there is increasing awareness of the connection between diabetes, depression, and burnout, the symptoms can go unnoticed. People may be really struggling with adhering to the recommendations but not be able to figure out why, despite their efforts, they cannot manage diabetes. We know that blood

---

24 Holt, R. I. and Golden, S. (2014) "Diabetes and depression." *Current Diabetes Reports 14*, 6, 491.

25 Joseph, J. J. and Golden, S. H. (2017) "Cortisol dysregulation: the bidirectional link between stress, depression, and type 2 diabetes mellitus." *Annals of the New York Academy of Sciences 1391*, 20–34.

26 Lloyd, C., Smith, J. and Weinger, K. (2005) "Stress and diabetes: a review of the links." *Diabetes Spectrum 18*, 2, 123–124.

sugars have a huge impact on the development of depression and the perception of stress. Severe blood sugars tax the body and mind's most vital reserves. However, if we look at the symptoms of depression and the symptoms of high blood sugars, we will see a great similarity. I bring this up simply to consider it in greater detail. As yoga therapists, we are often thinking about where to start. What will be the easiest thing to impact that will create other improvements? Do we address depression, stress, or hyperglycemia first? All of these have a physiological effect on the ANS and HPA axis, as well as psychological effects that impact mood and subsequent behavior. It is not all black and white; there are many layers of grey.

Table 11.1 Symptomatology comparison

Depression	Hyperglycemia
Muscle aches and joint pain	Sharp pain and cramps
Headaches	Headaches
Trouble concentrating	Trouble concentrating
Fatigue	Fatigue
Weight loss/weight gain	Weight loss/weight gain
Sleep issues, restlessness	Sleep issues, pain/cramps at night
Reduced activity	Increased thirst
Changes in appetite	Blurred vision
GI distress	GI distress

In the case of T2D, depression can also be a contributing factor in the development of diabetes. The risk factors for depression are similar to the risk factors for T2D: less physical activity, increased daily calorie intake, smoking, increased BMI index, and inflammation are all common in depressive symptoms and also in T2D.

As we delve deeper into the connection between diabetes, depression, and yoga as an intervention strategy, please keep in mind that the intervention strategies employed by both the medical and yoga therapy perspectives are the same for diabetics with depression and non-diabetics with depression. The negative clinical implications are greater for people with diabetes, because depression negatively impacts glucose metabolism, self-care behaviors, and quality of life.[27]

There are many reasons to employ yoga as an auxiliary or even replacement

27 Joseph, J. J. and Golden, S. H. (2017) "Cortisol dysregulation: the bidirectional link between stress, depression, and type 2 diabetes mellitus." *Annals of the New York Academy of Sciences 1391*, 20–34.

treatment for diabetes burnout and some types of depression (*that being said, chemical imbalances often need adjunctive allopathic treatment*). Yoga practices may produce potentially beneficial changes in the neurotransmitter systems, neuroendocrine system (HPA axis), inflammatory responses, and emotions associated with thought and behavior.[28]

Psychological stress can lead to an imbalance of the ANS with decreased parasympathetic nervous system activation and increased SNS activity associated with the underactivity of the GABA system's production of inhibitory neurotransmitters that put the brakes on anxious thinking. This physiological response puts pressure on a variety of organ systems and tissues and can be a contributing factor in the onset of T2D and depression. Yoga-based practices not only support anxiety, but also help people manage depression by increasing parasympathetic activity and increasing GABA levels that correlate with improved mood.

Yoga practice may lead to beneficial changes to the neurotransmitter systems, the HPA axis, and the immune system by reducing inflammatory responses. The practice of yoga (āsana, prāṇāyāma, and meditation) combined with increased self-reflective capabilities, inspired by the psychology and philosophy of yoga, provides a framework for yoga as an adjunct therapy in diabetes care, potentially reducing the onset of depression, diabetes, or both.

Increased HPA-axis activity, as seen by cortisol levels throughout the day, is a biological indicator of stress.[29] Studies show that yoga may have a direct neurological effect at the level of the hypothalamus on its production of cortisol, helping to reduce depression.[30] Also, there is a positive correlation between yoga and reduced plasma levels of cortisol, although much more research is needed as there are conflicting studies that say yoga has no effect.[31] However, other studies have shown inconclusive results on the effects of yoga on cortisol levels. The silver lining here is that where there was no reduction, yoga participants

28 Uebelacker, L., Lavretsky, H. and Tremont, G. (2016) "Yoga Therapy for Depression." In S. B. S. Khalsa, L. Cohen, T. McCall and S. Telles (eds) *The Principles and Practice of Yoga in Healthcare*. Pencaitland: Handspring Publishing. p.74.

29 Uebelacker, L., Lavretsky, H. and Tremont, G. (2016) "Yoga Therapy for Depression." In S. B. S. Khalsa, L. Cohen, T. McCall and S. Telles (eds) *The Principles and Practice of Yoga in Healthcare*. Pencaitland: Handspring Publishing. p.74.

30 Thirthalli, J., Naveen, G. H., Rao, M. G., Varambally, S., Christopher, R. and Gangadhar, B. N. (2013) "Cortisol and antidepressant effects of yoga." *Indian Journal of Psychiatry* 55, Suppl 3, S405–S408.

31 Uebelacker, L., Lavretsky, H. and Tremont, G. (2016) "Yoga Therapy for Depression." In S. B. S. Khalsa, L. Cohen, T. McCall and S. Telles (eds) *The Principles and Practice of Yoga in Healthcare*. Pencaitland: Handspring Publishing. p.73.

did not have an increase in their level of depression, suggesting that yoga has some impact on the development of the depression.[32]

The Psychology of Yoga Therapy for Mental Health

Now that you are well educated about the causes and risks of mental health problems with diabetes and how they impact metabolic control, self-care, and quality of life, let's get right into how to practice for improved mental health with diabetes. For yoga therapy to be transformative, a practice should target the triggers that exacerbate stress and encourage qualities that buffer the risk. We need effective and potent problem-solving skills that will support us in the heat of the moment. We do that through self-awareness and self-regulation. But it is not easy. There are acute and chronic stress responses with diabetes. Often, we need help in the middle of an acute stress response but are too overwhelmed by the moment to apply strategies and we revert to impulses. The tools we develop when not in a heightened state of sympathetic overdrive help us respond more appropriately when we are in that state.

There are some differences between the pathways for diabetes distress, anxiety, and depression, but the ability to stop a psychologically triggered stress response is critical in all three. Breath-centric āsana reduces physical tension associated with emotional tension, while an emphasis on breathing in āsana and seated prāṇāyāma will regulate the ANS. Meditation and profound relaxation techniques help to implant new neural pathways for cognitively differentiating stress from non-stressors.[33] Yoga Sūtra 1.41 reminds us how prāṇāyāma helps to purify the mind's lens, washing from our personal windshield the accumulated dirt that inhibits a clear perspective. From a calm and clear vantage point, we can reevaluate our thoughts and responses. We can ask questions of ourselves like: Is this real? Is this an appropriate response?

We learned how stress is both an actual response to a threat and psychologically created. The information that we take in from our senses (as impressions) is evaluated by the limbic system, which discerns threat from non-threat. Yoga Sūtra 2.16 reminds us that suffering can be avoided and that

32 Saeed, S. A., Cunningham, K. and Bloch, R. M. (2019) "Depression and anxiety disorders: benefits of exercise, yoga, and meditation." *American Family Physician* 99, 10, 620–627.

33 Krishnakumar, D., Hamblin, M. R. and Lakshmanan, S. (2015) "Meditation and yoga can modulate brain mechanisms that affect behavior and anxiety: a modern scientific perspective." *Ancient Science* 2, 1, 13–19.

often the sources of pain come from our own mind's perception of reality. The lived experience of a disease like diabetes, with the highs and lows of BG extremes and its influence on the physiological stress responses, impacts a person's perception of reality just as much as their perception influences their physiology. It is all interconnected, and the starting point in transforming mental health and attitudes really depends on where you can find a doorway in. Is it through the physiology or the mind? Undoubtedly, when the ANS is in balance, stress responses are blunted and people perceive more clearly, therefore responding in a way that stops a stress response. It is one thing to access this from actual practice, but what if a person can perceive clearly amidst an acute stress response? This is the real skillset.

Praktipaṣa bhāvanā—Cognitive Reappraisal

Our ability to influence emotions is an integral part of mental health resilience. In Yoga Sūtra 2.33, Patañjali says, "Upon having an awareness of negative thoughts, counteract them with positive thoughts." The act of transforming the perception of a negative thought into a positive, a threat into a non-threat, is called praktipaṣa bhāvanā. It means "to cultivate the opposite." The ability to do this amid acute and chronic stressors is a superhuman power, perhaps what Patañjali referred to as one of the siddhis (special powers) achieved through yoga practice. Praktipaṣa bhāvanā is a way of practicing viyoga and saṁyoga, separating from sources of suffering and consciously linking with sources of positivity.

Psychologists call this cognitive reframing or benefit-finding. I have always found it challenging to explain this principle to others, because it can sound, at times, as if you are making it up, denying, or lying to yourself. It is not that at all. It can be hard to find a positive when all you see are negatives. Being able to abide in both the good and the bad is better than just focusing on the good. In fact, benefit-finding is associated with better long-term outcomes than just focusing on the positive.[34] In teens with diabetes, benefit-finding has been found to reduce the risk of depression and make them more likely to follow through on self-care.[35]

34 McGonigal, K. (2015) *The Upside of Stress: Why Stress Is Good for You (and How to Get Good at It)*. New York: Penguin Random House. p.203.

35 McGonigal, K. (2015) *The Upside of Stress: Why Stress Is Good for You (and How to Get Good at It)*. New York: Penguin Random House. p.202.

We have learned that suffering (avidyā) is contingent on the fundamental misunderstanding that we are the changing circumstances and conditions surrounding us. Diabetes adds an extra layer of difficulty to navigate in the ocean of potential suffering—because of both its symptoms and management requirements.

The ability to witness a trigger and recognize that we have the power to choose how we respond is the starting point for resilience. T. K. V. Desikachar notably said that the first step in yoga is the recognition of suffering and the desire to improve.[36] With time, the practice purifies the mind, senses, and perception, and balances autonomic function, allowing us to see ourselves and our patterns in a new light. We can be more proactive and awake to our experiences, actively choosing what and how we give our energy.

Praktipaṣa Bhāvanā Steps

1. **Recognition:** Through self-awareness, we can begin to identify what we are feeling, thinking, and doing in response to triggers. The first step of "cultivating the opposite" is to simply recognize it. You don't even need to know what to do with it. Even T. K. V. Desikachar said that the first stage of clarity is the recognition of confusion.[37] Consider the connections between what you are thinking, feeling, and doing in response to a trigger. Am I feeling this way because I am really anxious or is it because I am worried that my BG is going to fall low?

2. **Flip it:** Whatever you are thinking or experiencing, consider the opposite. This is not lying to yourself; it is simply accepting that there is more than one way of seeing things. If you are fretting about going to the doctor, recall all the things that you have done right and try to diffuse the worry. If you are angry about eating a meal and the result is a BG number you do not like, try to recall all the times you did it right. Our minds like to gravitate towards the negative over the positive.

36 Desikachar, T. K. V. (1999) *The Heart of Yoga: Developing a Personal Practice* (Rev. ed.). Rochester, VT: Inner Traditions International. p.13.

37 Desikachar, T. K. V. (n.d.) *A-Z Quotes*. Accessed on 10/07/20 at: www.azquotes.com/quote/1522676.

3. **Let it go**: With training, you will learn to find new ways of looking towards the positive when experiencing the negative. Over time, it will become easier to replace a negative circumstance and transform it into something else. We can see monsters if they are what we are hardwired to believe in, but with practice we see that the monsters are only trees, and beautiful ones at that.

Vicāra

Another way of generating the technique of praktipaṣa bhāvanā is through the practice of vicāra. Vicāra is a method of svādhyāya or *self-inquiry*, where you have an honest conversation with yourself—about yourself and what causes you stress. In this process you look objectively at the sources of suffering as they manifest as thoughts, emotions, and behaviors.

As in viyoga, the root meaning of the word vicāra is the prefix "vi," meaning to *separate*. Any process of separation, vi, is to look at the pieces separately to see where the missing link is. It is to ask yourself important questions like: Why do I think this way? Why do I behave this way? Are there motivations? Do I have a choice?

When our brain receives information and assesses threat and non-threat, the information goes into the repository of the memory. We accumulate memories for experiences, and whether they are good or bad, or positive or negative, will determine our beliefs about our impressions. Beliefs are wrapped up in the stories that we tell ourselves about ourselves, and determine our perception of reality.

When you look back far enough to the origin of beliefs, you will find that most of them are unfounded. Most beliefs go back to the causes of avidyā, the kleśa-s: asmitā (ego), rāga (aversion), dveṣa (attachment), and abhiniveśa (fear). Vicāra can help people see with more clarity what is actually aversion and what is attachment, and then, with clarity, change their perception of reality. They are empowered to take charge of their emotions and implement conscious shifts.

I recommend practicing vicāra as an object of meditation regularly, but it is probably not a good idea to do it at the height of an acute stress response. Do it when you have more composure, and with regular practice it will help to attenuate the acute stress responses. In the Yoga Sūtra-s, vicāra is an object of meditative focus; in a yoga therapy context, it is a tool of viyoga. It is a way to have deeper, more meaningful conversations with oneself about beliefs and attitudes. In vicāra, we can understand the practice of praktipaṣa bhāvanā on a more profound level. You can reflect on the following questions.

Vicāra on Thoughts

What type of thoughts come to mind when I reflect on a diabetes stressor? Do specific words come to mind?

Vicāra on Emotion and Mood

When I reflect on the negative thought, is there an emotion, a feeling, or a visceral sensation attributed to the thoughts?

Vicāra on Behavior

When I reflect on thoughts, emotions, and physical sensation, is there a behavioral pattern? Or does a behavioral pattern trigger types of thoughts and/or emotions? Look for the connection.

Goal: To witness diabetes as an observer. To create a spaciousness where one can observe diabetes without identification with the periphery of change.

This is not:

- denial
- disassociation
- disconnection
- putting on a pretty face.

This is:

- wholeness
- connection
- response
- awareness
- mindfulness.

By reflecting on beliefs, thoughts, and impulses, we can progressively purify the intellect (buddhi) and achieve higher states of awareness (viveka) and freedom of choice. The concept of free will is an integral part of human evolution, and an overarching goal of yoga is to become *svātantrya*, the self-director of all dharma. Reflecting on the beliefs that a person holds about diabetes helps them separate from the false identification with diabetes and practice saṁyoga with the beneficial qualities of self-efficacy.

Vicāra Meditation

This can be applied to any practice to transform perception and behavior.

Goal: To increase self-reflective capacity, to reflect on the sources of distress (Vicāra), and to nullify triggers with cognitive reframing (praktipaṣa bhāvanā).

Follow the steps of prāṇa dhāraṇā (Chapter 5) to arrive in a state of calm, spacious awareness. Once established, reflect on a current diabetes challenge. Take a moment to locate what it is and any events leading up to it without obsessing on the story.

Examine the situation on the level of thought, emotion, and behavior.

Thought: When you think about the situation, what thoughts arise? Are there words and names associated with them? What causes your mind to waver? What is the source of the thoughts? Do they have any basis? *Behind all thoughts is only space.*

Emotion: Reflect on the quality of your emotions and physical sensations that come up in the body when you reflect on this situation. Where do these emotions and sensations come from? *Can you be with them while at the same time rest as a calm witness? Does this diffuse the sensations?*

Behavior: Consider your actions when you are stressed out by diabetes. Are there any patterns you can identify? Are the behaviors a result of a thought? Or a feeling? Which behaviors are helpful and which are unhelpful? What can you commit to doing differently? Or not doing at all?

Rest in awareness of the natural breath. Feel it at almost a complete standstill in the mid-brain.

Reflect on anything you have learned and anything you can take responsibility for. Commit to changing things on the level of thought, emotion, and behavior. Sometimes that is adding something; other times it is subtracting. What can you commit to?

Yoga Therapy for Diabetes-Related Stress and Anxiety

We will be focusing on a *chronic* state of diabetes stress and anxiety. Āyurveda classifies the mental state of *anxiety* as rajo-guṇa, a state of excess, agitation, vigilance, and worry. When rajas is predominant, the mind is challenged to settle down and turn off. There are many stages of anxiety ranging from chronic worry, to *diabetes distress*, to obsessive-compulsive disorder (OCD), to complete panic attacks. We can generalize rajasic emotion with qualities of agitation, apprehension, compulsion, dread, fear, insecurity, nervousness, phobia, wariness, and worry.[38]

Any state of anxiety will activate a fight-or-flight stress response via the sympathetic branch of the ANS. The physical symptoms of this are increased heart rate, sweating, tightness in the chest, shortness of breath, and insomnia.[39] Our focus for these practices is for sub-clinical management of *diabetes-related stress*, a psychological disorder; this is distinct from a clinical biological disorder represented by GAD, OCD, panic attacks, and PTSD. When assessing a treatment path, it is essential to recognize the difference between acute and chronic stress. Treating an individual amid acute stress is challenging, as these moments are represented by panic and overwhelm; however, working with chronic stress can help an individual respond more appropriately to acute stress.

There are two main pathways for working with distress and anxiety. One is to create a physiological rebalancing of the ANS, down-regulate the fight-or-flight response, and move into deeper states of relaxation. The other is through self-inquiry. When we ask ourselves honest questions about our own patterns of thought, emotion, and behavior in a state of calm, focused presence, it can help us uncover what is at the source of our suffering.

Some people with distress and anxiety will be physically and mentally agitated; others will be almost catatonic and internalize their stress. Each of these states requires a different starting point and practice. A general rule of thumb is: If a person is physically sedentary and mentally anxious, it is best to work with a laṅghana to bṛṁhaṇa to laṅghana orientation; starting slow, building up, and relaxing again. If a person is physically overactive and mentally anxious, the strategy is to move from bṛṁhaṇa to laṅghana.

---

38 Kraftsow, G. (1999) *Yoga for Wellness: Healing with the Timeless Teachings of Viniyoga*. New York: Penguin/Arkana. p.309.

39 Kraftsow, G. (1999) *Yoga for Wellness: Healing with the Timeless Teachings of Viniyoga*. New York: Penguin/Arkana. p.309.

Breathing is our primary strategy to consciously regulate the ANS and awaken svādhyāya, our self-reflective capacity. A useful orientation is diaphragmatic belly breathing, and progressively lengthening the exhalation helps to reduce sympathetic arousal. But the breath can also be a trigger for hypervigilance and create additional anxiety. If you notice a student is having trouble with breathing and is creating more tension, a helpful strategy is to work with the body and let the breath follow naturally. Once a sense of comfort arrives in a pose, the mind is at ease and you can begin the process of directing the breath. That being said, powerful kriyās like bhastrikā and kapālabhātī are contraindicated.

Although the goal of working with stress and anxiousness is equanimity, when you support someone with high levels of anxiety, restorative and calming postures can be agitating. In stillness, people are required to be with their worries rather than run away. I suggest meeting these types with a bṛṁhaṇa orientation first. It is like two negatives meet a positive: a hyper-aroused state cannot be asked to relax without preliminary activation and stimulation. Give these individuals tasks that will distract and focus their minds, like balance and alternate arm and leg movements. This will diffuse the physical hyperactivity and mental agitation before moving towards a laṅghana orientation.

Paradoxically, a yoga nidrā practice is a very effective way of reducing anxiety. Systematically rotating awareness throughout the body, guiding specific areas of the body to relax, and circulating consciousness between polarities (hot and cold, heavy and light, love and fear, joy and sadness) facilitate the direct experience of effortlessness and surrender. This is a useful skillset for people who experience *diabetes-related stress and anxiety.*

The following sequence shows an example of what a practice for diabetes-related distress could look like, although practices do vary in their application from person to person. A vicāra practice can be added, once a person is established in calm and stability.

It is oriented to the former orientation of physical and mental hyper-arousal, starting with a bṛṁhaṇa and moving to a laṅghana orientation with an emphasis culminating in the navel center. This helps the mind withdraw from its externalizing and saṁskāra of searching for danger, and rest within the self.

The breathing practice is an intermediate adaptation of śītalī, or śītkārī for those who cannot curl the tongue, with an alternate nostril exhale (anuloma ujjāyī). This is an interesting balance of a two-part inhale with slight retention, coupled with cooling from the śītalī and calming from the alternate nostril exhale. It is one of my personal favorites. Should it be too advanced, you could consider an ujjāyī prāṇāyāma ratio of 1:1:2:0 or even 1:1:2:1. A vicāra self-reflection practice could be added once a person is established in physical and mental calm and stability.

A Practice for Diabetes Distress and Anxiety

Primary goals: Reduce physical hyperactivity and mental agitation. Cultivate a space for introspection and observation, become less attached to and swayed by external stimuli.

Method: Bṛṁhaṇa to laṅghana orientation to activate the mind and body, modulate physiological hyper-arousal through breath-centric āsana, move towards a laṅghana orientation, introducing longer holds to create physical and mental stability and a continuity of calm.

Theme: Link with the innate source of stability and courage.

Breath-centric āsana: Begin with dynamic movement focusing on larger-class muscle groups and short inhale retention to meet mental and physical hyperactivity. Once the mind and body are more at ease, move towards a laṅghana orientation with longer-held forward bends and inversions (head below the heart will encourage the mental guṇa of sattva), and seated postures for grounding. Hold poses with the head below the heart to calm rajas and awaken self-reflective capacities—the ability to witness sensation and remain at ease.

Prāṇāyāma: Two-part śītalī or śītkārī inhale with anuloma alternate nostril exhale.

Meditation: At the navel, the center of stability, courage, and integration.

1	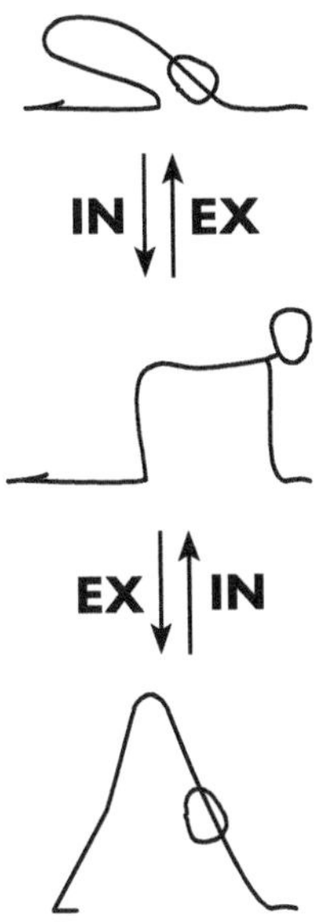	**Cakravākāsana and Adho Mukha Śvānāsana combo:** To strengthen the arms, stretch the hamstrings, promote axial extension (length) in the spine, and prepare for standing postures.	Start in a kneeling position with the abdomen on the thighs, and arms extended in front. Inhale: Lift up to the hands and knees, stack the shoulders over the wrists and the knees over the hips, lengthen the sternum from the navel, and broaden the collarbone. Exhale: Tuck the toes, press into the hands, and lift the knees off the ground, moving into downward facing dog (Adho Mukha Śvānāsana) while lengthening the spine. Inhale: Return to hands and knees. Exhale: Lower the hips to the heels, the torso to the thighs, soften the elbows, and return to the starting position. Repeat six times.
2		**Utthita Trikoṇāsana:** To awaken, energize, and stretch the body, one side at a time, in service of inhalation.	Stand with the feet wider than the shoulders. Have the left foot forward and right foot back and turned slightly in. Open the arms wide and turn the palms to face up. Exhale: Keeping the torso in the same plane, laterally bend, lowering the left hand to the left shin. Turn the right side of the navel and the right shoulder to the ceiling, while looking at the left foot. Inhale: Extend the right arm overhead, looking up at the right hand, stretch the right side body. Exhale: Reach the right arm back, and slightly behind the body, with palm facing up. Look down at the left foot while turning the right side of the abdomen to the ceiling. Progressively lengthen the inhale: Twice each of five, six, seven, and eight seconds. Stay in Utthita Trikoṇāsana with the arm extended overhead for six breaths; maintain an eight-second inhalation.

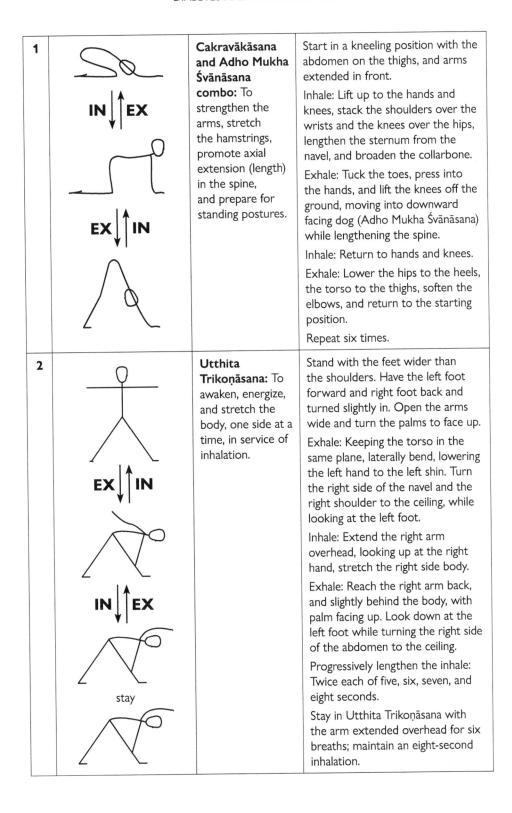

<table>
<tr>
<td>3</td>
<td>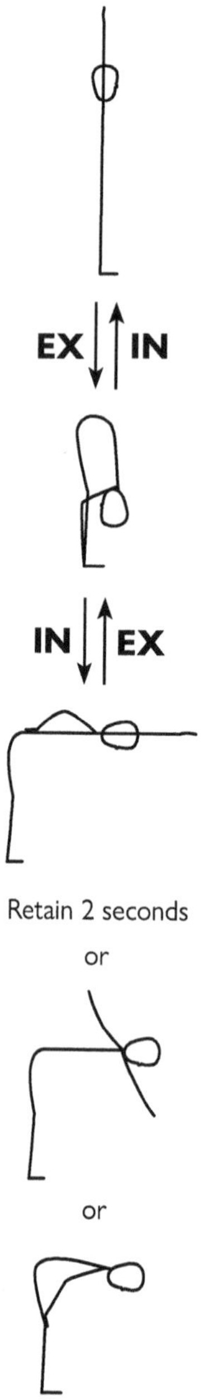
</td>
<td>Uttānāsana and Ardha Uttānāsana combo: To stretch the posterior legs, strengthen the low back, and retain the inhalation.</td>
<td>Start with the feet hip-width apart and arms overhead.
Exhale: Bend forward with slight flexion in the knees, bringing the chest to the thighs and the hands to sides of the feet.
Inhale: Lift the torso parallel to the ground, modify the arm position to make it more or less challenging. Keep the back flat, chin in, and spine long.
Retain: Two seconds.
Exhale: Bend forward with slight flexion in the knees, bringing the chest to the thighs and the hands to sides of the feet.
Inhale: Return to the starting position with a flat back.
Repeat six times.</td>
</tr>
</table>

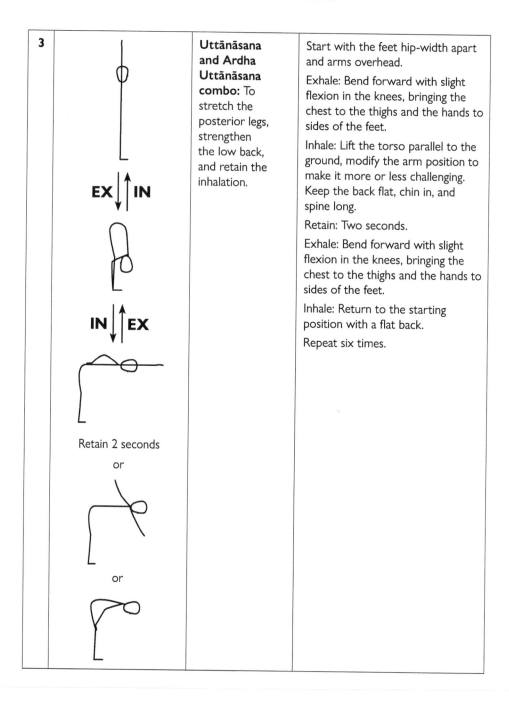

4	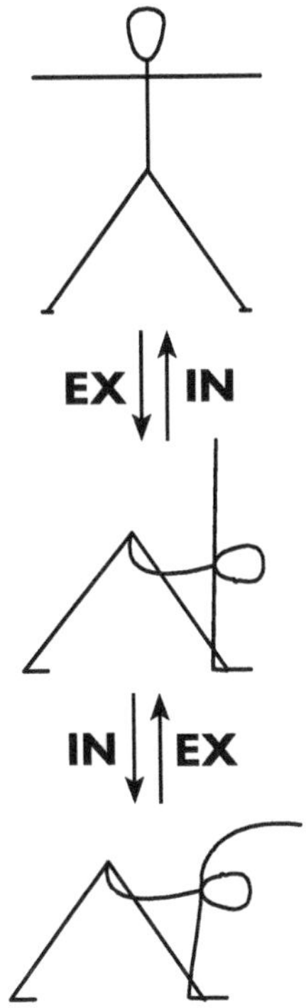	**Parivṛtti Trikoṇāsana with arm sweep:** To stretch the torso, mobilize the shoulders and upper back, and compress the abdomen. On a more subtle level, the intensity of the pose helps establish non-reactive awareness.	Stand with the feet wider than the shoulders and parallel, and the arms out to the sides, level with the floor. Exhale: Twist to the left, place the right hand on the floor outside of the left foot, reach the left arm up to vertical, and twist the navel to the left, gazing down at the bottom hand. Try to stack the right shoulder over the right wrist, bending the left knee more as needed. Inhale: Stay in the twist, extend the left arm overhead, lengthening the left side body, and gaze up at the left hand, keep the chin in. Exhale: Return to the previous position, with the left arm vertical. Gaze down, and twist the navel to the left. Inhale: Return to the starting position. Repeat six times, alternating sides.
5	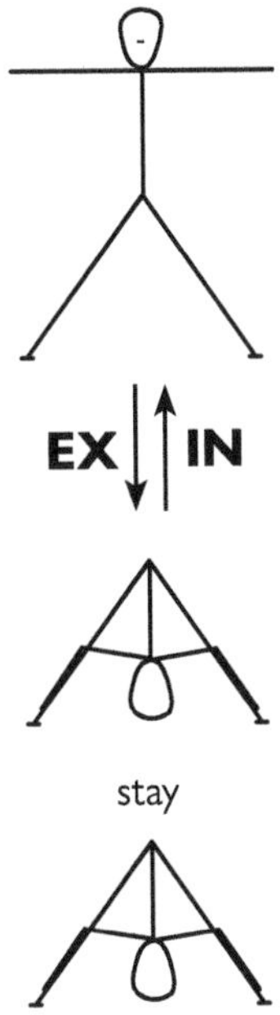	**Prasārita Pādottānāsana:** To counter pose from standing twist, introduce a longer pause for non-reactive awareness, and bring the head below the heart (Viparīta Karaṇī) for mental calm and stability.	Stand with the feet wider than the shoulders and parallel, and the arms out to sides, level with the floor. Exhale: Bend forward, with a slight bend in the knees, gliding the hands to the ankles. Inhale: Return to the starting position, with length in the spine. Repeat three times, and then stay in the pose for a minimum of one minute. Watch the mind move, and sensations move, yet remain established in non-reactive awareness.

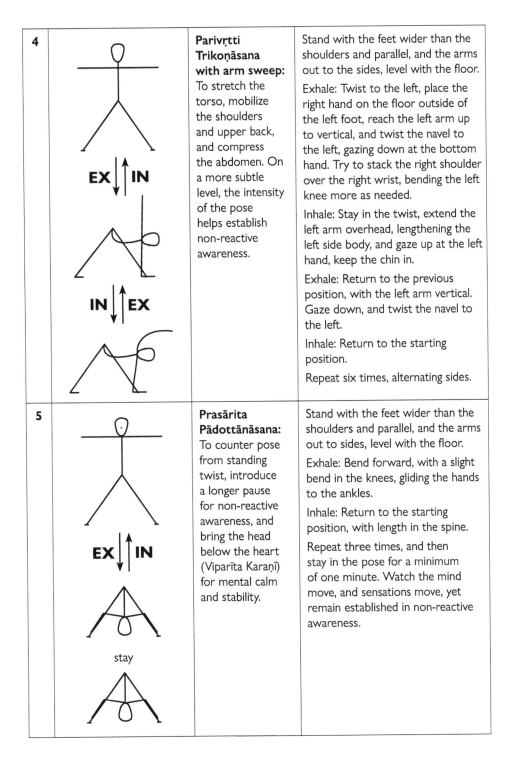

6	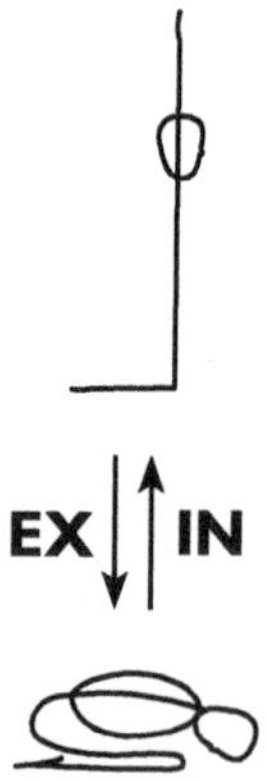 suspend 2s	**Vajrāsana:** To transition to the floor and introduce exhale suspension.	Start in a kneeling position with both arms overhead. Exhale: Bend forward and sweep the arms wide and behind the body while lowering the torso to the thighs and the forehead to the ground. Rest the hands at the low back with the palms facing up. Suspend exhale: Two seconds. Inhale: Return to the starting position. Repeat six times.
7	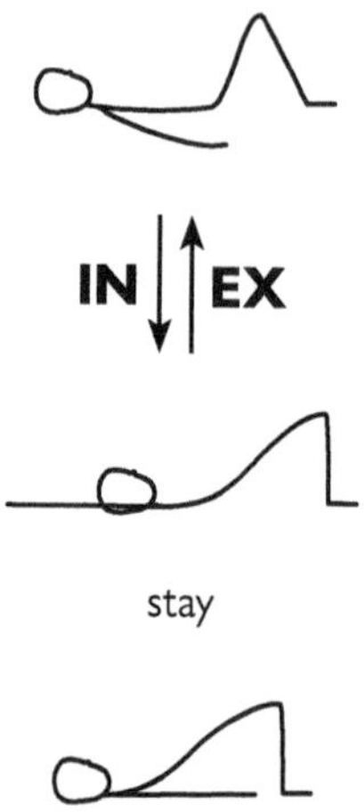	**Dvipāda Pītham:** To prepare the body for shoulder stand.	Lie on the back with the feet hip-width apart and arms by the sides. Inhale: Press into the feet and lift the hips off the ground while reaching the arms up and behind the head to the floor. Exhale: Lower the hips and arms, returning to the starting position. Repeat six times, and then stay in the pose, with the arms underneath the torso for six breaths. Lengthen the low back and maintain equal breath in and out.
8	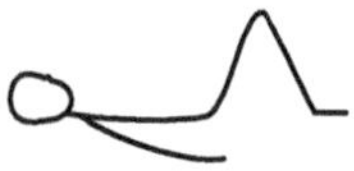	**Rest:** One minute; to prepare for shoulder stand.	

9	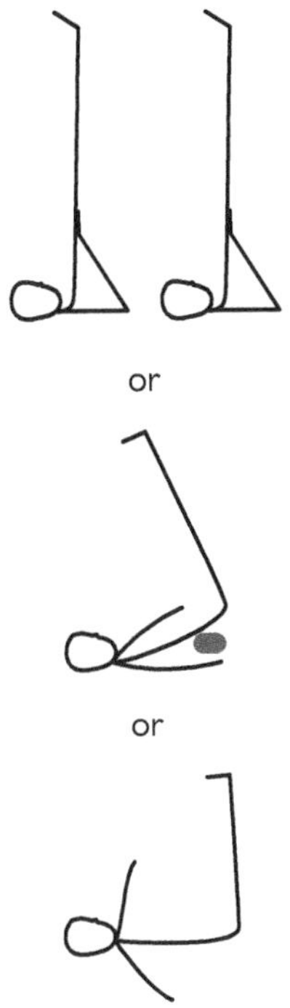	**Sarvāṅgāsana or modified Viparīta Karaṇī with block:** To create an active reversal effect (Viparīta Karaṇī), promoting physiological balance. On a more subtle level, the active reversal effect reduces mental rajas and promotes mental sattva. The physical challenge can be an opportunity to cultivate non-reactive awareness. The adaptation of Sarvāṅgāsana is a three-quarter lift to decrease the risk of hyper-compression of the cervical spine.	Lie on the back, and lift the legs overhead, elevating the pelvis. Place the hands at the low back, with the palms facing in. Powerfully energize the legs and feet up, draw the buttocks into the body. Allow for space between the chin and the throat. To lift into the modified position, come up into bridge pose and slide a block under the sacrum. Resting the pelvis securely on the sacrum, lift the legs to vertical and adduct the inner thighs together. Stay for 12 breaths.
10	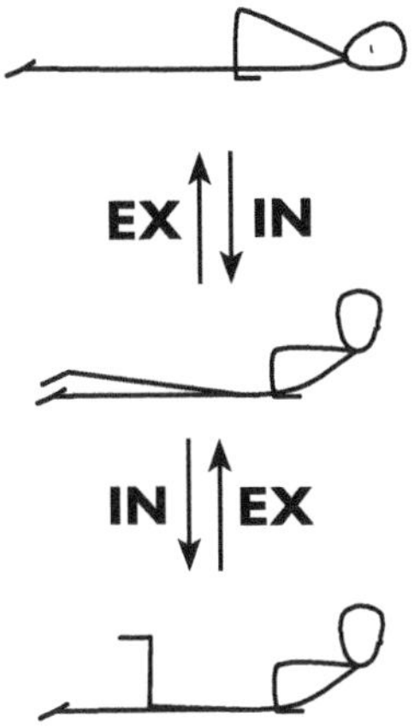	**Ardha Śalabhāsana variation:** To compensate for Sarvāṅgāsana and bring awareness down into the lower body.	Lie on the belly, turn the head to one side, have the hands under the shoulders. Inhale: Lift the chest and the right leg simultaneously, turning the head to center. Exhale: Bend the right knee. Inhale: Straighten the right leg, lengthen the spine, and lift the chest from the back muscles. Exhale: Release, return to the starting position, turning the head to the opposite side. Alternate legs, four times each side.

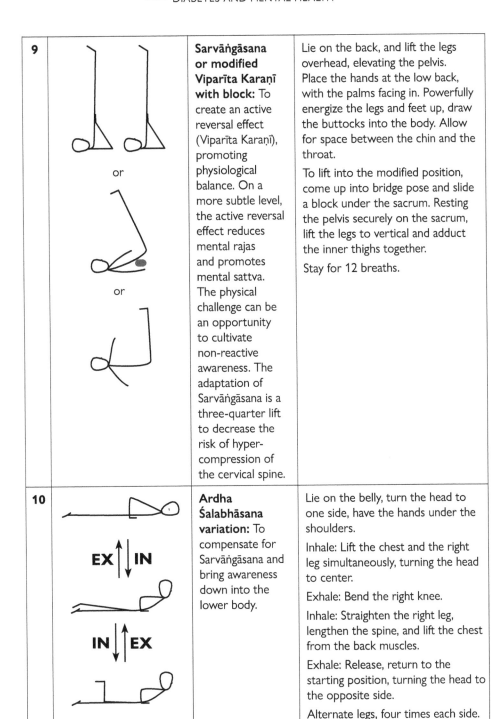

11	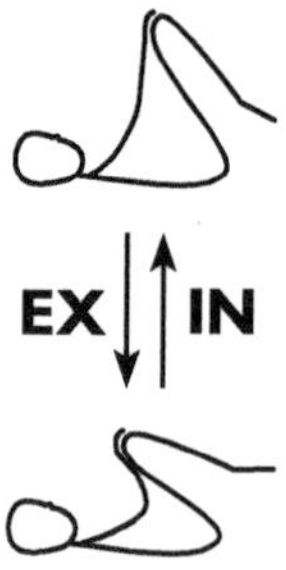	**Apānāsana:** To counter pose by stretching the low back, compressing the abdomen, and suspending exhalation.	Lie on the back, bend the knees into the body. Place the hands on the knees. Exhale: Gently pull both legs into the body. Suspend exhale: Two seconds. Inhale: Return to the starting position, straightening the elbows. Repeat six times.
12	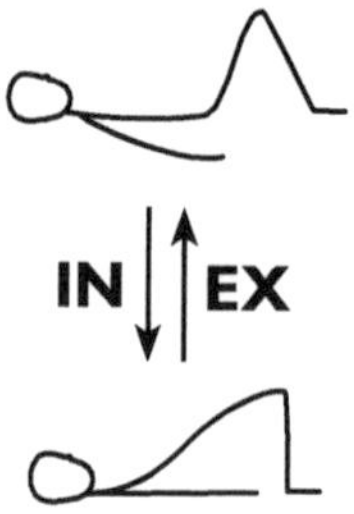	**Dvipāda Pītham:** To unwind the spine, free up the breath, and prepare for a seated pose.	Lie on the back with the feet hip-width apart and arms by the sides. Inhale: Press into the feet, lift the hips off the ground while reaching the arms up and behind the head to the floor. Exhale: Lower the hips and arms, and return to the starting position. Repeat six times.
13	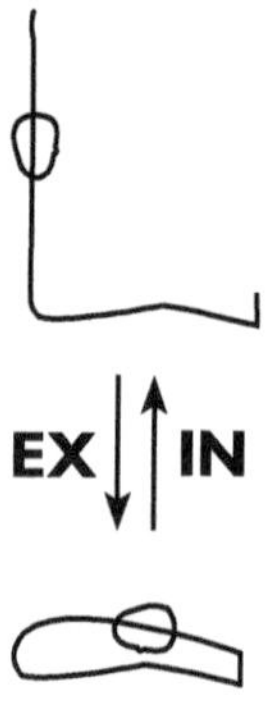 suspend exhale	**Paścimatānāsana:** To stretch the low back and legs, lengthen the exhale, suspend the exhale.	Sit upright with the legs forward, a slight bend in the knees, and the arms overhead. Exhale: Bend forward, lengthening the front of the torso until it reaches the thighs, place the hands on the feet. Suspend exhale: Four seconds. Relax the body and mind into the pause. Inhale: Lift the arms and torso, and with a flat back return to the starting position. Repeat six times.

14	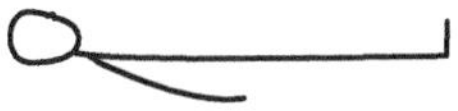	**Śavāsana:** To rest and orient the mind in the navel center, the pause between the breath, the pause between thought and reaction.	Lie on the back, and cover the eyes with a light cloth. Relax the body into the earth. Feel the earth holding the body in full support. Breathe into the abdomen, watch the rise and fall. Exhale: Allow the body to relax into the earth. Inhale: Feel the earth rising up to meet the body in full support. After a few minutes, relax all conscious shaping of the breath; the breath becomes natural. Rest the body and mind in the feeling of being held and supported by the earth for a minimum of five minutes.
15	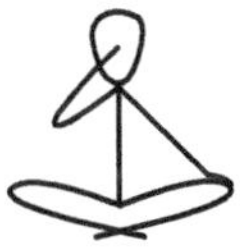	**Two-part śītalī or śītkārī with anuloma ujjāyī (alternate nostril exhale):** An interesting combination of bṛṁhaṇa and laṅghana orientation specialized for anxiety. To nourish, calm, and soothe the body and mind.	Sit in a comfortable position. Curl the tongue (śītalī) or rest the tongue where the teeth and upper gums meet (śītkārī). Inhale: Four seconds, lift the chin slightly. Pause: Four seconds. Inhale: Four seconds, lift the chin just beyond parallel. Pause: Four seconds. Tuck the tongue back, lower the chin. Lift the right hand into mṛgī mudrā (Chapter 5), close the right nostril, valve the left, and exhale through the valved left nostril. Lower the hand. Repeat the two-part inhale with śītalī or śītkārī. Then lift the hand and repeat the steps, exhaling through the valved right nostril. Repeat 12 times in total, alternating each nostril on exhale.

16	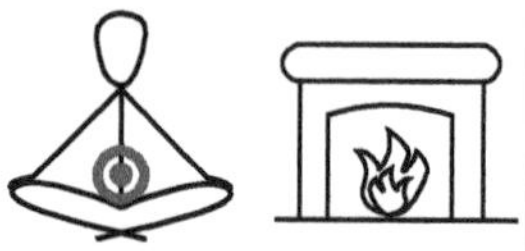	**Navel meditation—niṣṭhā dhāraṇā:** First, establish present awareness at the navel center by placing the breath and the mind in the abdomen. Sense or feel a presence, like a hearth, a fire, or a familiar warmth, like returning home. It is okay if this is hard to link with; it can take time to develop awareness. Just placing your attention in the region is sufficient.	Inhale: Sense, feel, imagine the warmth or light at the navel growing brighter and expanding outwards from the center. Exhale: Witness the golden hue being reabsorbed into the center from where it originated. Maintain this breath awareness for some time, making sure to keep your breath subtle and natural. Then, relax the technique and rest your attention in the hearth of the abdomen, your eternal home. Sense a feeling of deep stability, courage, and integration. Stay in this space for some time.

Yoga Therapy for Diabetes Burnout and Depression

In this practice, we will focus on diabetes burnout, depressive-like-symptoms resulting from the cumulative effect of diabetes overwhelm, and their implication on diabetes self-care. Again, these practices are descriptive and are not prescriptive. There is so much variance when working with mental health, especially when we add the psychological impact of disease into the mix.

Depression-like symptoms, as represented by diabetes burnout, are characterized by inaction, aversion, and denial. Tamo-guṇa is the force of stability represented by inertia and dullness. Tamo-guṇa is obstructive, and its veil of inertia covers the light of hope. Because of its inherent blocking energy, there is little inspiration to do anything. To counteract this, the mind needs brightening to reveal its own intrinsic source of joy. We can help dissipate tamas by moving it through rajas towards sattva.

When working on diabetes burnout and depressive-like symptoms as they relate to diabetes, we want to inspire a person to remember their innate strength and willpower to overcome obstacles and influence change in how they feel. There is a fine line between how far a person will go and when they will start to feel overwhelmed and want to give up. Therefore, practices should be short and concise and build upon each other progressively, encouraging self-confidence, self-efficacy, and inner strength. Small yogic "snacks" or short interventions throughout a person's day will help. The overwhelm of doing it all is what sparks the aversion, so giving people small and attainable challenges builds them up. Try eating one healthy thing today; go for a ten-minute walk around the block; do just one breathing practice. It does not have to be "big" to be transformative. With time, people will build upon their successes and become less fearful of failure.

Chronic activation of the stress responses leads to cortisol deficiency and burnout. Although some forms of depression and burnout co-produce sympathetic activation and symptoms of anxiety, when people are burnt out they most often experience a state of sympathetic suppression, represented by fatigue, lethargy, and inactivity.[40] There is a pervasive sense of hopelessness, despair, and lack of motivation. A practice for burnout should help to nourish and regulate the ANS to progressively lift energy and stimulate interest, willpower, and confidence. Whereas a practice for distress has a calming/reducing orientation, a practice for burnout/depression is *generally* a stimulating and nourishing practice. We want to encourage an attitude and feeling of "I've got this," of being powerful and capable of taking on diabetes.

Many people suffering from diabetes burnout and depressive-like symptoms can also experience anxiety. They may be physically manic but mentally depressed, and have trouble concentrating and remembering.[41] A bṛṁhaṇa to laṅghana to bṛṁhaṇa orientation can be useful. With mental agitation, we want to be cautious not to create a psychological trigger that will only set back self-confidence. A useful prāṇāyāma strategy is a staggered inhalation (in two or three parts). This can be applied in seated practice or specific postures, should they not aggravate the mind. If people have trouble with breathing, you can try to have them "sip" in the air from three to ten sips.[42] This can be done seated or in a supine position. Once this has been achieved without tension, you can try to do the same with their exhalation.

---

40 Kraftsow, G. (2020) "Yoga for depression: an integrated practice." *Yoga International.* Accessed on 10/07/20 at: https://yogainternational.com/article/view/yoga-for-depression-an-integrated-practice.

41 Butkiewicz, E., Carbone, A., Green, S., Miano, A. and Wegner, E. (2016) "Diabetes Management." In M. A. Burg and O. Oyama (eds) *Behavioral Health Specialist.* New York: Springer Publishing Company. p.91.

42 Butkiewicz, E., Carbone, A., Green, S., Miano, A. and Wegner, E. (2016) "Diabetes Management." In M. A. Burg and O. Oyama (eds) *Behavioral Health Specialist.* New York: Springer Publishing Company. p.93.

Others are physically depleted and mentally depressed. We see this orientation more frequently with burnout, as it shows up with the inactivity and unresponsiveness to diabetes self-management. For these individuals, use a practice that first grounds them and then progressively nourishes and awakens their body and intellect, a laṅghana to bṛṁhaṇa orientation. A gentle emphasis on chest openings encouraged by chest inhales and brief retention reverses the physical posture of depression (hunched over and kyphotic) to an attitude of open and vibrant confidence. Restorative and supportive backbends like Supta Baddha Koṇāsana and supine backbends with a gentle inhale breath emphasis are helpful. Backbends on the stomach can be favorable because of the grounding and assimilative properties of being on the abdomen, but for some this is anxiety provoking and uncomfortable.

Sometimes a laṅghana orientation has a bṛṁhaṇa effect just as a bṛṁhaṇa orientation may promote a laṅghana/reducing effect, like we see in the case of anxiety. We tend to conceptualize bṛṁhaṇa with inhale and standing postures like backbends and lateral bends, but another way to conceive of a practice strategy is by building ojas, the vital essence. In sympathetic suppression the cause is the overactivation of the sympathetic responses, leading to exhaustion and fatigue. We can sometimes achieve a bṛṁhaṇa quality with yoga nidrā. Let's be honest, there is not much that yoga nidrā is contraindicated for. With burnout, we run the risk of overdoing it and disempowering people. Sometimes people are, frankly, too exhausted to do anything physical and yoga nidrā is an extremely efficacious way of increasing ojas, which in this application has a nourishing (bṛṁhaṇa) quality.

Please be mindful that when there is excessive tamo-guṇa, as there is in burnout and depression, there can be a tendency to "bypass" the witnessing and fall asleep. Educate your student on the difference between sleeping and conscious rest. The ability to abide in the observer and consciously rest is a powerful tool that can spark more positivity and energy. Make sure to give the mind plenty of things to focus on so that it does not fall prey to the dull sleepiness of tamas. Over time, their capacity to hold restful attention will also illumine their awareness of the darkness that covers their inner light.

Infusing saṁkalpa or intention into a practice engenders a deeper sense of drive and purpose (dharma). Intention is refined with self-awareness, but an initial affirmation of "Let this practice be beneficial" as a sort of open-ended goal is a useful motivational tool.

Meditation is where wisdom and mental processes unite. Meditation is one of the most powerful tools for transforming perception and diffusing burnout, but it is not always appropriate when a person is acutely burnt out on diabetes or in a depressed state.[43] It can be challenging to sit in the pain and witness the darkness especially with self-reflective practices like vicāra. Mantra-based meditation is an excellent alternative strategy, as is meditating on the source of innate light and joy. Strong and wrathful deities like Kali and Rudra help to destroy the darkness, waken inner confidence, and embody a feeling of: I can influence my own condition; I can rise above this.

A Practice for Diabetes Burnout and Chronic Depression

Primary goals: Reduce sympathetic suppression by progressively activating the SNS, decrease mental dullness, and improve self-esteem. The longer-term goal is to awaken inner strength to improve one's conditions, and spark interest and joy in self-care.

Method: A laṅghana to bṛṁhaṇa orientation to progressively build and nourish the physiological responses (sympathetic suppression) and brighten the mind towards sources of inspiration. Start with a calming and grounding practice, and increase energy to activate and nourish the body and mind. It is about linking or creating a personal "source of inspiration." There is an asymmetrical focus to help orient the mind from distraction to attention, building up to longer holds to train willpower and strength.

Theme: To open the space of the heart, dispel darkness, and awaken qualities of inspiration, determination, and self-efficacy; a feeling of "I've got this."

Breath-centric āsana: Simple postures that will lengthen the spine, open the chest, and increase inhale capacity like extension and lateral bends. Progressively hold poses for longer periods of time to build willpower (for example, hold one breath, two breaths, three breaths, four breaths), to lengthen the inhale and inhale retention. This practice builds up to a five-breath stay in Mahāmudrā. Mahāmudrā was considered by Krishnamacharya to be the greatest accomplishments of hatha yoga. The intensity of this pose creates many sensations in the lower regions of the body that are said to be related to the lower mind, and swayed by impulse and survival. By working with this area, one develops mastery over the lower mind, impulse, and reactivity.

43 Butkiewicz, E., Carbone, A., Green, S., Miano, A. and Wegner, E. (2016) "Diabetes Management." In M. A. Burg and O. Oyama (eds) *Behavioral Health Specialist*. New York: Springer Publishing Company. p.91.

Prāṇāyāma: Two-part inhale krama with an emphasis on the chest and heart space.

Meditation: Heart kriyā and mantra: Om jyotir ahaṁ.

I am that light of pure awareness.

1	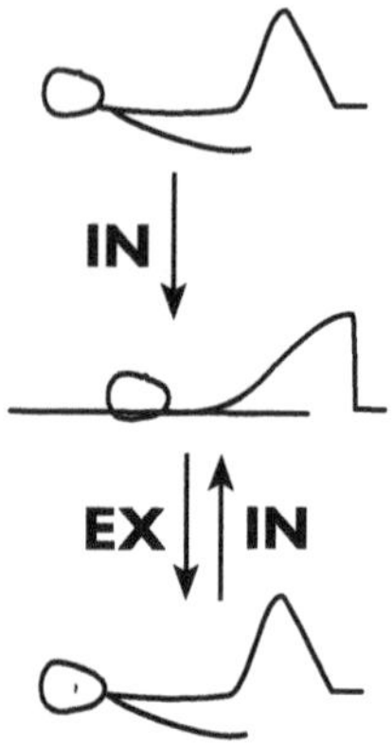	**Dvipāda Pītham variation:** To stretch the body, one side at a time, and focus the mind with alternate arm and head movements.	Lie on the back with the feet hip-width apart and arms by the sides. Inhale: Press into the feet, lift the hips off the ground, while reaching the right arm up and behind the head to the floor, and gaze up at the ceiling. Exhale: Lower the hips and the right arm, while simultaneously turning the head to the left, and return to the starting position. Repeat six times, alternating the arm and head rotation.
2	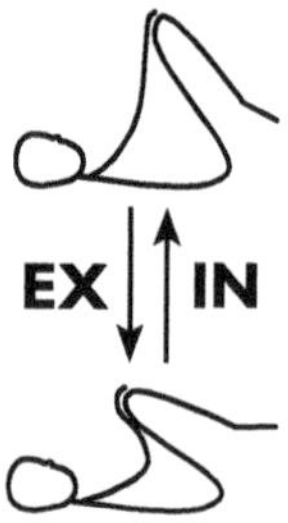	**Apānāsana:** To stretch the low back, compress the abdomen, and create a laṅghana effect by chanting on exhale.	Lie on the back, bend the knees into the body. Place the hands on the knees. Exhale: Chant Om jyotir ahaṁ, while gently pull both legs into the body. Inhale: Return to the starting position. Repeat six times.
3	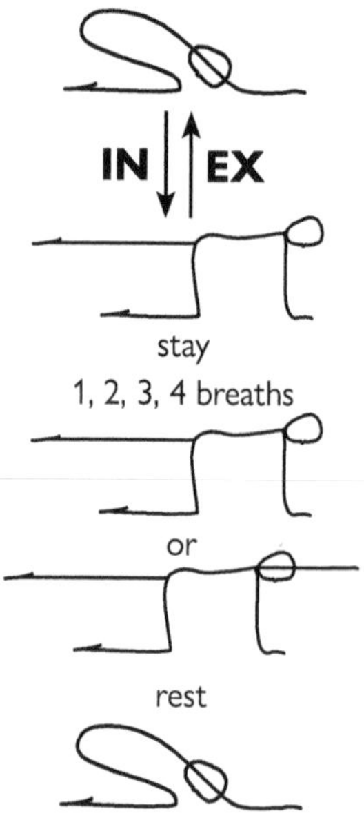	**Cakravākāsana variation (bird-dog):** To asymmetrically strengthen the body and introduce longer holds for mental stability.	Start in kneeling forward bend position, with the abdomen resting on the thighs, knees hip-width apart, and arms extended in front with the hands on the ground. Inhale: Lift the torso to hands and knees, while reaching the right leg back, lifting the foot off the ground, and optionally extending the left arm forward, with the thumb facing up and gaze neutral. Exhale: Return to the kneeling position, lowering the hand and knee to the ground and lowering the torso to the thighs. Repeat three times, alternating sides, and progressively stay on each side for one, two, and three breaths.

4	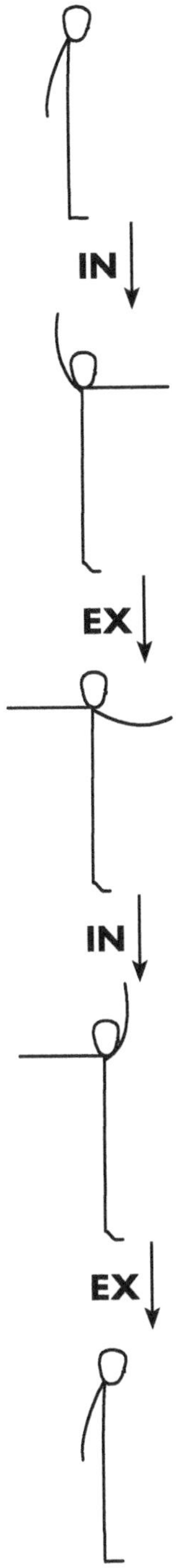	**Tāḍāsana variation with alternate arm movements:** To bring attention, balance, and stability to the body and mind.	Start in a standing position, with the feet slightly separated and arms by the sides. Inhale: Lift both arms and the heels. When the arms are shoulder height, continue lifting the right arm overhead. Exhale: Lower the right arm and heels halfway. Inhale: Lift the heels and left arm overhead. Exhale: Lower the arms and heels simultaneously. Equal inhale to equal exhale: 1:1 (for stability). Repeat six times.

5	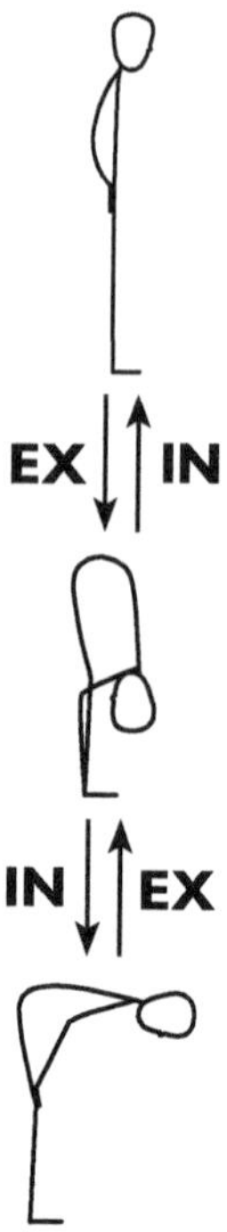 chant on exhale	**Uttānāsana and Ardha Uttānāsana combo:** To stretch the posterior legs, strengthen the low back, and create a laṅghana effect by chanting on exhale.	Start with the feet hip-width apart and hands on the backs of the legs. Exhale: While chanting *Om jyotir ahaṁ*, bend forward with slight flexion in the knees, gliding the hands down the legs to the ankles, and the chest to the thighs. Inhale: Lift the torso parallel to the ground, with the hands on the shins, back flat, chin in, and spine long. Exhale: While chanting *Om jyotir ahaṁ*, bend forward with slight flexion in the knees, gliding the hands down the legs to the ankles, and the chest to the thighs. Inhale: Return to the starting position with a flat back. Repeat six times.
6	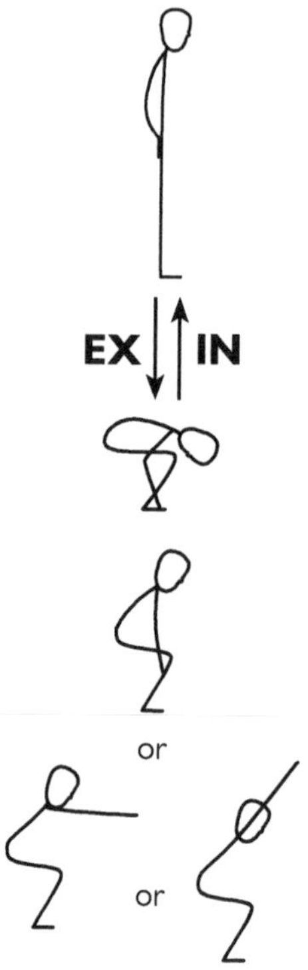 stay 1, 2, 3, 4 breaths	**Ardha Utkaṭāsana and Utkaṭāsana combo:** To strengthen the back, open the chest, and introduce longer holds for mental stability.	Stand with the feet hip-width apart and the hands on the backs of the legs. Exhale: Sit the hips back, bring the torso to the thighs and the hands on the ground by the sides of the feet. The hips should be just slightly higher than the knees. Inhale: Lift the torso into Utkaṭāsana, keeping the hips low, until the chest cannot lift any higher. Continue straightening the legs and return to the starting position. Repeat three times, then progressively stay in Utkaṭāsana for one, two, three, and four breaths. Stay with your arm variation of choice.

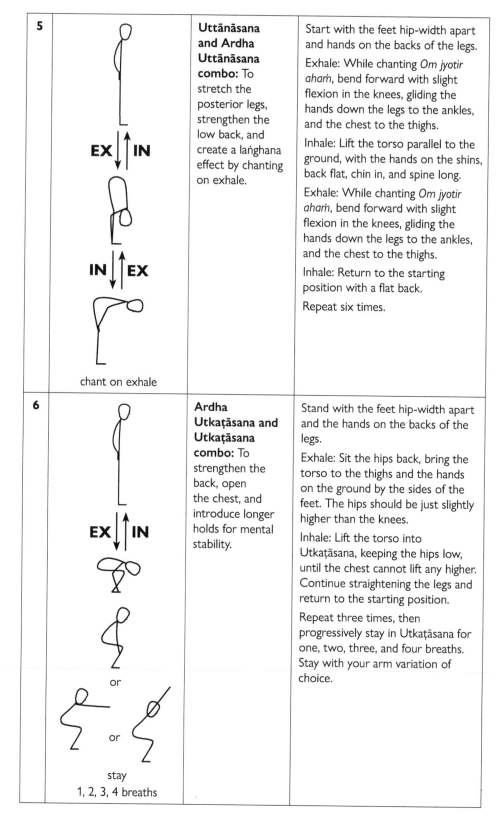

7	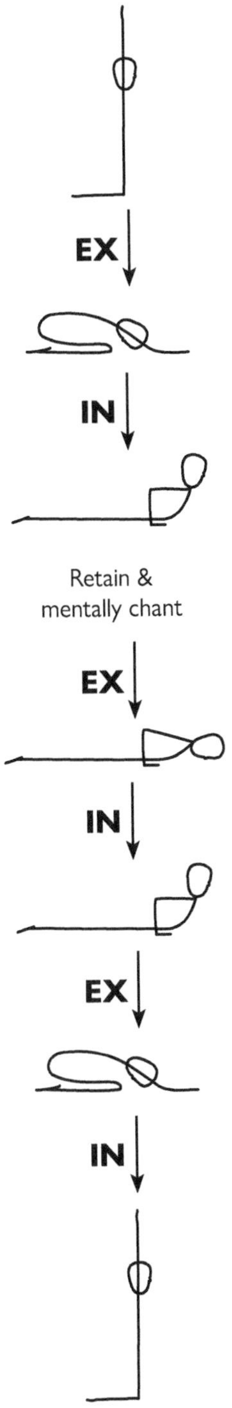 	**Vajrāsana, Bālāsana, and Bhujaṅgāsana combo:** To transition from standing to the floor, open the chest, and introduce inhale retention.	Start in a kneeling position with the knees hip-width apart and arms overhead. Exhale: Bend forward, reach the arms forward, sit the hips back to the heels, and slowly lower the torso to the thighs and hands to the ground. Inhale: Glide forward into cobra pose, with the belly on the ground, hands under the shoulders, elbows bent, torso in gentle extension, and neck long. Retain inhale, mentally chant *Om jyotir ahaṁ* at the heart. Exhale: Lower the torso to the ground. Inhale: Return to cobra pose and retain inhale, mentally chant *Om jyotir ahaṁ* at the heart. Exhale: Return the hips to the heels and torso to the thighs. Extend the arms with the hands on the ground. Inhale: Return to the starting position, using the back body to lift. Repeat six times.

8	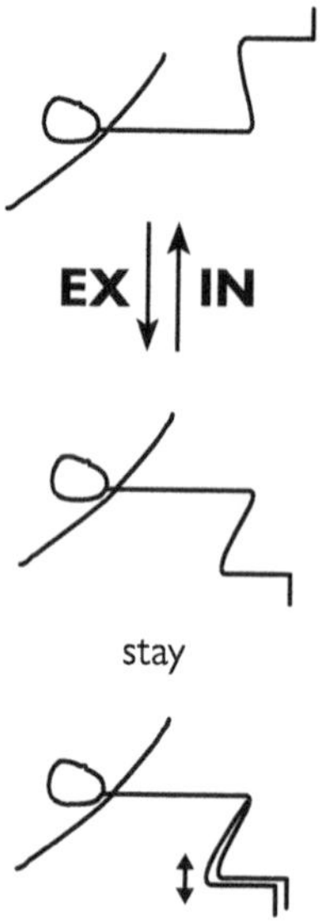	**Jaṭara Parivṛtti:** To strengthen the outer hip in preparation for Mahāmudrā.	Lie on the back with both arms wide and the knees bent into the chest. Exhale: Twist, gradually contract the abdomen, bring the legs over to the left side, and turn head to the right. Inhale: Return to the starting position. Repeat six times, alternating sides, and then twist the knees to the left and stay. Lift the right knee and foot until parallel with the ground. Press through the right knee, activating the outer hip muscles. Stay for five breaths, and then repeat on the other side.
9	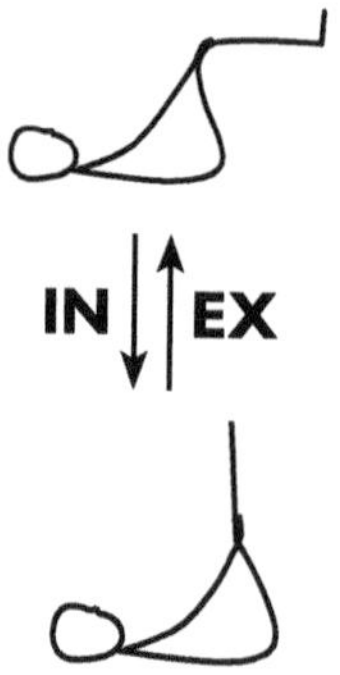	**Ūrdhva Prasārita Pādāsana:** To counter pose the spine from the twist with a symmetrical movement, lengthen the spine, and stretch the low back and hamstrings in preparation for seated postures.	Lie on the back with both knees lifted towards the chest, feet off the floor, and hands behind knees. Inhale: Extend the legs towards the ceiling, and flex the ankles. Exhale: Bend the knees, squeeze the abdomen, draw the thighs into the navel, and keep the sacrum on the ground. Repeat six times.

10	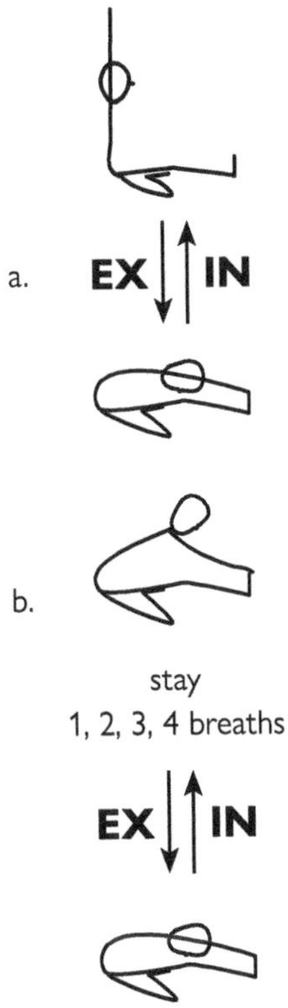 stay 1, 2, 3, 4 breaths	**Jānu Śīrṣāsana and Mahāmudrā:** The apex of the practice. To work with progressive stay, and build mental stability and willpower.	Sit with the right knee bent, right heel to the inner left thigh, left leg extended forward, and arms overhead. a. *Jānu Śīrṣāsana and Mahāmudrā* Exhale: Bend forward, bring the belly and chest to the left leg and hands to the foot. Inhale: Holding the foot with both hands, lean back, lift the torso as far away from the thigh as possible, keeping the chin in and spine long. Exhale: Bend forward, bring the belly and chest to the left leg and hands to the foot. Inhale: Return to the starting position. Repeat three times. b. *Mahāmudrā with progressive stay* Exhale: Bend forward, bring the belly and chest to the left leg and hands to the left foot. Inhale: Holding the foot with both hands, lean back, lift the torso as far away from the thigh as possible, keeping the chin in and spine long. Stay for one, two, three, four, and five breaths. Return to *Jānu Śīrṣāsana* between each round of stay.
11	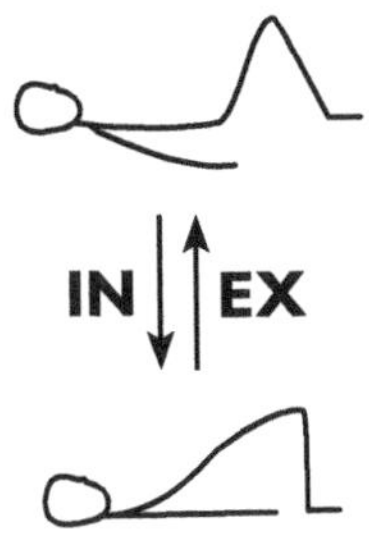	**Dvipāda Pītham:** To counter pose for Mahāmudrā and prepare for Śavāsana.	Lie on the back with the feet hip-width apart and arms by the sides. Inhale: Press into the feet and lift the hips off the ground while reaching the arms up and behind the head to the floor. Exhale: Lower the hips and arms and return to the starting position. Repeat six times.
12	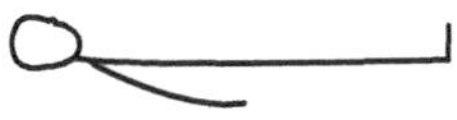	**Śavāsana:** To rest in spacious awareness and inner light.	Strategically relax the whole body down the back and up the front. Relax all shaping of the breath. Feel that the chest is open, clear, and spacious like a desert sky and rest.

Establish a natural breath flow:

Inhale chest	Pause	Inhale navel	Pause	Exhale	Number of times
3 seconds	3 seconds	2 seconds	2 seconds	6 seconds	4
4 seconds	4 seconds	3 seconds	3 seconds	8 seconds	4
5 seconds	5 seconds	4 seconds	4 seconds	10 seconds	4
6 seconds	6 seconds	5 seconds	5 seconds	12 seconds	4
6 seconds	–	–	–	8 seconds	2
4 seconds	–	–	–	6 seconds	2

Inhale: Feel, see, or sense the light in the heart expand and brighten.

Exhale: Feel, see, or sense that very light be reabsorbed back into the center of the heart space.

Maintain this awareness for several minutes, being as effortless as possible. Then relax the technique and rest in the spacious, clear, and nourishing light in the heart for some time.

Repeat the mantra *Om jyotir ahaṁ* from the heart space, sensing your inner effulgence diffusing all darkness, sadness, disappointment, and doubt. The light awakens a fervent love and compassion for oneself and a remembrance that life is a sacred gift.

13	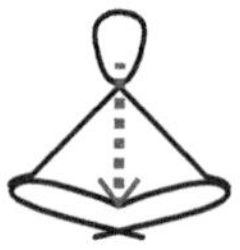	**Prāṇāyāma:** Two-part inhale krama: To create a balanced and nourishing bṛṁhaṇa effect and bring attention to the heart space.	Sit up tall. Bring attention to the spine.
14	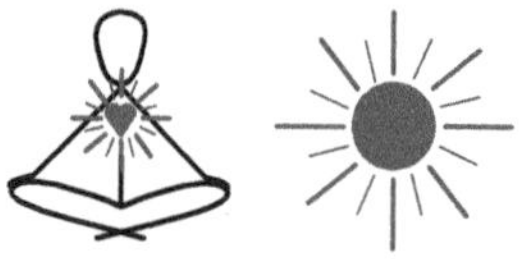	**Heart kriyā and mantra:** To experience the light of the heart.	Relax the shaping of the breath and bring attention to the heart space somewhere in the chest. See or feel the image of the sun at the heart. Consider this as your innate light, the light of the universe, the light that absorbs all sorrow.

CHAPTER 12

Above and Beyond Diabetes

As we near the end of this book, I want to leave you with a message from my heart and lived experience with diabetes. Life is sacred, and diabetes is an opportunity to empower you to rise to your own greatness. The risk factors are exactly why you rise above the world full of change and achieve the potential that you set out to fulfill.

We are born with a full vessel of *pranic* potential. Somewhere along the way, life happens and we veer off course, forgetting that our aim as humans is to know the self. Diabetes is a stain that can result in a long chain of sadness, grief, and anger. We begin to believe that life is just a series of injustice, abuse, and turmoil.[1] Simple causes need simple cures. The bigger the stain, the more detergent we need.

To remove the stain, we need powerful methods. Pandit Rajmani Tigunait, my grand-teacher, says that the greatest of all arts and sciences is *self-empowerment*, and that is precisely what we are doing when we practice for diabetes. We are cultivating the power to remove the obstacles of illness and transform adversity into an advantage. We are saying: Let us rise to greatness not in spite of diabetes but *because* of diabetes. Let us do everything in our ability to make the most of our limited time on earth. It is our right as humans.

So how do we create such power? Well, practice of course! That is essentially what the book is about—how to create the most resilient container of *pranic* potential so that we have the energy needed to remove the stains of diabetes and live our best life possible. Health, longevity, and resilience are all synonyms for *self-mastery*, the ultimate aim of the sacredness of life.

---

1 Tigunait, P. J. (n.d.) *Seminar Lotus of the Heart.* Honesdale, PA: Himalayan Institute.

Empowered Resilience—the Power to Bounce Back

The strength of an organism is dependent upon its protective coatings that buffer risk and reduce deterioration. Like a nerve cell has a myelin sheath, and a DNA strand possesses a protective cap known as a telomere, yoga practices create a layer that protects against diabetes risk factors. When deprived of these protective mantles, an organism's health deteriorates. Without a myelin sheath, a nerve cell will no longer conduct electrical impulses. A telomere keeps a DNA strand from unraveling, which protects it from the negative expression of genes. Given the opportunity to regenerate, a nerve cell will regrow its sheath. A healthy lifestyle maintains genes, which inhibit predispositions and risk factors.

The vessel of health should be as vital as possible so that all the regulatory systems can function properly, our immunity can bring us back when we are sick, and we can live in positive relationship with the world. Risk is anything that chips away at the vitality of the vessel and compromises its resilience to bounce back. Think about the concept of allostasis and allostatic load. Stress chips away at it, compromising the function of neuroendocrine responses. Psychological stress and actual stress from diabetes effects (BG levels) and health complications, either as a result of compromised self-care or the duration of a disease, all increase risk. Depression, anxiety, and burnout all compromise how we see the world, ourselves, and our potential as humans. Although T1D and T2D are separate conditions with distinct origins, both are precipitated by lifestyle factors like nutrition, physical activity, thoughts and emotions, relationships, sleep, and relaxation. The result can either increase risk or promote resilience.[2]

Yoga therapy is a protective process that acts as a buffer against diabetes risks by offering self-applied intervention strategies to reduce risk. The shield is ojas and sattvic living—a protective layering that offsets the energetic deficit from diabetes effects and supports learning and change.[3] The best part of it is that yoga and yoga therapy are not a pill that someone takes, they comes from within and continue to evolve from within. The practice of yoga in the individual is a dynamic relationship, just like diabetes. With an active, dynamic process that is completely modifiable by the practitioner to treat whatever

2 M. A. Burg and O. Oyama (eds) (2016) *Behavioral Health Specialist.* New York: Springer Publishing Company. p.268.

3 Anderson, R., Funnell, M., Carlson, A., Saleh-Statin, N., *et al.* (2005) "Facilitating Self-Care Through Empowerment." In F. J. Snoek and C. T. J. Skinner (eds) *Psychology in Diabetes Care.* Second edition. Chichester: Wiley & Sons Ltd. p.71.

deficiency or adversity is present, the individual is able to look at diabetes from a distinct perspective. No longer the victim, they can make changes. With time, their reserves increase. They can sustain deficits but can bounce back faster because they have a surplus of vitality.

While the risk of poor diabetes outcomes is well researched, there is less information about the processes of achieving positive outcomes. In the Western model of health, research on the relationship between resilient health outcomes and positive self-management processes is increasing; however, the research recommendations lack the dynamism and personalization that empower individuals to truly overcome their biggest obstacles to self-care.[4] We see this time and again when looking at the stats of how few people actually achieve the recommended parameters of glycemic control and in the numbers of people who suffer with burnout and depression because of diabetes. Endocrinologists and behavioral psychologists will confirm that the antidote to diabetes is resilience. Pandits and gurus will say that the remedy to all of life's suffering is self-empowerment. There is no difference; they are one and the same. Resilience is defined by a positive outcome in one or more areas of life, despite exposure to significant risk or adversity.[5]

There are plenty of people with diabetes who do exceptionally well. What makes these people different from those who are always bogged down by diabetes is their perception of diabetes stress. These individuals are resilient and empowered by diabetes. They have acquired personal tools to enable them to be involved in and responsible for their diabetes management. They possess effective behavioral strategies and attitudes to buffer the impact of diabetes risks. For example, a resilient person may adapt to a situation by reframing it in a positive light or eliciting support from others.[6] They are more likely to see a number as feedback rather than a threat. They know that although they have diabetes, they also are in charge of their health and wellbeing.

It is accurate that yoga and its practices of āsana, prāṇāyāma, and meditation empower diabetes resilience by improving glycemic control and autonomic

4 Hilliard, M. E., Harris, M. A. and Weissberg-Benchell, J. (2012) "Diabetes resilience: a model of risk and protection in type 1 diabetes." *Current Diabetes Reports 12*, 6, 739–748.

5 Hilliard, M. E., Yi-Frazier, J. P., Hessler, D., Butler, A. M., Anderson, B. J. and Jaser, S. (2016) "Stress and A1c among people with diabetes across the lifespan." *Current Diabetes Reports 16*, 8, 67.

6 Hilliard, M. E., Yi-Frazier, J. P., Hessler, D., Butler, A. M., Anderson, B. J. and Jaser, S. (2016) "Stress and A1c among people with diabetes across the lifespan." *Current Diabetes Reports 16*, 8, 67.

function.[7] Yoga āsanas strengthen muscles and organs. Breathing practices promote heart rate variability and vagal tone, and down-regulate the HPA axis, reducing stress hormones. Yoga psychology awakens perception and behavioral modifications. Meditation increases white and grey matter,[8] supporting memory, cognition, and mood. But despite all of the measurable benefits, the most important advantage of personal practice is empowered resilience. This is the ability to influence the direction of change and bounce back from imbalances. It is the power to sway outcomes, the wisdom to let go of mistakes and also to learn from them.

The most exceptional individuals are resilient to seemingly insurmountable challenges, and the challenges transform them for the better. Yoga outlines a pathway with specific methods and protective processes to offset individual risk factors. These individuals take a seat as the driver of their own chariot, empowered by personal choice and clarity of perception. With time, their understanding of diabetes changes, and they are more confident and hopeful.

Resilience is achieved through a dynamic process of engagement with surmounting risks (self-care). The most powerful mechanisms of resilience are practices that relate to a specific risk factor.[9] These factors are enduring—they will not go away—but we have the power to influence change with practice. Resilience with diabetes means learning to regulate—physically, mentally, and emotionally—when off balance. Empowered resilience (as yoga therapy) is a self-administered *protective process* designed to buffer the impact of diabetes with an ultimate aim of mastering all of life with and beyond diabetes.

There are three qualities of empowered resilience:

- self-awareness
- self-regulation
- self-efficacy.

---

7 Singh, S., Malhotra, V., Singh, K. P., Madhu, S. V. and Tandon, O. P. (2004) "Role of yoga in modifying certain cardiovascular functions in type 2 diabetic patients." *The Journal of the Association of Physicians of India* 52, 203–206.

8 Posner, M. I., Tang, Y. Y. and Lynch, G. (2014) "Mechanisms of white matter change induced by meditation training." *Frontiers in Psychology* 5, 1220.

9 Hilliard, M. E., Harris, M. A. and Weissberg-Benchell, J. (2012) "Diabetes resilience: a model of risk and protection in type 1 diabetes." *Current Diabetes Reports* 12, 6, 739–748.

Self-Awareness

People with diabetes are required to make thousands of decisions every day concerning their diabetes care. Without self-awareness, a person may lack sensitivity to hypoglycemia cues, be unaware of the connection of emotion and blood sugar, or eat the whole kitchen when low. Self-awareness acts as a shield to diabetes risks, empowering the individual to have a deeper relationship with diabetes and with themselves. The profundity of such a relationship provides tools for making more empowered choices regarding their diabetes care. Sensitization to the body and emotions awakens new awareness for diabetes. Without sensitivity, a person cannot understand their diabetes. Studies show that self-awareness interventions improve metabolic control and behavioral integration in T1D.[10]

At the age of 17, I walked into my first yoga class, just four years into a diabetes diagnosis. At the time, I did not understand the concept of suffering, nor did I possess the self-awareness to correlate diabetes-related stress with how positively or negatively I felt about myself. All I remember was how uncomfortable I felt in my skin all of the time. Highly explosive emotionally, I regularly used unhealthy coping mechanisms to numb my discomfort. I started yoga for purely physical reasons: I wanted to look better.

Through practice, I developed self-awareness. The first was proprioceptive, the physical awareness of my body and limbs and how to move them in and out of different shapes. The increased movement developed interoceptive knowledge, the ability to sense my bodily systems and emotional states as an object of my attention. This understanding helped me to see that there was no difference between the discomfort of holding a pose, experiencing an uncomfortable emotion, or abiding with lousy blood sugar. None of these temporary experiences were me, and I always had a chance to show up in every moment.

This self-awareness did not occur intentionally or all at once but was a result of the practice. The transformation was progressive, but with regular, consistent training, I experienced more freedom in my life with and beyond diabetes. But what was it that sparked my initial interest in practice? Curiosity for sure and, more profound than that, it was a *desire to change*. I did not know what I wanted to change, but my passion was to move from where I was to

10 Hernandez, C. A., Hume, M. R. and Rodger, N. W. (2008) "Evaluation of a self-awareness intervention for adults with type 1 diabetes and hypoglycemia unawareness." *Canadian Journal of Nursing Research 40*, 3, 38–56.

somewhere better. Something informed a desire in me, albeit subconsciously, to discover whether there was more to life than I knew. Cultivating self-awareness awakens this inner guide, and it becomes more audible and prevalent in every moment of our lives.

Self-awareness moves a person from ignorance to self-empowerment by awakening them to the possibility of change and the knowledge of how much better it will be to change, rather than stay the same. To move from ignorance to awareness, there has to be a catalyst—something that opens the mind to a different way of seeing things. It is not as simple as: Here's some information, please awaken now. Behavioral psychologists call the awareness of this process "the transition from precognition to cognition." Precognition is like the darkness just before the dawn. Cognition is when a person recognizes his or her role in diabetes management and makes an *intention* change. Self-awareness acts as the starting point for empowered decisions and resilience against the physical and mental challenges of diabetes management.

We cannot develop self-awareness without recognition that there is suffering. Avidyā is the fundamental misunderstanding obscuring the individual self (ego) from experiencing the universal self, who is impervious to suffering, the part of each person who is untouched by sorrow, fear, and illness. It is this inherent misunderstanding that the true, lasting, and innately joyous self is the transient grief, sorrow, pain, and fear. What removes the causes of all suffering is *viveka*, discriminative discernment or self-awareness. The translation of Sanskrit into English often lacks the emotive qualities of a word, and viveka as self-awareness is more than the power to see the difference, it is the knowledge that arises from clear perception. We've seen vi as the root of a word a lot in this book: viyoga, vicāra, viveka. You might begin to say that the definition of yoga is separation to get to union. To separate is to *identify* the source of suffering and then to have the *discipline* to *change* (*self-regulation*) by replacing old and dysfunctional patterns with *new* and more productive ones. However, before this can happen, the individual must first recognize that there is suffering and be open to changing it.

Self-awareness can only be achieved when the person is open to it and practices methods for refining it. Although you can assess and guide the process, the work must be done by the individual. By strengthening the relationship a person has with their emotions and actions through self-awareness practices, they begin to feel more in control of their diabetes care and have a better quality of life.

Self-Regulation

Self-regulation is the conscious ability to apply practices and interventions to bounce back and adapt in response to adversity and/or stressful circumstances in a way that conserves our vitality.[11] It empowers resilience because it is self-administered and not beholden to anyone but the individual. We are more likely to live more fully when we know that we can make ourselves feel better.

Science is discovering that resilience is a matter of physiology and not just psychology.[12] They are, however, interconnected. Physiology is the mediator of perception, just as perception is the mediator of physiology. Self-regulation is to balance both body and mind. By regulating the ANS through various yogic techniques, we can gain more agency of choice and recover faster from the impact of diabetes risk.

When you have diabetes, there are no extra reserves; you have to build them by making empowered decisions. Stress compromises the ANS, and jeopardizes mental health and diabetes management. Self-regulation balances the ANS, promotes mental stability, and encourages improved diabetes management because it *is* diabetes management.

The breath is the controller of the mind and physiology. A mind purified by prāṇāyāma sees clearly, promoting *adaptability* and resilience in the face of change. Yogis have known this for thousands of years, and how they discovered all of this wisdom through practice is a testament to direct experience as knowledge. Now science is taking note, and there seems to be infinite research on the connection that the breath makes between Eastern philosophy/practice/spiritualism and Western medicine/psychology. Studies show that breathing practices like prāṇāyāma and kriyā can reestablish the autonomic function and rewire the stress response. Autonomic implies "automatic," but our breath allows us to consciously regulate our respiration to elicit different energetic states that impact the way a person feels about themselves. For me, self-regulation means that I have the power. I try my best to maintain my BG within range, but sometimes I miscalculate. When my BG is off, it impacts my energy levels, and when this happens, I do not feel well. I feel like giving up or playing the victim card. Poor me! It is easy to say you can't do it because of diabetes;

---

11 Sullivan, M. B., Erb, M., Schmalzl, L., Moonaz, S., Noggle Taylor, J. and Porges, S. W. (2018) "Yoga therapy and polyvagal theory: the convergence of traditional wisdom and contemporary neuroscience for self-regulation and resilience." *Frontiers in Human Neuroscience 12*, 67.

12 McGonigal, K. (2012) *The Willpower Instinct: How Self Control Works*. New York: Penguin Random House. p.31.

it is harder to say you can do it because of diabetes. Obviously, the latter takes more work.

Sometimes we need to calm down and prepare for sleep. All of our digestion is done in a parasympathetic state. At other times we need to wake up and energize. In general, what we all need is balance. A balanced nervous system is more resilient to stressors because it can activate and respond just as efficiently as it can turn off and wind down. A skillful practitioner recognizes their imbalances and understands how to apply different practices to adjust their energetic condition for specific needs, restoring balance and increasing resilience.

In effect, self-regulation is turning yourself into a science experiment. A little dash of this, a splash of that—we become pranic shape-shifters learning to restore balance when it's off and to use that as an asset for health and longevity. A lot of people don't have to think about this stuff until it's too late. Diabetes is a blessing because it *requires* us to be this aware of how we feel so we can do something about it. That is what self-regulation provides: empowerment.

Self-Efficacy

The third rung in the resilience ladder is self-efficacy. Self-efficacy is defined as a personal judgment of how well one can accomplish tasks required to deal with prospective situations.[13] Self-efficacy is to feel confident in one's ability to simultaneously manage diabetes tasks and manage life. When people feel confident in their ability to do something well, they are more likely to rise up to the challenge and be less weighed down by the fear of adverse outcomes. The confidence outweighs the fear and judgment of mistakes. Fear of failure is the death of self-efficacy and the precursor to the more pervasive and life-threatening challenges of uncontrolled diabetes.

In diabetes, situations can be life threatening, so self-efficacy is of the utmost importance. Self-efficacy is not only the perception of how well one can execute a task, but also how well they can do it under immense pressure. Self-efficacy on one level is the ability to complete an *action*; on another level, it is an action rooted in a *belief* that you can do something and do it well. If past experiences are negative, and continuously so, people are more likely to

13 Wikipedia (2020) *Self-Efficacy*. Accessed on 06/07/20 at: https://en.wikipedia.org/w/index.php?title=Self-efficacy&oldid=955458399.

perceive their efforts as ineffective[14] and behave in a way that disempowers resilience.

Self-awareness and self-regulation teach self-efficacy, the belief that you can do it even if you make mistakes along the way. That your power to persevere is stronger than the adversity you are up against. That you've got this, and even if you take one step forward and then two steps back, you are still moving forward. Self-efficacy is about behaviors and beliefs. When people are confident in their ability to take care of themselves, they are more likely to adhere to health-promoting practices. If a person lacks confidence or is too attached to their goals, they are less likely to adhere to health-promoting behaviors. All adverse reactions are in response to learned triggers. To change the pattern is to disrupt and dissolve the triggers that elicit disempowered responses. When a person can do this, they will have more sovereignty in their decisions and, in turn, replace negative experiences with positive ones, progressively learning that they *can* take care of themselves.

Yoga may increase self-efficacy and the inherent motivation to make healthier decisions and improve mental health symptoms. It is found that these relationships are reciprocal, meaning that when a person's perception is clearer, they make better choices, and when they make better choices, they feel better.[15]

The motivation to act is steeped in goals, but it is the non-attachment to the goals that constitutes the resilience of self-efficacy. The action of self-care is improved with self-efficacy; however, if the goal is motivated only by a BG number, the individual will find disappointment. The discriminating (self-aware) yogi understands that any gratification in a number is fleeting. Sooner or later, diabetes will throw a curveball, and then the satisfaction of the number is gone. The most resilient are those who are confident in their ability to act and remain unattached to the fruits of their efforts. When it is only about the number, a person sets themselves up for disappointment, binding them to an endless cycle avidyā.

It is found that people with diabetes are more successfully motivated by intrinsic motivators than by extrinsic motivations. This is fascinating because intrinsic motivation is sourced from within. It is self-satisfaction in

---

14 Van Der Ven, N., Chatrou, M. and Snoek, F. J. (2009) "Cognitive Behavioral Group Training." In F. J. Snoek and C. T. J. Skinner (eds) *Psychology in Diabetes Care*. Chichester: Wiley & Sons Ltd. p.214.

15 Martin, E. C., Dick, A. M., Scioli-Salte, E. R. and Mitchell, K. S. (2015) "Impact of a yoga intervention on physical activity, self-efficacy, and motivation in women with PTSD symptoms." *Journal of Alternative and Complementary Medicine 21*, 6, 327–332.

the act of doing something. It is to work for the sake of working, to read for the purpose of learning, to take care of diabetes for the enjoyment of taking care of oneself. An example of an intrinsic motivator is the enthusiasm to take care of one's health and wellbeing because of the act of doing it, not because of anything else. An extrinsic motivator is a grade, let's say an A1c test or a doctor's praise. It is shown that individuals with diabetes are more successfully motivated by their desire to take care of themselves for their own sake than by receiving a gold star for their efforts. The key is figuring out how to awaken self-motivation in those deeply affected by negative past experiences, formed in their beliefs and options about themselves and diabetes. It is challenging to find a way to awaken their desire to know more or improve their quality of life if they are stuck in a cycle of suffering. Sometimes it is easier to remain in the discomfort of what is not working than to move towards the uncertainty of something potentially better.

Beyond Diabetes

When all three of these qualities are combined, we achieve *self-mastery*: the lifetime skill of empowered resilience. I reflect on what this actually means to me as a person living with diabetes. It means that I live with diabetes, completely connected with diabetes, and yet I live beyond it. I am more established in the part of me that is untouched by change, and therefore I gain autonomy over my condition. It is more a feeling of being than a thought. In fact, yoga therapy is just the preparation for the true aim of self-mastery: to know thyself. Sanskrit calls the person who has achieved independence svātantrya,[16] one who exists in the world yet rises above its conditionality. A svatantra is free from burden, while remaining wholly engaged in life.[17] This is the goal of a spiritual practice. Many may hear the word *spiritual* and recoil in fear, but there is no dogma in a spiritual connection. It is the essence of healing and mastery. It imbues us with the remedy to sickness, disease, and suffering, an antidote that comes from qualities of love, devotion, and trust. The remembrance that all of nature flows through us—that we are inextricably connected to the greater whole—guides and nurtures us forever. Without this, our lives lose meaning; we are identified

16 Wisdom Library (n.d.) *Svatantrya, Svātantrya: 12 Definitions*. Accessed on 11/05/20 at https://www.wisdomlib.org/definition/svatantrya.

17 Stryker, R. (2016) "Tantra Shakti: The Power of the Radiant Soul of Yoga." In *Para Yoga Manual.* pp.8–9.

with our suffering with no end in sight; most of us are sick because we have lost or never shown the gem of our heart. Our health shrivels up, and so does our child-like curiosity to know, discover, and experience more of life. Living with diabetes and beyond diabetes is to view all of life as a quest for self-knowledge. Disease is a tool for understanding what makes us tick and what brings us joy, so that we can link with that higher source and rise above diabetes.

A Practice to Rise Above and Beyond Diabetes

We have now merged beyond the application of yoga therapy for a specific condition into yoga as therapy. The yoga therapy for diabetes physical and mental practices serve as the foundation for the life-practice that is yoga.

1	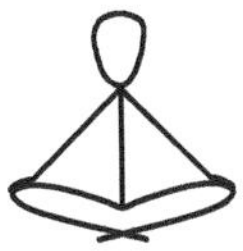	**Sukhāsana:** To check-in, present awareness, and set intention.	Sit in a comfortable position so that the spine can be straight. Take a moment to check-in. Become more aware of your awareness. Deepen and lengthen your breath to a 1:1 even breath. Consider that life is a sacred gift. Reflect on how you are more than the highs and lows of diabetes; you are an awareness untouched by change.
2	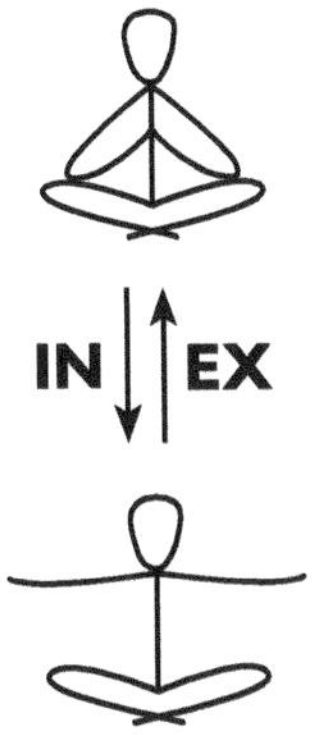 retain chant on exhale	**Sukhāsana with arm variation and sound:** To expand awareness.	Remain in a comfortable seat. Inhale: Open your arms, lift the chin slightly. Retain: Sense presence and awareness expanding from the chest to the fingertips and beyond. Exhale: Chant *Om* while bringing the hands to the heart. Repeat six times.

3	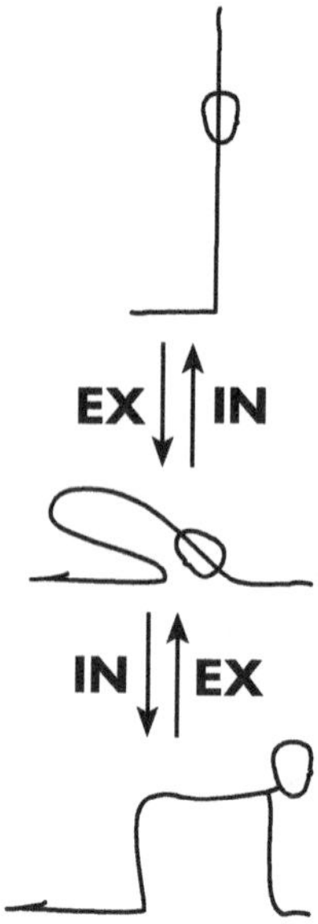	**Vajrāsana and Cakravākāsana combo:** To strengthen and stretch the body and prepare the breath.	Stand on the knees with the arms overhead. Exhale: Bend forward, lower the torso to the thighs, and the forehead and hands to the ground. Inhale: Come up to hands and knees. Exhale: Return the hips towards the heels, lower the torso to the thighs, bend the elbows, and rest the forehead on ground. Inhale: Return to the starting position. Repeat six times.
4	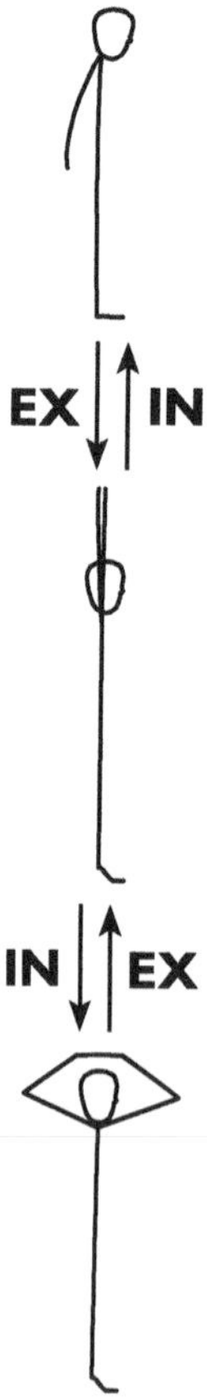 chant on exhale	**Tāḍāsana variation:** To focus the mind with balance and lengthen the exhale through the use of sound.	Stand with the feet hip-width apart and the arms by the sides. Inhale: Lift the heels, bring the arms overhead, interlace the fingers, turn the palms to face upward, and straighten the elbows. Exhale: Bend the elbows, lowering the backs of the hands to the crown of the head, and lower the heels halfway. Inhale: Restraighten the arms, and lift the heels up. Exhale: Return to the starting position. Do this twice. Do this twice more while chanting *Om.* Do this twice more while chanting *Om So Ham.*

5	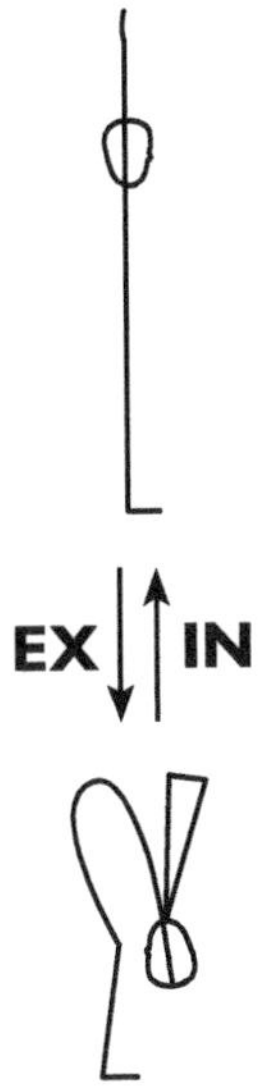 stay one breath	**Uttānāsana variation:** To stretch the back, and open the chest and shoulders.	Start by standing with the feet hip-width apart and arms overhead. Exhale: With a slight flexion in the knees, bend forward, lower the torso to the thighs, and place the hands at sacrum. Inhale: Stay, and interlace the hands and lift them away from the low back, opening the chest. Exhale: Stay, and deepen the forward bend. Inhale: Return to the starting position. Repeat six times.
6	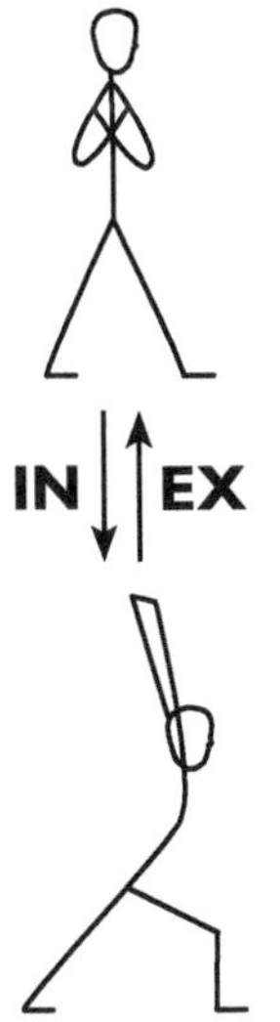 Retain & mentally chant 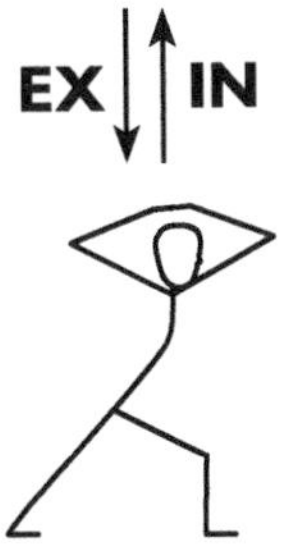	**Vīrabhadrāsana variation:** To stretch and open the chest, retain the inhale, and infuse sound and meaning in the body. Chant on exhale.	Start by standing with the left foot forward, the right foot back, and the hands placed on the heart. Inhale: Bend the left knee, extend both the arms overhead, interlace the hands with the palms face up, straighten the elbows, lengthen the low back, and lift the chest. Retain: Mentally recite *Om So Ham.* Exhale: Keep the palms facing up, bend the elbows, and lower the backs of the hands towards the crown of the head. Chant *Om So Ham.* Inhale: Restraighten the arms, keeping the palms up. Retain: Mentally recite *Om So Ham.* Exhale: Return to the starting position, chanting *Om So Ham.* Repeat six times on each side.

<table>
<tr>
<td>7</td>
<td>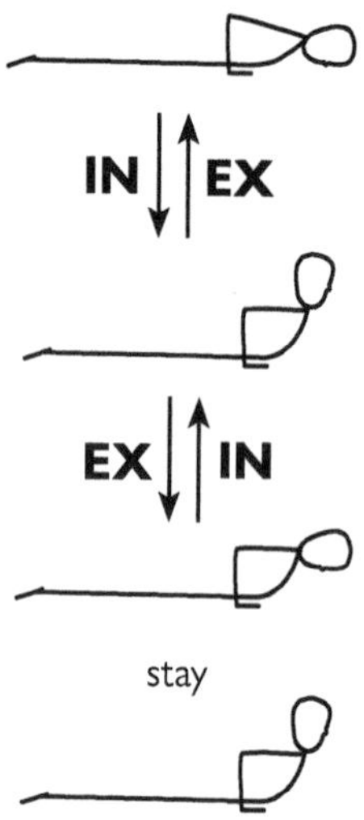

Retain & mentally chant</td>
<td>Bhujaṅgāsana variation: To transition from standing, contract the back, and open the chest through backbend and inhale retention.</td>
<td>Lie on the belly, with the hands under the shoulders and the elbows bent.
Inhale: Lift the chest by contracting the back, lengthen the low back, flatten the upper back, and lift the chin slightly.
Exhale: Lower halfway, contracting the abdomen, and lower the chin.
Inhale: Return to the lift, traction the hands, inhale into the chest, and lift the chin slightly.
Exhale: Return to the starting position.
Repeat six times.
Stay in the pose for six breaths, and mentally recite Om So Ham on inhale retention.</td>
</tr>
<tr>
<td>8</td>
<td>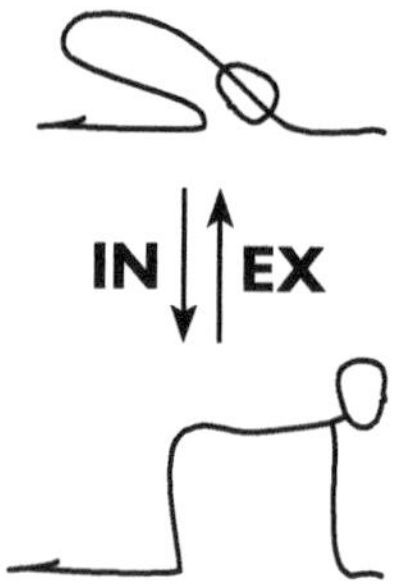
</td>
<td>Cakravākāsana: To counter pose from the backbend and give the breath a rest.</td>
<td>Start in a kneeling position with the abdomen on the thighs and the arms extended in front.
Inhale: Pull back on the hands, and rise to hands and knees. Stack the shoulders over the wrists and the knees over the hips. Lift the chest slightly, broadening the collarbone.
Exhale: Draw the hips towards the heels, bend the elbows, and lower the torso to the thighs, returning to the starting position.
Repeat six times.</td>
</tr>
<tr>
<td rowspan="2">9</td>
<td>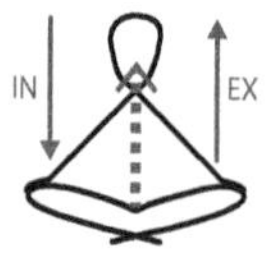
</td>
<td>Central channel breathing with retention at the heart: To awaken awareness beyond diabetes.</td>
<td>a. Come to a comfortable seated position.
b. Deepen and lengthen your breath: equal inhale to equal exhale.
c. Scan awareness down the front of the body, up the back of the body, and then down the center of the spine.</td>
</tr>
<tr>
<td colspan="3">d. Inhale from the crown of the head to the heart for the count of 8.
e. Retain the inhale at the heart for the count of 4.
f. Exhale from the heart to the crown of the head for the count of 8. Repeat 12 times.
<table>
<tr><td>Inhale</td><td>Hold (retention)</td><td>Exhale</td><td>Hold (suspension)</td><td>#</td></tr>
<tr><td>8</td><td>4</td><td>8</td><td>0</td><td>12 times</td></tr>
<tr><td>Crown to heart</td><td>Hold at the heart</td><td>Heart to crown</td><td></td><td></td></tr>
</table>
e. Relax the breath completely</td>
</tr>
</table>

10	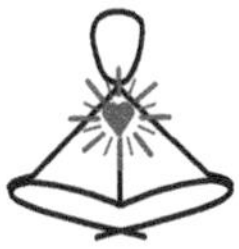	**Meditation beyond diabetes:** To connect with a part of the self that is beyond diabetes.	Become aware of the natural breath presiding at the nostrils. Follow the steps of prāṇa dhāraṇā (Chapter 5) for several minutes. Once you feel like the mind is prepared and established in the presence of prāṇa, move on to the next step. Consider a memory of a time when you experienced joy and delight. It could be a moment in time, an experience, a thing, a taste, or an object. Notice where you feel that joy in your body. Spend some time with this and direct the awareness of your natural breath to the location. Consider that all the joy you seek outwardly is already within you and has always been with you. Bring that "feeling" into the heart. It is like you are looking at it, you are in it, it is all around you. Recall that this feeling is the same as the feeling of innate joy, an inborn, inherent quality untouched by disease, suffering, cause, and effect. Becoming is remembering. Recall that this presence is who you really are: infinite, boundless joy. Now rest in the light and space of the heart. While remaining as effortless as possible, feel the mantra emerge with the natural rhythm of the breath. Exhale: *So.* Inhale: *Ham.* Return slowly, grateful for the gift that is your life.

Subject Index

Sub-headings in *italics* indicates figures.

Author Index

Page numbers refer to footnotes.